Diabetes

For Elsevier
Senior Content Strategist: Jeremy Bowes
Content Development Specialist: Sheila Black
Project Manager: Srividhya Vidhyashankar
Designer: Miles Hitchen
Illustration Manager: Jennifer Rose
Illustrator: Antbits Ltd

CHURCHILL'S POCKETBOOKS

Diabetes
Second Edition

Sujoy Ghosh MD(General Medicine)
DM(Endocrinology) MRCP(UK) MRCPS(Glasgow)
Assistant Professor, Department of Endocrinology
and Metabolism, Institute of Post Graduate
Medical Education and Research, Calcutta, India

Andrew Collier BSc MD FRCP(Glasgow & Edinburgh)
Professor of Diabetes Care; Honorary Senior
Lecturer and Consultant Physician, University
Hospital Ayr, Ayr, UK

Foreword by
John Pickup BM BCh MA DPhil FRCPath
Professor of Diabetes and Metabolism, King's College
London School of Medicine, Guy's Hospital, London, UK

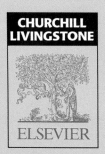

CHURCHILL
LIVINGSTONE

ELSEVIER

EDINBURGH LONDON NEW YORK OXFORD
PHILADELPHIA ST LOUIS SYDNEY TORONTO 2012

CHURCHILL LIVINGSTONE
ELSEVIER

© 2012 Elsevier Ltd. All rights reserved.

First edition 2000
Second edition 2012

ISBN 978-0-443-10081-9

British Library Cataloguing in Publication Data
A catalogue record for this book is available from the British Library

Library of Congress Cataloging in Publication Data
A catalog record for this book is available from the Library of Congress

Notices
Knowledge and best practice in this field are constantly changing. As new research and experience broaden our understanding, changes in research methods, professional practices, or medical treatment may become necessary.

Practitioners and researchers must always rely on their own experience and knowledge in evaluating and using any information, methods, compounds, or experiments described herein. In using such information or methods they should be mindful of their own safety and the safety of others, including parties for whom they have a professional responsibility.

With respect to any drug or pharmaceutical products identified, readers are advised to check the most current information provided (i) on procedures featured or (ii) by the manufacturer of each product to be administered, to verify the recommended dose or formula, the method and duration of administration, and contraindications. It is the responsibility of practitioners, relying on their own experience and knowledge of their patients, to make diagnoses, to determine dosages and the best treatment for each individual patient, and to take all appropriate safety precautions.

To the fullest extent of the law, neither the Publisher nor the authors, contributors, or editors, assume any liability for any injury and/or damage to persons or property as a matter of products liability, negligence or otherwise, or from any use or operation of any methods, products, instructions, or ideas contained in the material herein.

Printed in China

CONTENTS

FOREWORD

The practice and the science of diabetes, and the patients who suffer from this disease, have never remained the same. When I was beginning to learn about diabetes at medical school, about 40 years ago, insulin was of course extracted from animal pancreases (though highly purified, 'monocomponent' insulin was being introduced at that time). Glass syringes and needles had to boiled to sterilize them and monitoring of diabetes control was by urine testing. Beds on the medical ward were frequently occupied by diabetic patients, many with gangrenous feet. Within just a decade, when I was well into my career as a diabetologist, injected insulin was of human sequence and made by semi-synthesis or recombinant DNA technology, disposable plastic syringes and needles had been introduced (after a long fight), insulin 'pens' were appearing and even insulin pumps had been in use for five years. Patients monitored their own metabolic control using capillary blood samples and portable meters and not by urine testing. Type 2 diabetes was no longer called 'mild diabetes', though we thought it was a disease of the middle aged and elderly.

Change in diabetes has shown no signs of diminishing in the last decade, and in fact it is accelerating. Scientific advances in the understanding of diabetes and its complications are being translated into improved clinical practice at ever faster rates. But the increasing prevalence, costs and human suffering associated with diabetes have produced a global health nightmare which challenges us to do better – in public health, scientific and clinical research, clinical care and social policy.

What has changed recently? The relentless increase in obesity and inactivity amongst all age groups has caused the emergence of this type of diabetes in children and adolescents, as well as adults. Type 2 diabetes is now increasingly recognised as a disorder of the immune system, though it seems to be a disease of activated innate immunity. Rapid- and long-acting insulin analogues are now the insulins of choice for many people with diabetes, and newer insulins are just around the corner – analogues with even longer duration for better basal replacement, and rapid-acting formulations with even faster absorption for meal-time use. New technologies such as smart insulin pumps and continuous glucose monitoring are playing an increasing part in the management of selected patients with type 1 diabetes and sub-optimal glycaemic control. In type 2 diabetes, new blood glucose-lowering drugs such as gliptins and GLP-1 agonists are proving effective, and in the grossly obese patient with diabetes, bariatric surgery is becoming a recognised treatment option. In the everyday diabetes clinic, management of hypertension and lipids are now seen as being as integral to diabetes care as blood glucose control. And many more advances could be mentioned.

Diabetes is common, costly, complex and constantly changing. There is much to learn. The management of people with diabetes is not the same today as it was even a few years ago. Sujoy Ghosh and Andrew Collier have produced in this book a clear, up-to-date guide to modern diabetes and its management that will help all practitioners. I am sure it will make a substantial contribution both to our understanding of diabetes and to improving the care of the patients who suffer from it.

London 2012   John Pickup

PREFACE

The incidence of diabetes is increasing at epidemic proportions worldwide. The first *Pocketbook of Diabetes* was published in 2000 and the structure of this edition follows similar lines. However, diabetes expertise has moved on considerably, with greater understanding of aetiopathogenesis of the different types of diabetes, the emerging roles of novel pharmacological agents, and the importance of multidisciplinary team working and multi-risk-factor treatment.

Re-writing this book was easy and difficult at the same time. Our predecessor, Professor Andrew Krentz, who wrote the previous edition, had done a wonderful job and hence it was incredibly difficult to improve upon his work. At the same time his work provided us with a platform to update the book, keeping in view the advances in knowledge.

The emphasis of this book is on clinical management and the aim has been to provide a balanced view of current clinical practice. This book is not meant to be an alternative to time tested exhaustive text-books on diabetes. This pocketbook is meant to be a be a concise companion for all health professionals involved in diabetes management, providing easily accessible information and guidance.

Finally no words of praise are enough for the constant help and support that we received from our publishers, especially Sheila Black, for bearing with the unbearable!

Calcutta and Ayr, 2012

Sujoy Ghosh
Andrew Collier

ABBREVIATIONS

4 S Scandinavian Simvastatin Study

AAP atypical antipsychotic

ABPI ankle : brachial pressure index

AC abdominal circumference

ACCORD Action to Control Cardiovascular Risk in Diabetes

ACE angiotensin converting enzyme

ACR albumin/creatinine ratio

ACT acceptance and commitment therapy

ADA American Diabetes Association

ADOPT A Diabetes Outcome Progression Trial

ADVANCE Action in Diabetes and Vascular Disease: Preterax and Diamicron MR Controlled Evaluation

AED antiepileptic drug

AER albumin excretion rate

ALLHAT Antihypertensive and Lipid-Lowering Treatment to Prevent Heart Attack Trial

ARB angiotensin receptor blocker

ARI aldose reduction inhibitor

ASCOT Anglo-Scandinavian Cardiac Outcomes Trial

ASH alcoholic steatohepatitis

ASSIGN Assessing cardiovascular risk using SIGN guidelines to assign preventive treatment

ATP adenosine triphosphate

BDI Beck Depression Inventory

BERTIE Bournemouth Type 1 Intensive Education

BGAT Blood Glucose Awareness Training

BHS British Hypertension Society

BITES Brief Intervention in Type 1 Diabetes – Education for Self-efficacy

BMD bone mineral density

BMI body mass index

BMS bare metal stents

BNF British National Formulary

BP blood pressure

BSA body surface area

BUN blood urea nitrogen

CABG coronary artery bypass grafting

CAPD continuous ambulatory peritoneal dialysis

CARDS Collaborative Atorvastatin Diabetes Study

CARE Cholesterol and Recurrent Events

CBT cognitive behavioural therapy

CCB calcium channel blocker

CES-D Centre for Epidemiological Studies – Depression Scale

cGMP cyclic guanosine monophosphate

CHD coronary heart disease

CHF congestive heart failure

CI confidence interval

CKD chronic kidney disease

CMG continuous monitoring of interstitial glucose

CoA coenzyme A

COC combined oral contraceptive

COPD chronic obstructive pulmonary disease

CRP C-reactive protein

CSI continuous subcutaneous insulin infusion

CSMO clinically significant macular oedema

CT computed tomography

CTG cardiotocography

CVD cardiovascular disease

DAFNE Dose Adjustment for Normal Eating

DCCT Diabetes Control and Complications Trial

DES drug-eluting stents

DESMOND Diabetes Education and Self-Management for Ongoing and Newly Diagnosed

DHAP dihydroxy acetonephosphate

DIGAMI Diabetes mellitus, Insulin-Glucose infusion in Acute Myocardial Infarction

DISH diffuse idiopathic skeletal hyperostosis

DISN diabetes inpatient specialist nurse

DKA diabetic ketoacidosis

DPP dipeptidyl peptidase

DR diabetic retinopathy

DRS Diabetic Retinopathy Study

DSME diabetes self-management education

DVLA Driver and Vehicle Licensing Agency

ED erectile dysfunction

EDHF endothelium-derived hyperpolarizing factor

ER endoplasmic reticulum

ESRD end-stage renal disease

FDA Food and Drug Administration

FFA fundus fluorescein angiography

FIELD Fenofibrate Intervention and Event Lowering in Diabetes

FLD fatty liver disease

FPG fasting plasma glucose

FSH follicle-stimulating hormone

GA3P glyceraldehyde 3-phosphate

GAD glutamic acid dehydrogenase

GDM gestational diabetes mellitus

GFR glomerular filtration rate

GHbSD standard deviations of glycosylated haemoglobin

GI glycaemic index

GIP glucose-dependent insulinotropic peptide

GLP-1 glucagon-like peptide-1

GLUT glucose transporter

GnRH gonadotropin-releasing hormone

GP general practitioner

HAATT Hypoglycaemia Anticipation, Awareness and Treatment Training

HADS Hospital Anxiety and Depression Scale

HAPO Hyperglycaemia and Adverse Pregnancy Outcome

HbA1c glycated haemoglobin

HDL high density lipoprotein

HF heart failure

HHS hyperosmolar hyperglycaemic state

HIV human immunodeficiency virus

HLA human leukocyte antigen

HNF hepatocyte nuclear factor

HOMA homeostasis model assessment

HONK hyperosmolar non-ketotic (coma)

HOPE Heart Outcomes Prevention Evaluation

HOT Hypertension Optimal Treatment

HPS Heart Protection Study

HR hazard ratio

HTA Health Technology Assessment

IDF International Diabetes Federation

IFCC International Federation of Clinical Chemistry and Laboratory Medicine

IFG impaired fasting glucose

IGT impaired glucose tolerance

IPF insulin promoter factor

IPPV intermittent postive-pressure ventilation

IRMA intraretinal microvascular anomaly

IRS insulin receptor substrate

IUD intrauterine device

IUGR intrauterine growth restriction

IUS intrauterine systems

IV intravenous

JBS 2 Joint British Societies' guideline

LADA latent autoimmune diabetes in adults

LCD low calorie diet

LDL low density lipoprotein

LED low energy diets

LH luteinizing hormone

LVSD left ventricular systolic dysfunction

MDI multiple daily injections

MDRD Modification of Diet in Renal Disease

MELAS mitochondrial myopathy, encephalopathy, lactic acidosis and stroke-like

MI myocardial infarction

MNT medical nutrition therapy

MODY maturity-onset diabetes of the young

MR modified release

MRI magnetic resonance imaging

NAD nicotinamide adenine dinucleotide

NASH non-alcoholic steatohepatitis

NCEP National Cholesterol Education Program

NDH non-diabetic hyperglycaemia

NGSP National Glycohemoglobin Standardization Program

NHS QIS NHS Quality Improvement Scotland

NICE National Institute for Health and Clinical Excellence

NPDR non-proliferative diabetic retinopathy

NPH neutral protamine Hagedorm

NPWT negative pressure wound therapy

NYHA New York Heart Association (classification)

OCT optical coherence tomography

OGTT oral glucose tolerance test

OR odds ratio

PAD peripheral arterial disease

PAID Problem Areas in Diabetes

PCI percutaneous coronary intervention

PCOS polycystic ovary syndrome

PCR protein/creatinine ratio

PCT porphyria cutanea tarda

PDR poliferative diabetic retinopathy

PHQ Patient Health Questionnaire

PPR peroxisome proliferator-activated receptor

PROactive PROspective pioglitAzone Clinical Trial In macroVascular Events

PUFA omega-3 polyunsaturated fatty acids

PVD peripheral vascular disease

QALY quality-adjusted life year

QOF quality outcomes framework

QoL quality of life

QUICKI quantitative insulin sensitivity check index

RAAS renin–angiotensin–aldosterone system

RARS refractory anaemia with ringed sideroblasts

RCT randomized controlled trial

RR relative risk

RRT renal replacement therapy

SBP systolic blood pressure

SCID Structured Clinical Interview for DSM-IV-TR

SD standard deviation

SE standard error

SGA small for gestational age

SGLT sodium–glucose co-transporter inhibitor

SHBG sex hormone-binding globulin

SIGN Scottish Intercollegiate Guidelines Network

SMBG self-monitoring of blood glucose

SMD standardized mean difference

SMUG self-monitoring of urine glucose

SREBP sterol regulatory element-binding protein

SSRI selective serotonin reuptake inhibitor

SU sulphonylurea

TCA tricyclic antidepressant

TG triglycerides

TSH thyroid-stimulating hormone

TZD thiazolidinedione

UGDP University Group Diabetes Program

UKPDS UK Prospective Diabetes Study

VADT Veterans Affairs Diabetes Trial

VEGF vascular endothelial growth factor

VLCD very low calorie diet

VLED very low energy diet

WHO World Health Organization

DIAGNOSIS, CLASSIFICATION, EPIDEMIOLOGY AND BIOCHEMISTRY

THE SYNDROME OF DIABETES MELLITUS

Diabetes mellitus is defined as a metabolic disorder of multiple aetiology characterized by chronic hyperglycaemia with disturbances of carbohydrate, protein and fat metabolism resulting from defects in insulin secretion, insulin action, or both. The clinical diagnosis of diabetes is often indicated by the presence of symptoms such as polyuria, polydipsia and unexplained weight loss, and is confirmed by documented hyperglycaemia.

The clinical presentation ranges from asymptomatic type 2 diabetes to the dramatic life-threatening conditions of diabetic ketoacidosis (DKA) or hyperosmolar non-ketotic coma (HONK)/ hyperosmolar hyperglycaemic state (HHS). The principal determinants of the presentation are the degrees of insulin deficiency and insulin resistance, although additional factors may also be important. In addition, pathological hyperglycaemia sustained over several years may produce functional and structural changes within certain tissues. Patients may present with macrovascular complications that include ischaemic heart disease, stroke and peripheral vascular disease, whereas the specific microvascular complications of diabetes include retinopathy, nephropathy, neuropathy.

DIAGNOSTIC CRITERIA FOR DIABETES MELLITUS

Assigning a type of diabetes to an individual often depends on the circumstances present at the time of diagnosis, and many diabetic individuals do not easily fit into a single specific type. An example is a person who has acquired diabetes because of large doses of exogenous steroids and who becomes normoglycaemic once the glucocorticoids are discontinued. In addition, some patients may present with major metabolic decompensation yet can subsequently be treated successfully with oral agents. Thus, for the clinician and patient, it is less important to label the particular type of diabetes than it is to understand the pathogenesis of the hyperglycaemia and to treat it effectively.

The American Diabetes Association (ADA, 2011) gives the following **criteria for the diagnosis of diabetes:**

- A1C $\geq 6.5\%$. The test should be performed in a laboratory using a method that is certified by the National Glycohemoglobin Standardization Program (NGSP) and standardized to the Diabetes Control and Complications Trial (DCCT) assay, or

- fasting plasma glucose (FPG) ≥ 126 mg/dL (7.0 mmol/L). Fasting is defined as no caloric intake for at least 8 h, or
- 2-h plasma glucose ≥ 200 mg/dL (11.1 mmol/L) during an oral glucose tolerance test (OGTT). The test should be performed as described by the World Health Organization (WHO), using a glucose load containing the equivalent of 75 g anhydrous glucose dissolved in water
- in a patient with classic symptoms of hyperglycaemia or hyperglycaemic crisis, a random plasma glucose ≥ 200 mg/dL (11.1 mmol/L)
- in the absence of unequivocal hyperglycaemia, the result should be confirmed by repeat testing.

The symptoms of thirst, polyuria, polyphagia and weight loss, coupled with a raised plasma glucose level, are diagnostic. In the absence of symptoms two abnormal results (i.e. two raised fasting levels) or an abnormal OGTT result is diagnostic. However, the OGTT is influenced by many factors other than diabetes, including age, diet, state of health, gastrointestinal disorders, medications and emotional stress.

> **Tip box**
>
> Chronic hyperglycaemia is the sine qua non of diabetes mellitus.

CATEGORIES OF INCREASED RISK FOR DIABETES (PRE-DIABETES): IMPAIRED FASTING GLUCOSE (IFG)/IMPAIRED GLUCOSE TOLERANCE (IGT)

The ADA criteria introduced the category of impaired fasting glucose, defined as fasting venous plasma level of 5.6–6.9 mmol/L. The diagnosis of impaired glucose tolerance can be made only using a 75-g oral glucose tolerance test; a 2-h glucose measurement points to the diagnosis of impaired glucose tolerance when the plasma glucose is found to be greater than 7.7 mmol/L but less than 11.1 mmol/L. Recently another category, impaired glycated haemoglobin, HbA1c (A1C 5.7–6.4%), has been added.

Categories of increased risk for diabetes (pre-diabetes) (ADA, 2011)

FPG 100–125 mg/dL (5.6–6.9 mmol/L): IFG
or

2 h plasma glucose in the 75-g OGTT 140–199 mg/dl
(7.8–11.0 mmol/l): IGT
or
A1C 5.7–6.4%

Tip box

Impaired fasting glycaemia and glucose tolerance are usually asymptomatic.

The diagnosis of impaired glucose tolerance relies on glucose tolerance testing (see below) and denotes an intermediate stage between normality and diabetes. Patients with impaired glucose tolerance, although not at direct risk of developing chronic microvascular disease, may be detected following the development of macrovascular complications:

- ischaemic heart disease
- cerebrovascular disease
- peripheral vascular disease.

The presence of one of these conditions should therefore alert the clinician to the possibility of undiagnosed impaired glucose tolerance or type 2 diabetes, even in the absence of osmotic symptoms.

Oral glucose tolerance test

The ADA (1997) proposed measurement of fasting glucose as the principal means of diagnosing type diabetes. The WHO (1998) placed emphasis on the oral glucose tolerance test as the 'gold standard', with both fasting and 120-min values being taken into consideration. Only when an OGTT cannot be performed should the diagnosis rely on fasting levels.

The OGTT is the most robust means of establishing the diagnosis of diabetes. Glucose tolerance tests should be carried out under controlled conditions after an overnight fast.

Tip box

To avoid false-positive results, patients should receive an unrestricted diet containing adequate carbohydrate (> 150 g daily) for 3 days prior to an oral glucose tolerance test.

TABLE 1.1 Preparation for a fasting blood test

- The subject should refrain from consuming any food or drink from midnight before the morning of the test
- Water alone is permitted for thirst
- Regular medication can generally be deferred until the sample has been taken
- The appropriate sample is taken between 0800 and 0900 hours the following morning

The patient is prepared as detailed in Table 1.1:

- Anhydrous glucose is dissolved in 300 mL water; flavouring with sugar-free lemon and chilling increases palatability and may reduce nausea. The patient should sit quietly throughout the test.
- Blood glucose is sampled before (time zero) and 120 min after ingestion of the drink, which should be completed within 5 min.
- Urinalysis may also be performed every 30 min, although this is really of interest only if a significant alteration in renal threshold for glucose is suspected.

Interpretation of the results of a 75-g glucose tolerance test is presented in Table 1.2. Note that results apply to venous plasma: whole blood values are 15% lower than corresponding plasma values if the haematocrit is normal. For capillary whole blood, the diagnostic cut-offs for diabetes are ≥6.1 mmol/L (fasting) and 11.1 mmol/L (i.e. the same as for venous plasma). The range for impaired fasting glucose based on capillary whole blood is ≥5.6 and <6.9 mmol/L. Note that marked carbohydrate deprivation can impair glucose tolerance; the subject should have received adequate nutrition in the days preceding the test.

TABLE 1.2 Interpretation of 75-g oral glucose tolerance test

	Venous plasma glucose (mmol/L)		
	Fasting		120 min post-glucose load
Normal	≤5.6		<7.8
Impaired fasting glucose	5.6–6.9		<7.8
Impaired glucose tolerance	6.1–6.9	and/ or	7.8–11.0
Diabetes mellitus	≥7.0		>11.1

Tip box

In the absence of symptoms, diabetes must be confirmed by a second diagnostic test (i.e. fasting, random or repeat glucose tolerance test) on a separate day.

Tip box

To get blood glucose values in mg/dl multiply the values in mmol/L by 18

Intercurrent illness

Patients under the physical stress associated with surgical trauma, acute myocardial infarction, acute pulmonary oedema or stroke may have transient increases of plasma glucose that often settle rapidly without specific antidiabetic therapy. However, such clinical situations are also liable to unmask asymptomatic pre-existing diabetes or to precipitate diabetes in predisposed individuals. Such increases, which may have short- and longer-term prognostic importance, should not be dismissed; as a minimum, appropriate follow-up and retesting is indicated following resolution of the acute illness. If there is doubt about the significance of hyperglycaemia, the blood glucose level should be rechecked 30–60 min later and the urine tested for ketones.

If hyperglycaemia is sustained, treatment with insulin may be indicated. More marked degrees of hyperglycaemia, particularly with ketonuria, demand vigorous treatment in an acutely ill patient.

Non-diabetic hyperglycaemia

As detailed above, impaired fasting glycaemia (IFG) is defined as a fasting glucose > 5.6 and < 7.0 mmol/L, whereas impaired glucose tolerance (IGT) is defined as fasting glucose < 7 mmol/L and 2-h glucose > 7.8 and < 11.1 mmol/L. IGT and IFG are both associated with an increased risk of future diabetes. However, IFG and IGT appear to have different underlying aetiologies. IFG reflects raised hepatic glucose output and a defect in early insulin secretion, whereas IGT predominantly reflects peripheral insulin resistance. IGT is also associated with an increased risk of cardiovascular disease (CVD) independently of other risk factors. The magnitude of this increased risk varies between studies, but for cardiovascular disease mortality the odds ratio was 1.34 (95% CI 1.14–1.57) in the DECODE (2003) meta-analysis. IFG appears to have only a slightly increased risk of CVD independently of other factors.

The term 'pre-diabetes', which is sometimes used to refer to IGT and/or IFG, is no longer the preferred term because not all patients go on to develop diabetes. A significant proportion of individuals who have impaired glucose tolerance diagnosed by an OGTT

TABLE 1.3 Diagnostic criteria for diabetes mellitus and non-diabetic hyperglycaemia

	Fasting plasma glucose (FPG)	Random plasma glucose (RPG)	Oral glucose tolerance test	HbA1c
Diabetes	FPG >7.0 mmol/L on two occasions or with symptoms*	RPG >11.1 mmol/L on two occasions or with symptoms	2-h glucose >11.1 mmol/L	≥6.5%
Non-diabetic hyper-glycaemia	IFG: FPG >5.6 and <7.0 mmol/L		IGT: FPG <7 mmol/l and 2-h glucose >7.8 and <11.1 mmol/L	>5.7% and <6.5%

*Thirst, polyuria, nocturia.
HbA1c, glycated haemoglobin; IFG, impaired fasting glucose; IGT, impaired glucose tolerance.
Source: American Diabetes Association (2011). Reproduced with permission.

revert to normal glucose tolerance on retesting. Non-diabetic hyperglycaemia (NDH) is increasingly being used as a wider term that encompasses hyperglycaemia where the HbA1c level is raised but is below the diabetic range (Table 1.3).

Tip box

Testing for diabetes should be undertaken by clinical laboratories not at point of care. Bedside instruments such as glucometers should not be used to diagnose diabetes.

Glycated haemoglobin (HbA1c)
The ADA Joint Expert Committee has recommended HbA1c as a diagnostic tool with a cut-off ≥6.5% to diagnose diabetes. HbA1c is well established as a marker of glycaemic control in people with established diabetes as it reflects average plasma glucose over the previous 2–3 months. In addition, HbA1c has a number of advantages over fasting blood glucose or OGTT. HbA1c can be measured at any time of day and does not require special preparation such as fasting.

However, HbA1c testing is not widely available in many countries throughout the world and there are aspects of its measurement that are problematic. These include anaemia, abnormalities of haemoglobin, pregnancy and uraemia. Some of these problems may be a bigger problem in under-resourced countries owing to the high prevalence of anaemia and haemoglobinopathies.

CLASSIFICATION OF DIABETES MELLITUS

TYPE 1 DIABETES (β-CELL DESTRUCTION, USUALLY LEADING TO ABSOLUTE INSULIN DEFICIENCY)

Immune-mediated diabetes

The clinical presentation of type 1 diabetes in younger patients is usually acute with classical osmotic symptoms. In general, symptoms will have been present for only a few weeks with osmotic symptoms; weight loss predominates and gradually increases in intensity. Weight loss reflects:

- catabolism of protein and fat resulting from profound insulin deficiency
- dehydration if hyperglycaemia is marked.

Associated symptoms, particularly blurred vision, are not uncommon although generally less prominent. Although the islet β-cell destruction of type 1 diabetes is a process that occurs gradually over many years, it *was* very uncommon to detect type 1 diabetes during the early asymptomatic stages of the condition. In some patients, once symptoms appear, diagnosis may sometimes be expedited by awareness of symptoms in other family members with diabetes. Despite the presence of significant osmotic symptoms, some patients do not seek medical advice and a significant proportion (approximately 5–10%) of patients with type 1 diabetes continue to present in diabetic ketoacidosis (DKA).

 Approximately 5–10% of patients with type 1 diabetes present with DKA.

Diabetic ketoacidosis

At the time of diagnosis, patients may develop rapid metabolic decompensation in the presence of an intercurrent illness, such as infection, that is likely to expose the patient's limited, endogenous insulin reserve; an abrupt ascent in plasma glucose concentration

TABLE 1.4 Cardinal clinical features of diabetic ketoacidosis

- Marked polyuria and polydipsia
- Nausea and vomiting
- Dehydration
- Reduced level of consciousness
- Acidotic (Kussmaul) respiration

may ensue in concert with dehydration, ketosis, acidosis and electrolyte depletion.

DKA is a life-threatening medical emergency requiring hospitalization for treatment with intravenous fluids and insulin. Patients with the features listed in Table 1.4 along with the following features should be admitted promptly to hospital for further assessment and treatment:

- heavy glycosuria
- ketonuria (++ or greater).

The diagnosis and management of DKA are considered in more detail in Section 4.

 Patients with clinical features suggestive of DKA must be admitted to hospital without delay.

Type 1 accounts for only 5–10% of those with diabetes and was previously encompassed by the terms insulin-dependent diabetes or juvenile-onset diabetes. It results from a cellular-mediated autoimmune destruction of the β-cells of the pancreas. Markers of the immune destruction of the β-cell include islet cell autoantibodies, autoantibodies to insulin, autoantibodies to glutamic acid decarboxylase (GAD_{65}), and autoantibodies to the tyrosine phosphatases IA-2 and IA-2β. One or, usually, more of these autoantibodies are present in 85–90% of individuals when fasting hyperglycaemia is initially detected. In addition, the disease has strong human leukocyte antigen (HLA) associations, with linkage to the DQA and DQB genes, and it is influenced by the DRB genes. These *HLA-DR/DQ* alleles can be either predisposing or protective.

In this form of diabetes, the rate of β-cell destruction is quite variable, being rapid in some individuals (mainly infants and children) and slow in others (mainly adults). Some patients, particularly children and adolescents, may present with ketoacidosis as the first manifestation of the disease. Others have modest fasting hyperglycaemia that can change rapidly to severe hyperglycaemia and/or ketoacidosis in the presence of infection or other stress. Still others, particularly adults, may retain residual β-cell function sufficient to prevent ketoacidosis for many years. Immune-mediated diabetes commonly occurs in childhood and adolescence, but it can occur at any age, even in the eighth and ninth decades of life.

Autoimmune destruction of β-cells has multiple genetic predispositions and is also related to environmental factors that are still poorly defined. These patients are also prone to other autoimmune disorders such as Graves' disease, Hashimoto's thyroiditis, Addison's disease, vitiligo, coeliac disease, autoimmune hepatitis, myasthenia gravis and pernicious anaemia.

> **Tip box**
>
> Obese patients with type 1 diabetes may present earlier in the process with milder symptoms due to increased insulin resistance.

Pluriglandular syndrome

The pluriglandular syndrome type II should be borne in mind in patients presenting with features suggesting autoimmune type 1 diabetes, particularly in those who are known to be positive for islet cell antibodies. Consideration should be given to checking for other endocrine autoantibodies in the serum, particularly:

- thyroid microsomal and thyroglobulin antibodies
- adrenal antibodies.

Antibody positivity does not predict future autoimmune disease with certainty. However, the prevalence of autoimmune thyroid disease, Addison's disease and other non-endocrine autoimmune disorders such as pernicious anaemia, coeliac disease and premature menopause is increased in patients with type 1 diabetes. Vitiligo is a useful cutaneous marker of autoimmune disease. Periodic checks of target organ function, such as thyroid function tests or serum B_{12} level, are indicated even in the absence of clinical features. Coexisting endocrinopathies may adversely affect metabolic stability.

Idiopathic diabetes

Some forms of type 1 diabetes have no known aetiology. Some of these patients have permanent insulinopenia and are prone to ketoacidosis, but have no evidence of autoimmunity. Only a minority of patients fall into this category and most are of African or Asian ancestry. Individuals with this form of diabetes suffer from episodic ketoacidosis and exhibit varying degrees of insulin deficiency between episodes. This form of diabetes is strongly inherited, lacks immunological evidence for β-cell autoimmunity, and is not HLA associated. An absolute requirement for insulin replacement therapy in affected patients may come and go.

TYPE 2 DIABETES (RANGING FROM PREDOMINANTLY INSULIN RESISTANT WITH RELATIVE INSULIN DEFICIENCY TO PREDOMINANTLY AN INSULIN SECRETORY DEFECT WITH INSULIN RESISTANCE)

The majority of patients with type 2 diabetes are diagnosed at a relatively late stage of a long, pathological process that has its origins in the patient's genotype (or perhaps intrauterine experience), and develops and progresses over many years.

Tip box

Type 2 diabetes represents a late stage of a complex and progressive pathological process.

The presenting clinical features of type 2 diabetes range from none at all to those associated with the dramatic and life-threatening, hyperglycaemic emergency of the hyperosmolar non-ketotic syndrome (HONK)/hyperosmolar hyperglycaemic state (HHS). In many patients with lesser degrees of hyperglycaemia, symptoms may go unnoticed or unrecognized for many years; however, such undiagnosed diabetes carries the risk of insidious tissue damage. It has been estimated that patients with type 2 diabetes have often had pathological degrees of hyperglycaemia for several years before the diagnosis is made. For example, more than 5 million people in the USA alone may have undiagnosed diabetes.

Tip box

Approximately 50% of patients in the UK with type 2 diabetes are undiagnosed.

This form of diabetes, which accounts for about 90–95% of those with diabetes, previously referred to as non-insulin-dependent diabetes, type II diabetes or adult-onset diabetes, encompasses individuals who have insulin resistance and usually have relative (rather than absolute) insulin deficiency. At least initially, and often throughout their lifetime, these individuals do not need insulin treatment to survive.

There are probably many different causes of this form of diabetes. Islet mass is reduced with deposition of islet amyloid polypeptide; the latter produces striking histological changes within the islets, yet its role in the initiation and progression of type 2 diabetes is not known. Increased plasma levels of proinsulin-like molecules indicate β-cell dysfunction; this is an early feature, being demonstrable prior to the development of diabetes in high-risk groups. Autoimmune destruction of β-cells does not occur, and patients do not have any of the other causes of diabetes listed above or below.

Most patients with type 2 diabetes are obese, and obesity itself causes some degree of insulin resistance. The absence of weight loss reflects the presence of sufficient secretion of endogenous insulin to prevent catabolism of protein and fat. Patients who are not obese by traditional weight criteria may have an increased percentage of body fat distributed predominantly in the abdominal region. Ketoacidosis seldom occurs spontaneously in this type of diabetes; when seen, it usually arises in association with the stress of another illness, such as infection. Type 2 diabetic patients are at increased risk of developing macrovascular and microvascular complications. Whereas patients with this form of diabetes may have insulin levels that appear normal or increased, the higher blood glucose levels in these diabetic patients would be expected to result in even higher insulin values had their β-cell function been normal. Thus, insulin secretion is defective and insufficient to compensate for insulin resistance. Insulin resistance may improve with weight reduction and/or pharmacological treatment of hyperglycaemia, but is seldom restored to normal. The risk of developing type 2 diabetes increases with age, obesity and lack of physical activity. It occurs more frequently in women with previous gestational diabetes mellitus (GDM) and in individuals with hypertension or dyslipidaemia. Its frequency varies in different racial/ethnic subgroups. It is often associated with a strong genetic predisposition – more so than the autoimmune form of type 1 diabetes.

Aetiology of type 2 diabetes

There is a strong inheritable genetic connection in type 2 diabetes: having relatives (especially first-degree relatives) with type 2 diabetes increases substantially the risk of developing type 2 diabetes.

The genetics are complex and not completely understood, but presumably the disease is related to multiple genes. Only a handful of genes have been identified so far: genes for calpain-10, potassium inward-rectifier 6.2, peroxisome proliferator-activated receptor-γ and insulin receptor substrate-1. Evidence also supports inherited components for pancreatic β-cell failure and insulin resistance.

Considerable debate exists regarding the primary defect in type 2 diabetes mellitus. Most patients have insulin resistance and some degree of insulin deficiency. However, insulin resistance *per se* is not the *sine qua non* for type 2 diabetes because many people with insulin resistance (particularly those who are obese) do not develop glucose intolerance. Therefore, insulin deficiency is necessary for the development of hyperglycaemia. Insulin concentrations may be high, yet inappropriately low for the level of glycaemia. Several mechanisms have been proposed, including increased non-esterified fatty acids, inflammatory cytokines, adipokines and mitochondrial dysfunction for insulin resistance, and glucotoxicity, lipotoxicity and amyloid formation for β-cell dysfunction.

Presumably, the defects of type 2 diabetes occur when a diabetogenic lifestyle (excessive caloric intake, inadequate caloric expenditure, obesity) is superimposed upon a susceptible genotype. The body mass index (BMI) at which excess weight increases risk for diabetes varies with different racial groups. For example, compared with persons of European ancestry, persons of Asian ancestry are at increased risk for diabetes at lower levels of waist circumference/BMI. This can be seen from the adoption of the type 2 epidemiological pattern in those who have moved to a different environment in comparison with the same genetic pool of persons who have not, for instance in immigrants to Western developed countries compared with the lower incidence of countries of their origin.

Measures of insulin resistance (Table 1.5)

Homeostasis model assessment (HOMA) and quantitative insulin sensitivity check index (QUICKI) have been used to quantify degrees of insulin resistance and β-cell secretory capacity. HOMA uses fasting measurements of blood glucose and insulin concentrations to calculate indices of both insulin sensitivity and β-cell function. The principle of HOMA is that blood glucose and insulin concentrations are related by the feedback of glucose on β-cells to increase insulin secretion. The model assumes that normal-weight subjects aged less than 35 years have an insulin resistance (R) of 1 and 100% β-cell function.

TABLE 1.5 Measures of insulin resistance

HOMA (R) = [Insulin (mU/L) × glucose (mmol/L)]/22.5
HOMA β-cell function = [20 × insulin mU/L]/[glucose (mmol/L) − 3.5]
QUICKI employs the log of both blood insulin and glucose concentrations to quantify insulin resistance
HOMA and QUICKI measures of insulin resistance are usually in very close agreement
HOMA, homeostasis model assessment; QUICKI, quantitative proliferator-activated receptor.

OTHER SPECIFIC TYPES OF DIABETES

Genetic defects of the β-cell

Several forms of diabetes are associated with monogenetic defects in β-cell function. These forms of diabetes are frequently characterized by onset of hyperglycaemia at an early age (generally before age 25 years). They are referred to as maturity-onset diabetes of the young (MODY) and are characterized by impaired insulin secretion with minimal or no defects in insulin action. They are inherited in an autosomal dominant pattern. Abnormalities at over six genetic loci on different chromosomes have been identified to date. The most common form is associated with mutations on chromosome 12 in a hepatic transcription factor referred to as hepatocyte nuclear factor (HNF)-1α; MODY3 accounts for 70% of the MODY population A second form is associated with mutations in the glucokinase gene on chromosome 7p and results in a defective glucokinase molecule. Glucokinase converts glucose to glucose 6-phosphate, the metabolism of which, in turn, stimulates insulin secretion by the β-cell. Thus, glucokinase serves as the 'glucose sensor' for the β-cell. Because of defects in the glucokinase gene, increased plasma levels of glucose are necessary to elicit normal levels of insulin secretion. Patients with MODY2 present with a less severe form of hyperglycaemia that can be managed with medical nutrition therapy alone. The less common forms result from mutations in other transcription factors, including HNF-4α, HNF-1β, insulin promoter factor (IPF)-1 and NeuroD1 (Table 1.6). Up to 15% of patients with MODY present with clinical characteristics of MODY, but do not have any known mutation and are classified as MODY-X until further genetic loci have been explored.

TABLE 1.6 Aetiological classification of diabetes mellitus

I. Type 1 diabetes (β-cell destruction, usually leading to absolute insulin deficiency)

A. Immune-mediated
B. Idiopathic

II. Type 2 diabetes (may range from predominantly insulin resistance with relative insulin deficiency to a predominantly secretory defect with insulin resistance)

III. Other specific types

A. Genetic defects of β-cell function
  1. Chromosome 12, HNF-1α (MODY3)
  2. Chromosome 7, glucokinase (MODY2)
  3. Chromosome 20, HNF-4α (MODY1)
  4. Chromosome 13, insulin promoter factor-1 (IPF-1; MODY4)
  5. Chromosome 17, HNF-1β (MODY5)
  6. MODY7: mutation in carboxyl ester lipase
  7. Mitochondrial DNA
  8. Others: mutation in subunit of ATP-sensitive K channel
B. Genetic defects in insulin action
  1. Type A insulin resistance
  2. Leprechaunism
  3. Rabson–Mendenhall syndrome
  4. Lipoatrophic diabetes
  5. Others
C. Diseases of the exocrine pancreas
  1. Pancreatitis
  2. Trauma/pancreatectomy
  3. Neoplasia
  4. Cystic fibrosis
  5. Haemochromatosis
  6. Fibrocalculous pancreatopathy
  7. Others
D. Endocrinopathies
  1. Acromegaly
  2. Cushing syndrome
  3. Glucagonoma
  4. Phaeochromocytoma
  5. Hyperthyroidism
  6. Somatostatinoma
  7. Aldosteronoma
E. Drug or chemical induced
  1. Vacor
  2. Pentamidine
  3. Nicotinic acid
  4. Glucocorticoids
  5. Thyroid hormone
  6. Diazoxide
  7. β-adrenergic agonists
  8. Thiazides
  9. Dilantin

Continued

TABLE 1.6   Aetiological classification of diabetes mellitus—cont'd

    10. Interferon-γ
    11. Clozapine
    12. Protease inhibitors
    13. Others
F. Infections
    1. Congenital rubella
    2. Cytomegalovirus
    3. Others
G. Uncommon forms of immune-mediated diabetes
    1. 'Stiff man' syndrome
    2. Anti-insulin receptor antibodies
    3. Others
H. Other genetic syndromes sometimes associated with diabetes
    1. Down syndrome
    2. Klinefelter syndrome
    3. Turner syndrome
    4. Wolfram syndrome
    5. Friedreich ataxia
    6. Huntington disease
    7. Laurence–Moon–Biedl syndrome
    8. Myotonic dystrophy
    9. Porphyria
    10. Prader–Willi syndrome
    11. Others

IV. Gestational diabetes mellitus

Patients with any form of diabetes may require insulin treatment at some stage of their disease. Such use of insulin does not, of itself, classify the patient.
HNF, hepatocyte nuclear factor; IPF, insulin promoter factor; MODY, maturity-onset diabetes of the young.
Source: American Diabetes Association (2011). Reproduced with permission.

Molecular genetic testing

Knowledge of the genotype in the unaffected child of a patient with this syndrome offers the possibility of a firm diagnosis or, importantly, exclusion of the possibility of diabetes in later life. If the genetic testing is negative, no screening will be necessary and individuals and their families can be reassured. If an unaffected offspring is found to have a MODY2 mutation, then annual testing of fasting plasma glucose and, for females, awareness of the importance of excellent glycaemic control before conception and during pregnancy are required. Identification of a MODY1 or MODY3 genotype necessitates more rigorous, regular screening through childhood, adolescence and early adult life to detect the development of diabetes, as pharmacological treatment, including insulin, is likely to prove necessary. Such testing raises ethical issues and it has been suggested that it should be offered only after appropriate genetic counselling. Whether such knowledge will ultimately allow intervention to prevent or retard the appearance of diabetes is currently uncertain.

Point mutations in mitochondrial DNA have been found to be associated with diabetes mellitus and deafness. The most common mutation occurs at position 3243 in the tRNA leucine gene, leading to an A-to-G transition. An identical lesion occurs in the MELAS (mitochondrial myopathy, encephalopathy, lactic acidosis and stroke-like) syndrome; however, diabetes is not part of this syndrome, suggesting different phenotypic expressions of this genetic lesion.

Genetic abnormalities that result in the inability to convert proinsulin to insulin have been identified in a few families, and such traits are inherited in an autosomal dominant pattern. The resultant glucose intolerance is mild. Similarly, the production of mutant insulin molecules with resultant impaired receptor binding has also been identified in a few families. It is associated with an autosomal inheritance and only mildly impaired or even normal glucose metabolism.

Genetic defects in insulin action

There are unusual causes of diabetes that result from genetically determined abnormalities of insulin action. The metabolic abnormalities associated with mutations of the insulin receptor may range from hyperinsulinaemia and modest hyperglycaemia to severe diabetes. Some individuals with these mutations may have acanthosis nigricans. Women may be virilized and have enlarged, cystic ovaries. In the past, this syndrome was termed type A insulin resistance. Leprechaunism and the Rabson–Mendenhall syndrome are two paediatric syndromes that have mutations in the insulin receptor gene with subsequent alterations in insulin receptor function and extreme insulin resistance. The former has characteristic facial features and is usually fatal in infancy, whereas the latter is associated with abnormalities of teeth and nails plus pineal gland hyperplasia.

Diseases of the exocrine pancreas

Any process that injures the pancreas diffusely can cause diabetes. Acquired processes include pancreatitis, trauma, infection, pancreatectomy and pancreatic carcinoma. With the exception of cancer, damage to the pancreas must be extensive for diabetes to occur; adrenocarcinomas that involve only a small portion of the pancreas have been associated with diabetes. This implies a mechanism other than simple reduction in β-cell mass. If sufficiently extensive, cystic fibrosis and haemochromatosis (see p. 32) will also damage β-cells and impair insulin secretion. Fibrocalculous pancreatopathy may be accompanied by abdominal pain radiating to the back and by pancreatic calcifications identified on X-ray examination. Pancreatic fibrosis and calcium stones in the exocrine ducts have been found at autopsy.

A similar form of chronic calcific pancreatitis with diabetes is also noted in patients with chronic alcoholism, and is associated with diffuse small stones in smaller pancreatic ducts.

Endocrinopathies

Several hormones, such as growth hormone, cortisol, glucagon and adrenaline (epinephrine), antagonize insulin action. Excess amounts of these hormones (e.g. acromegaly, Cushing's syndrome, glucagonoma and phaeochromocytoma, respectively) can cause diabetes. This generally occurs in individuals with pre-existing defects in insulin secretion, and hyperglycaemia typically resolves when the hormone excess is resolved.

Somatostatinoma- and aldosteronoma-induced hypokalaemia can cause diabetes, at least in part by inhibiting insulin secretion. Hyperglycaemia generally resolves after successful removal of the tumour.

Drug- or chemical-induced diabetes

Many drugs can impair insulin secretion. These drugs may not cause diabetes by themselves, but they may precipitate diabetes in individuals with insulin resistance. Certain toxins such as that in Vacor (a rat poison) and intravenous pentamidine can permanently destroy pancreatic β-cells. Such drug reactions fortunately are rare. In such cases, the classification is unclear because the sequence or relative importance of β-cell dysfunction and insulin resistance is unknown. There are also many drugs and hormones that can impair insulin action. Examples include glucocorticoids and nicotinic acid. Patients receiving interferon-α have been reported to develop diabetes associated with islet cell antibodies and, in certain instances, severe insulin deficiency. Such drug reactions fortunately are rare. The list shown in Table 1.6 is not all-inclusive, but reflects the more commonly recognized drug-, hormone- and toxin-induced forms of diabetes.

Second-generation antipsychotic agents

Epidemiological studies suggest an increased risk of hyperglycaemia-related adverse events in patients treated with the atypical antipsychotics (AAPs). Precise risk estimates for hyperglycaemia-related adverse events are not available. Assessment of the relationship between AAPs and glucose abnormalities is complicated by an increased background risk of diabetes mellitus in patients with schizophrenia and the increasing incidence of diabetes mellitus in the general population. Given these confounders, the relationship between, as well as the mechanisms involved in, AAP use and hyperglycaemia-related adverse events is not completely understood. The mechanisms involved in the development of hyperglycaemia are unclear. A meta-analysis of observational studies showed that there was a 1.3-fold increased risk of diabetes in people with schizophrenia taking second-generation antipsychotics compared with the risk in those receiving a first-generation antipsychotic agent. Studies also indicate that the hyperglycaemia is not dose-dependent, is frequently reversible on cessation of treatment with AAPs, and frequently reappears on reintroduction of these therapies. Despite discontinuation of the suspect drug, some patients require continuation of antidiabetic treatment.

Patients with an established diagnosis of diabetes mellitus who are started on AAPs should be monitored regularly for worsening of glucose control. Patients with risk factors for diabetes mellitus (e.g. obesity, family history of diabetes, hypertension) who are starting treatment with AAPs should undergo fasting blood glucose testing/HbA1c measurements at the beginning of treatment and periodically during treatment. Patients should also be monitored for the osmotic symptoms of hyperglycaemia.

Infections

Certain viruses have been associated with β-cell destruction. Diabetes occurs in patients with congenital rubella, although most of these patients have HLA and immune markers characteristic of type 1 diabetes. In addition, Coxsackievirus B, cytomegalovirus, adenovirus and mumps virus have been implicated in inducing diabetes.

Uncommon forms of immune-mediated diabetes

In this category, there are two known conditions, and others are likely to occur. The 'stiff man' syndrome is an autoimmune disorder of the central nervous system characterized by stiffness of the axial muscles with painful spasms. Patients usually have high titres of the

GAD autoantibodies, and approximately one-third will develop diabetes.

Anti-insulin receptor antibodies can cause diabetes by binding to the insulin receptor, thereby blocking the binding of insulin to its receptor in target tissues. However, in some cases, these antibodies can act as an insulin agonist after binding to the receptor and thereby cause hypoglycaemia. Anti-insulin receptor antibodies are occasionally found in patients with systemic lupus erythematosus and other autoimmune diseases. As in other states of extreme insulin resistance, patients with anti-insulin receptor antibodies often have acanthosis nigricans. In the past, this syndrome was termed type B insulin resistance.

Ataxia telangiectasia, an autosomal recessive disorder, is found to be associated with an anti-insulin antibody-mediated insulin-resistant form of diabetes. Another form of autoimmune insulin syndrome with hypoglycaemia has been described in Japan, and is caused by polyclonal insulin-binding autoantibodies that bind to endogenously synthesized insulin. If the insulin dissociates from the antibodies several hours after a meal, hypoglycaemia ensues.

In plasma cell dyscrasias, such as multiple myeloma, the plasma cells may produce monoclonal antibodies against insulin, causing hypoglycaemia by a similar mechanism.

Other genetic syndromes sometimes associated with diabetes

Many genetic syndromes are accompanied by an increased incidence of diabetes mellitus. These include the chromosomal abnormalities of Down, Klinefelter and Turner syndromes. Wolfram syndrome is an autosomal recessive disorder characterized by insulin-deficient diabetes and the absence of β-cells at autopsy. Additional manifestations include diabetes insipidus, hypogonadism, optic atrophy and neural deafness. Other syndromes are listed in Table 1.6.

Lipodystrophic diabetes

These are enigmatic disorders that may be classified as either:

● congenital, or
● acquired (onset often in early childhood).

The principal phenotypic characteristic is partial or total absence of subcutaneous fat, variable degrees of insulin resistance, hyperlipidaemia (sometimes severe with risk of pancreatitis and atherosclerosis) and the metabolic syndrome. The paucity of adipose tissue leads to striking clinical appearances and ketosis-resistant diabetes. The molecular defects responsible await elucidation. Cirrhosis and mesangioproliferative glomerulonephritis are recognized features of some forms. Genetic forms include Berardinelli–Seip congenital lipodystrophy and Dunnigan familial partial lipodystrophy. More recently the acquired form, a human immunodeficiency virus (HIV)-related lipodystrophy in patients treated with highly active antiretroviral therapy has been recognized.

Alterations in the structure and function of the insulin receptor cannot be demonstrated in patients with insulin-resistant lipodystrophic diabetes. Therefore, it is assumed that the lesion(s) must reside in the postreceptor signal transduction pathways.

Gestational diabetes mellitus (GDM)

GDM is defined as any degree of glucose intolerance with onset or first recognition during pregnancy. The definition applies regardless of whether only diet modification or insulin is used for treatment, or whether the condition persists after pregnancy. It does not exclude the possibility that unrecognized glucose intolerance may have antedated or begun concomitantly with the pregnancy. GDM complicates 1–14% of pregnancies in the UK, depending on the population studied. GDM represents nearly 90% of all pregnancies complicated by diabetes.

Tip box

Deterioration of glucose tolerance occurs normally during pregnancy, particularly in the third trimester.

Testing for gestational diabetes

Risk assessment for GDM should be undertaken at the first prenatal visit. Previous recommendations included screening for GDM in all pregnancies. Women with clinical characteristics consistent with a high risk of GDM (marked obesity, personal history of GDM, glycosuria, or a strong family history of diabetes) should undergo oral glucose testing (OGTT; see below) as soon as feasible. If they are found not to have GDM at that initial screening, they should be retested between 24 and 28 weeks of gestation. Women of average risk should have testing undertaken at 24–28 weeks' gestation.

Confirmation of the diagnosis precludes the need for any glucose challenge. In the absence of this degree of hyperglycaemia, evaluation for GDM in women with average or high-risk characteristics should include a diagnostic OGTT.

TABLE 1.7 Screening for and diagnosis of gestational diabetes mellitus (GDM)

75-g OGTT, with plasma glucose measurement fasting, 1 h and 2 hrs, at 24–28 weeks of gestation in women not previously diagnosed with overt diabetes

The OGTT should be performed in the morning after an overnight fast of at least 8 h

The diagnosis of GDM is made when any of the following plasma glucose values are exceeded:
- Fasting >92 mg/dL (5.1 mmol/L)
- 1 h >180 mg/dL (10.0 mmol/L)
- 2 h >153 mg/dL (8.5 mmol/l)

OGTT, oral glucose tolerance test.

Following publication of the Hyperglycemia and Adverse Pregnancy Outcomes (HAPO) trial, the International Association of Diabetes and Pregnancy Study Groups (IADPSG), an international consensus group with representatives from multiple obstetrical and diabetes organizations, including ADA, developed revised recommendations for diagnosing GDM (Table 1.7):

- Perform a 75-g OGTT, with plasma glucose measurement fasting and at 1 and 2 h, at 24–28 weeks of gestation in women not previously diagnosed with overt diabetes. The OGTT should be undertaken in the morning after an overnight fast of between 8 and 14 h, after at least 3 days of unrestricted diet (≥150 g carbohydrate per day) and unlimited physical activity. The subject should remain seated and should not smoke throughout the test.
- The diagnosis of GDM is made when any of the plasma glucose values in Table 1.7 are exceeded.

EPIDEMIOLOGY

Diabetes is one of the most common forms of chronic diseases globally, affecting almost all ethnic groups. In 2011 it was estimated that in 366 million people worldwide suffered from diabetes, most of them living in developing nations (see appendix 1.1, figure 1.5). Globally, almost 6.6% of those aged 20–80 years were estimated to suffer from diabetes. Some 80% of people with diabetes live in low- and middle-income countries. This figure is estimated to increase to 552 million by 2030 (see appendix 1.1, figure 1.6), with the greatest increase in developing countries such as India and China; (see appendix 1.1, figure 1.7) 183 million people (50%) with diabetes are undiagnosed. Traditionally diabetes was thought to be a disease affecting people aged over 55 years. It is now increasingly appreciated that the age of onset of diabetes, especially in developing countries, is decreasing. In India it is estimated that 70% of all new-onset diabetes is in those aged less than 45 years of age.

Type 2 diabetes accounts for at least 90% of all diabetes worldwide. Rapid urbanization, increasing consumption of high-energy food, and sedentary lifestyles is leading to this rapid rise in the number of people suffering from diabetes. The increase in diabetes prevalence, especially in young adults, is likely to lead to an escalation of healthcare costs, and to increased mortality and morbidity along with loss of economic growth.

This rapid rise is occurring in parallel with the obesity epidemic. There is also a sharp rise in the number of patients with impaired glucose tolerance and impaired fasting glucose. This group of patients, with so-called pre-diabetes, is at increased risk of developing in diabetes in future and should be the target of preventive strategies.

The prevalence of type 1 diabetes is also stated to be rising, especially in Scandanavian countries. It tends to occur in genetically susceptible individuals. Some 10–20% of all newly diagnosed cases occur in those who have an affected first-degree relative. Viral infections and nutritional factors have been implicated in the development of type 1 diabetes.

TYPE 1 DIABETES

The incidence of type 1 diabetes shows considerable geographical variation. The highest rates are in Finland, Norway, Sweden and Denmark, with Japan having the lowest incidence amongst the developed countries. In the UK, Finland and Poland the incidence has been rising in recent years; other countries have also reported increasing rates. For example, in the young in Scotland, diabetes is the most common metabolic disease, with an annual incidence of 35 per 100 000 population in 2003 with a near quadrupling of new cases in the last 40 years.

Tip box

The incidence of type 1 diabetes in persons under the age of 16 years has doubled during recent years in the UK.

Variable incidence rates between and within populations are cited as evidence of pathogenetic environmental factors (e.g. viruses, toxins). Intrauterine factors may be important and affect early development. In particular, placental transmission of viruses leading to type 1 diabetes (e.g. rubella) is widely recognized. Possibly cereals, food toxins and enteroviruses trigger islet autoimmunity through intrauterine exposure during pregnancy. Some studies have shown positive associations between diabetes and duration of breastfeeding and the early introduction of cow's milk, whereas others have found no effect.

The peak age of presentation is 11–13 years; however, type 1 diabetes can affect any age group, even the very elderly. In some populations, up to 20% of patients diagnosed initially with type 2 diabetes prove to have evidence of autoimmune activity more typical of type 1 diabetes; such patients respond initially to oral antidiabetic agents but have an early requirement for insulin therapy. Reports of circulating antibodies directed to glutamic acid decarboxylase (GAD) in such patients point to progressive β-cell destruction. This form has been called 'latent autoimmune diabetes in adults' (LADA).

Tip box

Type 1 diabetes often has a long, asymptomatic, prodromal period during which β-cells are selectively destroyed.

Predicting type 1 diabetes

The increase in understanding of the pathogenesis of type 1 diabetes mellitus has made it possible to consider intervention to slow the autoimmune disease process in an attempt to delay or even prevent the onset of hyperglycaemia. Subjects who are at high risk of developing type 1 diabetes can be identified using a combination of immune, genetic and metabolic markers.

However, because only around 10% of patients have a first-degree relative with the disorder, general population screening is not feasible with present strategies. Moreover, prediction, even in higher-risk groups, is imperfect and the complex methodology is not available other than for clinical trials. For relatives of a patient with type 1 diabetes, approximate risks for developing the syndrome are as follows:

- sibling affected – 10% risk overall
- mother affected – 2–3% (risk to offspring varies with age at which mother developed diabetes – higher with younger-onset)

- father affected – 5–10%
- both parents affected – 30%.

Approximately 30–50% of identical (monozygotic) twins and up to 20% of non-identical (dizygotic) twins will ultimately develop type 1 diabetes if the other twin is affected. Experimental interventions to limit β-cell damage using potentially toxic immunosuppressive agents (e.g. ciclosporin) at diagnosis have proved to be, at best, only partially effective; this reflects the extensive and irreversible loss of β-cells by the time of presentation.

TYPE 2 DIABETES

The clinical and biochemical features of type 2 diabetes are presented in Table 1.8.

Diabetes is one of the most common forms of chronic disease, globally affecting almost all ethnic groups. It is estimated that 285 million people worldwide suffer from diabetes, most of them living in developing nations. It is estimated that almost 6.6% of those aged 20–80 years suffer from diabetes globally. This figure is estimated to increase to 438 million by 2030, with the greatest increase in developing countries such as India and China. Traditionally diabetes was thought to be a disease affecting people aged over 55 years. It is now increasingly appreciated that the age of onset of diabetes, especially in developing countries, is decreasing. In India it is

---

TABLE 1.8 Clinical and metabolic features of type 2 diabetes

- Presentation usually in middle age or later life
- Obesity common (present in >75%)
- Symptoms often mild, absent or unrecognized
- Relative rather than absolute insulin deficiency
- Insulin resistance common
- Ketosis-resistant
- Progressive disorder – even with antidiabetic therapy
- Insulin treatment often required to maintain long-term glycaemic control
- Other features of the 'insulin resistance syndrome' often present (e.g. hypertension, dyslipidaemia)
- High risk of macrovascular complications – main cause of premature death
- Tissue damage often present at diagnosis

estimated that 70% of all cases of new-onset diabetes are in those aged less than 45 years.

Type 2 diabetes accounts for at least 90% of all diabetes worldwide. Rapid urbanization, increasing consumption of high-energy food and sedentary lifestyles are leading to this rapid rise in the number of patients suffering from diabetes. The increase in diabetes prevalence, especially in young adults, is likely to lead to an escalation of health-care costs and to increased mortality and morbidity rates, along with loss of economic growth.

This rapid rise is occurring in parallel with the obesity epidemic. There is also a sharp rise in the number of patients with impaired glucose tolerance and impaired fasting glucose (Table 1.9). These patients, with so-called pre-diabetes, are at increased risk of developing diabetes in the future and should be the target of preventive strategies.

The lowest prevalence (< 3%) has been reported in the least developed countries; by contrast, the highest prevalence rates (30–50% of adults) are observed in populations (e.g. North American Indians, Pacific Islanders, Australian Aborigines) that have undergone radical changes from traditional to westernized lifestyles (see below). The Pima Indians of Arizona have the highest prevalence, with over 50% of adults aged 35 years or above having diabetes. The prevalence of diabetes is also high in migrant populations; for example, South Asians in the UK have a 4-fold higher rate than the indigenous white

TABLE 1.9 Diabetes and impaired glucose tolerance (IGT) for 2011 and 2030

	2010	2030
Total world population (billions)	7.0	8.3
Adult population (20–79 years, billions)	4.4	5.6
Diabetes and IGT (20–79 years)		
Global prevalence (%)	8.3	9.9
Comparative prevalence (%)	8.5	8.9
No. of people with diabetes (millions)	366	552
IGT		
Global prevalence (%)	6.4	7.1
Comparative prevalence (%)	6.5	6.7
No. of people with IGT (millions)	280	398

Source: International Diabetes Federation. IDF Diabetes Atlas, 5th edn. IDF, Brussels; 2011. Reproduced with permission.

population. Thus, type 2 diabetes represents an enormous, and rapidly expanding, global public health problem.

Global maps illustrating the projected increase from 2010 to 2030 in the prevalence of diabetes, by region, can be found in Appendix 1.1.

The increasing prevalence of type 2 diabetes depends on a number of factors:

- an increase in the levels of obesity. (Data from the Framingham study show that almost all of the increase in diabetes prevalence in the USA is due to obesity)
- demographic change – half of all people with diabetes are over 65 years old, so as the population ages the prevalence increases
- a fall in the age of onset of type 2 diabetes – people developing diabetes at an earlier age probably reflects weight gain compared with previous generations
- better survival with diabetes because of better control of blood glucose, blood pressure and hyperlipidaemia
- changes in the definition of diabetes, with the diagnosis made at a lower level of fasting
- better detection of diabetes due to opportunistic case-finding, practice-based screening and greater public awareness
- in developing countries, prevalence differs significantly owing to differences in diet, physical exercise and socioeconomic factors – the urban rate is generally assumed to be twice the rural estimate
- for the world as a whole there are more women than men with diabetes. The female excess is pronounced in the developed countries, but in developing countries the numbers are equal
- from 1995 to 2025 the adult population is predicted to increase by 64% and the prevalence of diabetes will increase by 35% (a real increase in the number of diabetic patients of 122%)
- in developed countries there will be an increase in the adult population of 11% with a 27% increase in the prevalence of diabetes
- in developing countries there will be an increase in the adult population of 82% with a 48% increase in the prevalence of diabetes (an increase in the number of diabetic patients of 170%).

PREDICTION AND PREVENTION

It is impossible accurately to predict who will develop type 2 diabetes. Major gaps in understanding of the aetiology of this heterogeneous disorder need to be filled before this will become feasible. However, it is possible to define groups at higher than average risk of developing type 2 diabetes. Factors that have been identified include:

- affected first-degree relative – parent or sibling
- ethnicity – high-risk populations
- middle age to elderly (earlier in high-risk ethnic groups)
- glucose intolerance ('pre-diabetes', non-diabetic hyperglycaemia)
- obesity (especially visceral adiposity)
- certain endocrinopathies
- treatment with diabetogenic drugs
- sedentary lifestyle
- cigarette smoking
- history of gestational diabetes
- other features of the insulin resistance syndrome
- low birth weight (fetal origins hypothesis).

Clinical studies have suggested that the risk of progression from a high-risk group such as impaired glucose tolerance to type 2 diabetes may be averted (or at least postponed) by measures such as dietary advice and supervised physical training (e.g. the Malmö Study in Sweden and the Diabetes Prevention Study in Finland). The US Diabetes Prevention Program showed a 58% reduction (with lifestyle changes) in risk of progression from impaired glucose tolerance to type 2 diabetes (versus 31% for metformin).

Change in lifestyle is the cornerstone of prevention:

- avoidance of obesity
- regular aerobic exercise
- avoiding smoking.

METABOLIC SYNDROME

There are multiple definitions of the metabolic syndrome. It consists of a clustering of cardiovascular risk factors that include central obesity, hypertension and dyslipidaemia, which are all associated with insulin resistance. The presence of the metabolic syndrome is considered an important risk factor for cardiovascular disease and mortality in non-diabetic subjects and patients with type 2 diabetes. The most recent definition of the metabolic syndrome is the consensus document from the International Diabetes Federation (IDF) (Table 1.10). The IDF metabolic syndrome criteria take into account ethnic differences in body fat distribution. The WHO, National Cholesterol Education Program (NCEP) and the Expert Panel on Detection, Evaluation, and

---

TABLE 1.10 Metabolic syndrome

Metabolic syndrome is indicated where central obesity is accompanied by any two of the following four factors:

- raised TG level: > 150 mg/dL (1.7 mmol/L), or specific treatment for this lipid abnormality
- reduced HDL cholesterol: < 40 mg/dL (1.03 mmol/L*) in males and < 50 mg/dL (1.29 mmol/L*) in females, or specific treatment for this lipid abnormality
- raised blood pressure: systolic BP > 130 mmHg or diastolic BP > 85 mmHg, or treatment of previously diagnosed hypertension
- raised FPG > 100 mg/dL (5.6 mmol/L), or previously diagnosed type 2 diabetes. If > 5.6 mmol/L or > 100 mg/dL, OGTT is strongly recommended but is not necessary to define presence of the syndrome

BP, blood pressure; FPG, fasting plasma glucose; HDL, high-density lipoprotein; TG, triglycerides; OGTT, oral glucose tolerance test.
Source: International Diabetes Federation (2006). Reproduced with permission.

Treatment of High Blood Cholesterol in Adults (Adult Treatment Panel (ATP) III) have each proposed different criteria for the diagnosis.

THE INTERNATIONAL DIABETES FEDERATION (IDF) DEFINITION

For a person to be defined as having the metabolic syndrome they must meet the criteria defined in Table 1.10.

Central obesity is most easily measured by waist circumference using the guidelines in Table 1.11, which are sex and ethnic group (not country of residence) specific.

The clinical value of using 'metabolic syndrome' as a diagnosis is contentious. There are different sets of conflicting criteria in existence. Recently published studies have used different criteria and followed subjects for varied lengths of time. Thus the magnitude of risk associated with the metabolic syndrome varies across studies. Generally, the development of CVD correlates with the number of features of the metabolic syndrome at baseline. Men with three or more features at baseline are at greater risk of developing CVD than those with none. However, when confounding factors such as obesity are accounted for, diagnosis of the metabolic syndrome *per se* has a negligible increased association with the risk of heart disease. The metabolic syndrome probably should not be regarded as a clinical entity, but as a clustering of cardiovascular risk factors, each of which requires treatment.

TABLE 1.11 Ethnic specific values for waist circumference

Country/ethnic group	Waist circumference (cm)	
	Male	Female
Europids	>94	>80
In the USA, the ATP III values (102 cm male; 88 cm female) are likely to continue to be used for clinical purposes		
South Asians	>90	>80
Based on a Chinese, Malay and Asian–Indian population		
Chinese	>90	>80
Japanese	>90	>80
Ethnic South and Central Americans	Use South Asian recommendations until more specific data are available	
Sub-Saharan Africans	Use European data until more specific data are available	
Eastern Mediterranean and Middle East (Arab) populations	Use European data until more specific data are available	

ATP, Adult Treatment Panel.
Source: International Diabetes Federation (2006). Reproduced with permission.

The metabolic syndrome is associated with increased risk of a variety of disease outcomes including diabetes, CVD, fatty liver and non-alcoholic steatohepatosis, polycystic ovary syndrome, gallstones, asthma, sleep apnoea and some malignant diseases. The biggest impact that metabolic syndrome has on health is the increased incidence of atheromatous vascular disease. The individual components of the metabolic syndrome – hypertension, dyslipidaemia and glucose intolerance – were all known individually to be associated with increased atheromatous vascular disease.

Central to the concept of metabolic syndrome is insulin resistance, which is strongly associated with non-diabetic hyperglycaemia and type 2 diabetes. It is uncertain whether insulin resistance is the fundamental metabolic defect that links these abnormalities together. However, there is considerable epidemiological and experimental evidence that insulin resistance syndrome confers an increased risk of cardiovascular disease. Importantly, the magnitude of the risk associated with a combination of factors is greater than would be expected by simple addition (i.e. the effects are synergistic).

Finally, there is evidence from longitudinal studies that these metabolic risk factors:

● worsen continuously across the spectrum of glucose intolerance
● may be present many years before the diagnosis of type 2 diabetes.

Again, depending on the study, the all-cause mortality rate is increased by 20–80% in individuals with the metabolic syndrome, with mortality from CVD increased by 60–280% and death from coronary heart disease increased by 70–330%. Presence of the metabolic syndrome confers an increased risk of death from coronary heart disease in women compared with that in men. Other studies have shown a relative risk of developing CVD for those with three or more features compared with that in those with two or fewer features of 1.3–1.7. For individuals with diabetes the relative risk is higher, with a 5-fold increased risk of CVD in those with the metabolic syndrome and diabetes versus those with diabetes without the metabolic syndrome.

Metabolic syndrome is classically associated with type 2 diabetes. However, obese patients with type 1 diabetes are also at risk of developing the metabolic syndrome. This combination is probably present in more than 30% of type 1 patients (depending on the background prevalence of metabolic syndrome). These patients:

● are more likely to develop macrovascular and microvascular complications, and have significantly higher morbidity and mortality rates
● have a higher insulin requirement
● need to be treated more aggressively (glycaemic control plus management of hypertension/dyslipidaemia)
● have a need for insulin sensitizers (e.g. metformin).

FATTY LIVER DISEASE

Fatty liver disease (FLD) is considered to be part of the metabolic syndrome and is due to defects in fat metabolism. Imbalance in energy consumption and its metabolism results in increased lipid storage. Lipid storage may also be a consequence of peripheral resistance to insulin, whereby the transport of fatty acids from adipose tissue to the liver is increased. Impairment or inhibition of the receptor molecules, peroxisome proliferator-activated receptor (PPAR)-α, PPAR-γ and sterol regulatory element-binding protein (SREBP)-1, that control the enzymes responsible for the oxidation and synthesis of fatty acids also appears to contribute to the accumulation of fat. Alcohol excess is known to damage mitochondria and other cellular structures, further impairing cellular energy mechanism. Non-alcoholic FLD may begin as an excess of unmetabolized energy in liver cells. Hepatic steatosis (retention of lipid) is considered to be reversible and to some extent non-progressive if there is cessation or removal of the underlying cause.

Severe fatty liver is often accompanied by inflammation, a situation that is referred to as steatohepatitis. Progression to alcoholic steatohepatitis (ASH) or non-alcoholic steatohepatitis (NASH) depends on the persistence or severity of the inciting cause. Pathological lesions in both conditions are similar. However, the extent of inflammatory response varies widely and does not always correlate with degree of fat accumulation.

Liver with extensive inflammation and high degree of steatosis often progresses to more severe forms of the disease. Hepatocyte ballooning and hepatocyte necrosis of varying degree are often present at this stage. Liver cell death and inflammatory responses lead to the activation of stellate cells, which play a pivotal role in hepatic fibrosis. The extent of fibrosis varies widely. Perisinusoidal fibrosis is most common, especially in adults, and predominates in and around the terminal hepatic veins. The progression to cirrhosis may be influenced by the amount of lipid accumulated, the degree of steatohepatitis, and a variety of other sensitizing factors. In alcoholic FLD the transition to cirrhosis related to continued alcohol consumption is well documented, but the process involved in non-alcoholic FLD is less clear.

Cirrhosis, secondary to FLD, is now very common, and as obesity/insulin resistance becomes more common cirrhosis will become an even bigger clinical issue.

HAEMOCHROMATOSIS ('BRONZE DIABETES')

Haemochromatosis is usually defined as iron overload with a hereditary/primary cause, or originating from a metabolic disorder. However, the term has often also been used more broadly to refer to any form of iron overload. The term haemosiderosis is generally used to indicate the pathological effect of iron accumulation in any given organ, which occurs mainly in the form of haemosiderin.

Hereditary haemochromatosis is the most common of several 'iron overload' diseases. It is the most common single-gene inherited disorder in Caucasians, with 1 in 10 persons carrying an abnormal gene. Haemochromatosis is caused by mutations in the *HFE* gene, inherited in an autosomal recessive manner. The two mutations identified in the *HFE* gene are C282Y and H63D.

As many as 1 in 200 Americans are believed to carry both markers of the gene for haemochromatosis, and it is estimated that about half will eventually develop complications. This will give a prevalence similar to that of type 1 diabetes but, as in type 2 diabetes, the condition appears to be relatively underdiagnosed.

Haemochromatosis causes the body to absorb excessive amounts of iron from the diet. The body lacks an efficient means of excreting this excess iron, and as a result excess iron is deposited in organs, mainly the liver, but also the pancreas, heart, endocrine glands and joints.

Haemochromatosis is characterized by the four main features:

- Increased pigmentation (slate-grey or brownish bronze) is seen in more than 90% of patients; it is often one of the first signs of the disease and may precede other signs by many years. Hyperpigmentation is most evident on sun-exposed skin, particularly the face. There may also be skin thinning and/or ichthyosis-like changes (scaling) with partial loss of body hair (pubic region most affected)
- Enlarged liver occurs in more than 95% of patients and is often accompanied by cirrhosis and liver failure
- Diabetes mellitus, often requiring insulin therapy, is seen in 30–60% of patients
- Heart failure due to cardiomyopathy.

SYMPTOMS

The condition is 10 times more common in males than in females, and usually presents between 40 and 60 years of age. Symptoms tend to occur in men between the ages of 30 and 50 years, and in women over the age of 50 years, with joint pain being the most common presentation:

- joint pain – commonly in the second and third metacarpophalangeal joints, and the interphalangeal and carpal joints
- fatigue
- lack of energy
- abdominal pain
- loss of sex drive.

INVESTIGATIONS

- Measurement of serum iron levels has no value in making the diagnosis.
- Transferrin saturation corresponds to the ratio of serum iron and total iron-binding capacity. Similar to iron, it is influenced by liver disease (other than haemochromatosis) and inflammation; therefore, it has limitations in the diagnostic workup.
  - Haemochromatosis is suggested by persistently raised transferrin saturation in the absence of other causes of iron overload. It is the initial test of choice.
  - The screening threshold for haemochromatosis is a fasting transferrin saturation of 45–50%.
  - Approximately 30% of women younger than 30 years who have haemochromatosis do not have increased transferrin saturation.
  - High transferrin saturation is the earliest evidence of haemochromatosis. A value greater than 60% in men and 50% in women is highly specific.
- Serum ferritin levels raised above 200 μg/L in premenopausal women and 300 μg/L in men and postmenopausal women indicate primary iron overload due to haemochromatosis, especially when associated with high transferrin saturation and evidence of liver disease.
  - Ferritin concentration can be high in other conditions, such as infections, inflammations and liver disease.
  - Ferritin concentration higher than 1000 μg/L suggests liver damage with fibrosis or cirrhosis.
  - Ferritin levels are less sensitive than transferrin saturation in screening tests for haemochromatosis.
- Genetic testing for the *HFE* mutation is indicated in patients with evidence of iron overload (e.g. raised transferrin saturation, high serum ferritin levels, excess iron staining or iron concentration on liver biopsy samples) and also in all first-degree relatives of patients with haemochromatosis. This is indicated particularly in patients with known liver disease and evidence of iron overload, even if other causes of liver disease are present.

  Liver biopsy:

- is useful to identify liver disease and to determine the presence or absence of cirrhosis, which directly affects prognosis.
- is indicated in the following cases:
  - raised liver enzymes in combination with hereditary haemochromatosis
  - serum ferritin level above 1000 μg/L.

MANAGEMENT

It is important to detect haemochromatosis as early as possible so that venesection can be instituted to prevent the build-up of iron and potential complications. Tiredness and abdominal pain should diminish, and increased pigmentation of the skin should fade. Once complications such as diabetes and cirrhosis have developed, they cannot be reversed. In addition, arthritis may fail to improve with venesection.

Haemochromatosis cannot be treated with a low iron diet alone. However, some foods affect the way the body absorbs iron. The following dietary tips may play a small part in reducing the symptoms of the disease:

- Minimize alcohol intake, particularly with meals – alcohol may lead to increased iron absorption and increase the risk of liver disease
- Reduce intake of liver, kidney and red meat – iron absorption from red meat is 20–30% compared with 1–20% for vegetables and grains
- Avoid vitamin supplements or tonics containing iron or vitamin C – vitamin C enhances the absorption of iron from the diet.

Treatment of haemochromatosis consists of regular venesection. Depending on the degree of iron overload, the procedure may initially be performed once weekly or once monthly. This regularity of treatment continues until serum ferritin levels return to normal; this may take up to 2 years. After this, lifelong maintenance therapy needs to be set in place as excess iron continues to be absorbed. On average, venesection is required every 3–4 months to prevent build-up and maintain normal levels. Regular monitoring of serum ferritin, transferrin saturation, haematocrit and haemoglobin is necessary throughout the treatment process.

Acquired haemochromatosis may be the result of blood transfusions, excessive dietary iron, or secondary to other disease.

- Alcoholic liver disease – patients include those who are heavy drinkers, perhaps of iron-containing fortified wines, and who have cirrhosis. Liver biopsy in these patients may show a modest increase in iron; however, contrary to patients with haemochromatosis, the hepatic iron levels are relatively normal.
- Ineffective erythropoiesis with marrow hyperplasia – patients with hyperplastic erythroid marrow absorb an increased amount of iron to the point where they may have clinical iron overload. Examples include the hereditary sideroblastic anaemias, severe

α- and β-thalassaemia, and the myelodysplastic syndrome variants, such as refractory anaemia with ringed sideroblasts (RARS).

- Iron overload associated with chronic anaemia – examples include hereditary spherocytosis and acquired sideroblastic anaemia, where patients have increased effective erythropoiesis and increased iron absorption.

- Multiple transfusions – hypertransfusion is performed in patients with β-thalassaemia major, sickle cell anaemia, refractory aplastic anaemia and myelodysplastic syndrome. Such patients may receive as much as 100 units of red cells.

- Porphyria cutanea tarda (PCT) – this is primarily a skin and liver disease that occurs in familial and sporadic forms. The cause of liver siderosis in sporadic PCT has not been established, but may be related to a mutation in the *HFE* gene.

POLYCYSTIC OVARY SYNDROME (PCOS)

PCOS is one of the most common female endocrine disorders, affecting approximately 5–10% of females of reproductive age (12–45 years). A majority of patients with PCOS have insulin resistance and/or are obese. Their raised insulin levels contribute to or cause the abnormalities seen in the hypothalamic–pituitary–ovarian axis that lead to PCOS.

Hyperinsulinaemia increases the gonadotropin-releasing hormone (GnRH) pulse frequency, luteinizing hormone (LH) over follicle-stimulating hormone (FSH) dominance, which increases ovarian androgen production, decreases follicular maturation, and decreases sex hormone-binding globulin (SHBG) binding; all of these steps lead to the development of PCOS. Insulin resistance is a common finding among patients of normal weight as well as overweight patients.

Hyperinsulinaemia in patients with PCOS has been found to be associated with an increased 17,20-lyase activity, leading to excess androgen production.

Adipose tissue possesses aromatase, an enzyme that converts androstenedione to oestrone, and testosterone to oestradiol. The excess adipose tissue in obese patients creates the paradox of having both excess androgens (which are responsible for hirsutism and virilization) and oestrogens (which inhibits FSH via negative feedback).

The principal features are:

- obesity
- anovulation – oligomenorrhoea, amenorrhoea (irregular, few, or absent menstrual periods)

- hirsutism – excessive mild symptoms of hyperandrogenism, such as acne or hyperseborrhoea, are frequently seen in adolescent girls and are often associated with irregular menstrual cycles. In most instances, these symptoms are transient and reflect only the immaturity of the hypothalamic–pituitary–ovarian axis during the first years following menarche.

Tip box

Not all women with PCOS have polycystic ovaries, nor do all women with ovarian cysts have PCOS.

The diagnosis is straightforward using the Rotterdam criteria (Table 1.12), even when the syndrome is associated with a wide range of symptoms.

History-taking should enquire specifically about:

- the menstrual pattern
- history of obesity
- hirsutism
- absence/presence of breast discharge.

These four questions can diagnose PCOS with a sensitivity of approximately 80% and a specificity of about 90%.

Investigations should include:

- Gynaecological ultrasonography – in PCOS there is 'follicular arrest', whereby several follicles develop to a size of 5–7 mm (pre-ovulatory size is 16 mm or more). According to the Rotterdam criteria, 12 or more small follicles (2–9 mm) should be seen in an ovary on ultrasound examination and/or the ovarian volume should be $> 10 \text{ cm}^3$ on either side.

TABLE 1.12 Diagnosis of polycystic ovary syndrome

In 2003 a consensus workshop sponsored by ESHRE and ASRM in Rotterdam indicated PCOS to be present when 2 of the following 3 criteria are met:
- oligo-ovulation and/or anovulation
- excess androgen activity
- polycystic ovaries (by gynaecological ultrasonography)
- exclusion of other endocrine disorders

ESHRE, European Society of Human Reproduction and Embryology; ASRM, American Society for Reproductive Medicine.

- Serum (blood) levels of androgens including androstenedione, testosterone and dehydroepiandrosterone sulphate may be raised. The free testosterone level is considered to be the best measure.
- Other blood tests are suggestive but not diagnostic. The ratio of LH : FSH is greater than 1 : 1, as tested on day 3 of the menstrual cycle. This pattern is not specific and is present in less than 50%.

Common assessments for associated conditions or risks include:

- fasting biochemical screen and lipid profile
- frank diabetes can be seen in 65–68% of women with this condition.

For exclusion of other disorders that may cause similar symptoms:

- prolactin to rule out hyperprolactinaemia
- thyroid-stimulating hormone (TSH) to rule out hypothyroidism
- 17-hydroxyprogesterone to rule out 21-hydroxylase deficiency (congenital adrenal hyperplasia).

Women with PCOS are at risk of the following:

- type 2 diabetes
- hypertension
- dyslipidaemia
- cardiovascular and cerebrovascular disease
- miscarriage
- acanthosis nigricans
- endometrial hyperplasia and increased risk of endometrial cancer. This appears to be due to over-accumulation of the uterine lining and also lack of progesterone, resulting in prolonged stimulation of uterine cells by oestrogen. It is, however, unclear whether this increased risk is directly due to PCOS or to the associated obesity, hyperinsulinaemia and hyperandrogenism
- [autoimmune thyroiditis].

DIFFERENTIAL DIAGNOSIS

Other causes of irregular or absent menstruation and hirsutism, include congenital adrenal hyperplasia, Cushing syndrome, hyperprolactinaemia and androgen-secreting neoplasms, as well as other pituitary or adrenal disorders.

PCOS has been reported in other insulin-resistant situations, such as acromegaly.

MEDICAL TREATMENT OF PCOS IS TAILORED TO THE PATIENT'S GOALS

In each of these areas, there is considerable debate as to the optimal treatment. One of the major reasons for this is the lack of large-scale clinical trials comparing different treatments. Broadly, these may be considered under four categories:

1. Lowering of insulin levels

Successful weight loss is the most effective method of restoring normal ovulation/menstruation. Reducing insulin resistance by improving insulin sensitivity through medications such as metformin and/or thiazolidinediones is often helpful.

2. Treatment of hirsutism or acne

The standard contraceptive pill may be effective in reducing hirsutism. A common choice of contraceptive pill is one that contains cyproterone acetate; in the UK/USA the available brand is Dianette/Diane. Cyproterone acetate is a progestogen with antiandrogen effects.

Other drugs with antiandrogen effects include flutamide and spironolactone, both of which can give some improvement in hirsutism. Spironolactone is probably the most commonly used drug in the USA. Metformin may reduce hirsutism, perhaps by reducing insulin resistance, and is often used when there are other features such as insulin resistance, diabetes or obesity that should also benefit from metformin. Eflornithine (Vaniqa) is a drug that is applied to the skin in cream form, often to the face. It is an irreversible inhibitor of ornithine decarboxylase, the enzyme that catalyses the rate-limiting step in folliculogenesis. Hence it inhibits hair growth directly. Individuals may vary in their response to different therapies, and it is usually worth trying other drug treatments if one does not work, but drug treatments do not work well for all individuals. For removal of facial hair, electrolysis or laser treatments are faster, more efficient, although expensive alternatives.

3. Restoration of fertility

Of course, not all women with PCOS have difficulty becoming pregnant. Treatment of infertility is not within the scope of this book.

4. Restoration of regular menstruation, and prevention of endometrial hyperplasia and endometrial cancer

If fertility is not the primary aim, menstruation can usually be regulated with a contraceptive pill. The purpose of regulating menstruation is essentially for the woman's convenience and perhaps sense of well-being; there is no medical requirement for regular periods, so long as they occur sufficiently often (at least every 3 months). Most brands of contraceptive pill result in a withdrawal bleed every 28 days if taken in 3-week intervals. Dianette is also beneficial for hirsutism, and is therefore often prescribed for PCOS.

If a regular menstrual cycle is not desired, then therapy for an irregular cycle is not necessarily required – if a menstrual bleed occurs at least every 3 months, the endometrium is being shed sufficiently often to prevent increased risk of endometrial abnormalities or cancer. If menstruation occurs less often or not at all, some form of progestogen replacement is recommended. Some women prefer a uterine progestogen implant such as the intrauterine system (Mirena) coil, which provides simultaneous contraception and endometrial protection for many years, although often with unpredictable minor bleeding. An alternative is an oral progestogen taken at intervals (e.g. every 3 months) to induce a predictable menstrual bleed.

BIOCHEMISTRY OF DIABETES

INSULIN

The hormone insulin is a primary regulatory signal in animals, suggesting that the basic mechanism is old and central to animal life (Figs 1.1 & 1.2). β-cells in the islets of Langerhans release insulin in two phases. In the first phase insulin release is triggered rapidly in response to increased blood glucose levels. The second phase is a sustained, slow release of newly formed vesicles that are triggered independently of glucose.

During the first phase of insulin release, glucose enters the β-cells through the glucose transporter (GLUT-2), and through glycolysis and the respiratory cycle multiple high-energy adenosine triphosphate (ATP) molecules are produced, leading to the ATP-controlled potassium channels (K^+) closing and the cell membrane depolarizing. On depolarization, voltage-controlled calcium channels (Ca^{2+}) open. An increased calcium level causes activation of phospholipase C, which cleaves the membrane

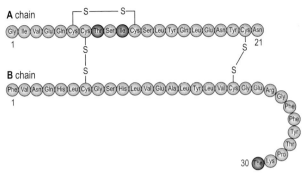

Figure 1.1 Primary structure (amino acid sequence) of human insulin.

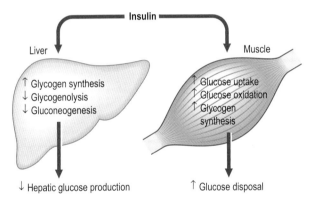

Figure 1.2 Regulation of glucose metabolism by insulin.

phospholipid, phosphatidylinositol 4,5-bisphosphate, into inositol 1,4,5-triphosphate and diacylglycerol. Inositol 1,4,5-triphosphate (IP3) binds to receptor proteins in the membrane of endoplasmic reticulum (ER), which allows the release of Ca^{2+} from the ER via IP3 gated channels, and further raises the cell concentration of calcium. The increased amount of calcium in the cells causes release of previously synthesized insulin, which has been stored in secretory vesicles.

Evidence of early impaired first-phase insulin release can be seen in the oral glucose tolerance test, demonstrated by a substantially raised blood glucose level at 30 min, a marked drop by 60 min, and a steady climb back to baseline levels over the following hourly time points.

Insulin secretion from the pancreas is not continuous, but oscillates within a period of 3–6 min, changing from generating a blood insulin concentration of more than about 800 pmol/L to less than 100 pmol/L. This is thought to avoid downregulation of insulin receptors in target cells and to assist the liver in extracting insulin from the blood.

Other substances known to stimulate insulin release include amino acids from ingested proteins and acetylcholine, released from vagus nerve endings (parasympathetic nervous system). Glucagon-like peptide (GLP) and glucose-dependent insulinotropic peptide (GIP), released by enteroendocrine cells of intestinal mucosa, also stimulate insulin release. Acetylcholine triggers insulin release through phospholipase C, whereas GLP and GIP act through adenylate cyclase. The three amino acids, alanine, glycine and arginine, which stimulate insulin secretion, act similarly to glucose by altering the membrane potential of β-cells.

The sympathetic nervous system (via α_2-adrenergic stimulation as demonstrated by the agonists clonidine or methyldopa) inhibits the release of insulin. However, circulating adrenaline (epinephrine) will activate β_2-receptors on the β-cells in the pancreatic islets to promote insulin release. This is important, as muscle cannot benefit from the raised blood sugar resulting from adrenergic stimulation (increased gluconeogenesis and glycogenolysis from the low blood insulin : glucagon state) unless insulin is present to allow for GLUT-4 translocation into the tissue.

When the glucose level comes down to the usual physiological value, insulin release from the β-cells slows or stops. If blood glucose levels drop lower, release of hyperglycaemic hormones (most prominently glucagon from islet of Langerhans' α-cells) forces release of glucose into the blood from cellular stores, primarily liver cell stores of glycogen. By increasing blood glucose levels, the hyperglycaemic hormones prevent or correct life-threatening hypoglycaemia. Release of insulin is strongly inhibited by the stress hormone noradrenaline (norepinephrine), leading to increased blood glucose levels during stress. The many roles of insulin are summarized in Table 1.13.

Tip box

Hepatic glucose production is the principal determinant of the fasting blood glucose concentration.

Tip box

Stimulation of glucose uptake (and subsequently metabolism or storage as glycogen) requires higher plasma insulin concentrations than are necessary for suppression of hepatic glucose production.

TABLE 1.13 Main physiological actions of insulin

- Increased glycogen synthesis – increases hepatic (and skeletal muscle/ adipose tissue) storage of glucose cells in the form of glycogen; lowered levels of insulin cause liver cells to convert glycogen to glucose and excrete it into the bloodstream
- Increased fatty acid synthesis – increased uptake of plasma lipids by adipose tissue; lack of insulin causes the reverse
- Increased esterification of fatty acids – increased adipose tissue production of triglycerides from fatty acid esters; lack of insulin causes the reverse
- Decreased proteolysis
- Decreased lipolysis – reduction in conversion of fat cell lipid stores into free fatty acids; lack of insulin causes the reverse
- Decreased gluconeogenesis – decreased production of glucose from non-sugar substrates; lack of insulin causes glucose production from assorted substrates in the liver and elsewhere
- Increased amino acid uptake – increased uptake of circulating amino acids; lack of insulin inhibits absorption
- Increased potassium uptake – increased cellular uptake of plasma potassium; lack of insulin inhibits absorption. Insulin's increase in cellular potassium uptake lowers potassium levels in blood
- Arterial muscle tone – induces arterial wall muscle relaxation, increasing blood flow, especially in microarteries; lack of insulin reduces flow by allowing these muscles to contract

Insulin degradation

Once an insulin molecule has docked on to the receptor and effected its action, it may be released back into the extracellular environment or it may be degraded by the cell. Degradation normally involves endocytosis of the insulin–receptor complex followed by the activation of the insulin degrading enzyme. Most insulin molecules are degraded by liver cells. It has been estimated that a typical insulin molecule is finally degraded approximately 70 min after its initial release into the circulation.

GLUCAGON

Glucagon is an important hormone involved in carbohydrate metabolism. Glucagon is synthesized and secreted from the α-cells of the islets of Langerhans. It is released when blood glucose levels start to fall too low, causing the liver to convert stored glycogen into glucose and release it into the bloodstream, raising blood glucose levels and ultimately preventing the development of hypoglycaemia.

The action of glucagon is thus opposite to that of insulin. However, glucagon also stimulates the release of insulin, so that newly available glucose in the bloodstream can be taken up and used by insulin-dependent tissues (Tables 1.14 & 1.15).

THE INSULIN RECEPTOR

The insulin receptor is a transmembrane receptor belonging to the large class of tyrosine kinase receptors (Fig. 1.3). Two α-subunits and two β-subunits make up the receptor. The β-subunits pass through the cellular membrane and are linked by disulphide bonds. Receptor activity is mediated by tyrosines phosphorylation within the cell. The 'substrate' protein for insulin receptor substrate (IRS)-1 is phosphorylated, leading to an increase in the high-affinity glucose transporter (GLUT-4) molecules on the outer membrane of insulin-responsive tissues. These tissues include muscle cells, adipose tissue and hepatocytes. This process leads to an increase in the uptake of glucose from blood into these tissues and a cascade of post-receptor signalling events still not fully elucidated. GLUT-4 is transported from cellular vesicles to the cell surface, where it mediates the transport of glucose into the cell. Other isoforms of glucose transporters (e.g. GLUT-1 at the blood–brain and blood–retinal barriers, GLUT-2 in islet β-cells) do not require insulin to transfer glucose into cells.

TABLE 1.14 Causes of increased and decreased secretion/inhibition of glucagon

Increased secretion of glucagon is caused by:	Decreased secretion/inhibition of glucagon is caused by:
• Decreased plasma glucose	• Somatostatin
• Increased catecholamines – nor-adrenaline (norepinephrine) and adrenaline (epinephrine)	• Insulin
• Increased plasma amino acids (to protect from hypoglycaemia if an all-protein meal is consumed)	• Increased free fatty acids and keto acids in the bloodstream
• Sympathetic nervous system	• Increased urea production
• Acetylcholine	
• Cholecystokinin	

TABLE 1.15 Metabolic actions of insulin and glucagon

	Insulin	Glucagon
Fatty acid uptake and release in fat	Stimulates synthesis TG from FFA; inhibits release of FFA from TG	Stimulates release of FFA from TG
Liver glycogen	Increases synthesis and thereby glucose uptake and storage	Stimulates glycogenolysis and glucose release
Liver gluconeogenesis	Inhibits; saves amino acids	Stimulates; glucose synthesized and released
Glucose uptake, skeletal muscle	Stimulates uptake, storage as glycogen and use in energy metabolism	No receptors, no effect
Glycogen, skeletal muscle	Stimulates synthesis	No receptors, no effect
Amino acid uptake	Stimulates and is necessary for protein synthesis	No receptors, no effect
Brain (hypothalamus)	Reduces hunger through hypothalamic regulation	No effect

FFA, free fatty acids; TG, triglycerides.

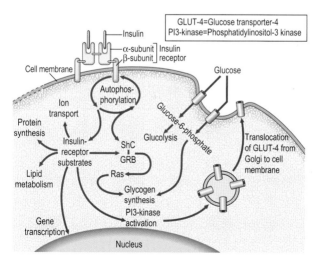

Figure 1.3 Cellular binding of insulin to its receptor and post-binding events. GLUT-4, glucose transporter-4; GRB, growth factor receptor-bound protein; PI3-kinase, phosphatidylinositol-3 kinase.

- Receptor defects – there may be a reduced number of insulin receptors or a reduction in their affinity for insulin. This may occur in response to chronic hyperinsulinaemia (so-called downregulation). Lesser degrees of obesity and glucose intolerance are associated with receptor defects that are largely reversible with treatment. Inherited severe receptor defects are rare.
- Post-receptor defects – defects in intracellular events distal to the binding of insulin account for insulin resistance in most patients with type 2 diabetes; the maximal response to insulin is impaired and is usually only partially reversible, even with insulin-sensitizing drugs. The precise nature of these defects has not yet been identified.

> **Tip box**
>
> Insulin receptor downregulation and post-receptor defects frequently coexist.

LIPOLYSIS

Lipolysis is the hydrolysis of lipids (Fig. 1.4). Metabolically it is the breakdown of triglycerides into free fatty acids within cells. When fats are broken down for energy, the process is known as

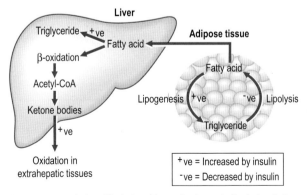

Figure 1.4 Regulation of lipolysis and ketone body metabolism by insulin (+ve = increased by insulin; −ve = decreased by insulin).

β-oxidation: ketones are produced and are found in large quantities in ketosis (a state in metabolism occurring when the liver converts fat into fatty acids and ketone bodies, which can be used by the body for energy). Lipolysis testing strips such as Ketostix are used to recognize urinary ketones.

The following hormones induce lipolysis: noradrenaline (epinephrine), noradrenaline (norepinephrine), glucagon, growth hormone and cortisol (although cortisol's actions are still unclear). These trigger G-protein-coupled receptors, which activate adenylate cyclase. This results in increased production of cAMP, which activates protein kinase A, which subsequently activate lipases found in adipose tissue.

Triglycerides are transported through the blood to appropriate tissues (adipose, muscle, etc.) by lipoproteins such as chylomicrons. Triglycerides present on the chylomicrons undergo lipolysis by the cellular lipases of target tissues, which yield glycerol and free fatty acids. Free fatty acids released into the blood are then available for cellular uptake. Free fatty acids not immediately taken up by cells may bind to albumin for transport to surrounding tissues that require energy. Serum albumin is the major carrier of free fatty acids in the blood. The glycerol also enters the bloodstream and is absorbed by the liver or kidney where it is converted to glycerol 3-phosphate by the enzyme glycerol kinase. Hepatic glycerol 3-phosphate is converted mostly to dihydroxyacetone phosphate (DHAP) and then glyceraldehyde 3-phosphate (GA3P), to rejoin the glycolysis and gluconeogenesis pathway.

While lipolysis is triglyceride hydrolysis, the process by which triglycerides are broken down, esterification is the process by which triglycerides are formed. Esterification and lipolysis are essentially reversals of one another.

GLUCOSE TOXICITY

Importantly, from a therapeutic standpoint, there is evidence that hyperglycaemia *per se* may adversely affect both insulin action and endogenous insulin secretion. These effects have been termed 'glucose toxicity'. The clinical implication is that reducing the level of hyperglycaemia (by non-pharmacological measures, oral agents or insulin) may produce secondary improvements in intermediary metabolism.

LIPOTOXICITY

Disturbed fatty acid metabolism has been documented in patients with type 2 diabetes and lesser degrees of glucose intolerance. Experimental data indicate that raised fatty acid concentrations may:

- impair insulin-mediated glucose disposal and oxidation (via the glucose–fatty acid or Randle cycle)
- accelerate hepatic glucose production
- inhibit endogenous insulin secretion
- contribute to hypertriglyceridaemia.

These effects may be regarded as evidence for a toxic effect of fatty acids. Under experimental conditions, fatty acids may induce apoptosis in islet β-cells. Tumour necrosis factor-α produced by adipocytes has also been implicated in the production of insulin resistance in glucose metabolism via inhibitory effects on insulin signalling. In addition, increased circulating fatty acid concentrations have been implicated in the pathogenesis of hypertension.

APPENDIX 1.1: PREVALENCE ESTIMATES OF DIABETES, 2011–2030

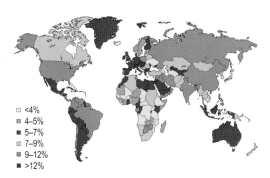

    □ <4%
    ■ 4–5%
    ■ 5–7%
    □ 7–9%
    ■ 9–12%
    ■ >12%

Figure 1.5 Prevalence (%) estimates of diabetes (20–79 years), 2010. (Source: International Diabetes Federation/IDF Diabetes Atlas, 5th edn. IDF, Brussels. © International Diabetes Federation 2011. Reproduced with permission.)

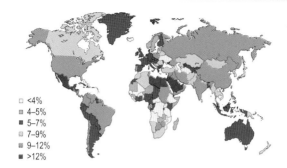

☐ <4%
▨ 4–5%
■ 5–7%
▨ 7–9%
▨ 9–12%
■ >12%

Figure 1.6 Prevalence (%) estimates of diabetes (20–79 years), 2030. (Source: International Diabetes Federation/IDF Diabetes Atlas, 5th edn. IDF, Brussels. © International Diabetes Federation 2011. Reproduced with permission.)

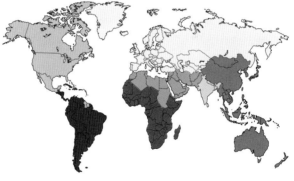

REGION	2011 Millions	2030 Millions	INCREASE %
■ Africa	14.7	28.0	90%
▨ Middle East and North Africa	32.8	59.7	83%
☐ South-East Asia	71.4	120.9	69%
■ South and Central America	25.1	39.9	59%
▨ Western Pacific	131.9	187.9	42%
▨ North America and Caribbean	37.7	51.2	36%
☐ Europe	52.6	64.0	22%
World	**366.2**	**551.8**	**51%**

Figure 1.7 International Diabetes Federation regions and global projections for the number of people with diabetes (20–79 years), 2010–2030. (Source: International Diabetes Federation/ IDF Diabetes Atlas, 5th edn. IDF, Brussels. © International Diabetes Federation 2011. Reproduced with permission.)

INITIAL MANAGEMENT AND EDUCATION

CLINICAL PRESENTATION OF DIABETES

The clinical presentation of diabetes is heterogeneous, ranging from asymptomatic type 2 diabetes to the dramatic life-threatening conditions of diabetic ketoacidosis (DKA) and hyperosmolar non-ketotic coma (HONK). Patients with type 2 diabetes are often detected by opportunistic screening such as urinalysis or routine blood glucose tests in general practice, at health insurance checks or during attendance at hospital for an unrelated problem. This heterogeneity in presentation reflects not only the relevant diagnostic category into which the patient falls (type 1 or type 2), but also the point in the natural history of the disorder at which the diagnosis is made. Patients may present with macrovascular complications or the specific microvascular complications of diabetes.

Tip box

The clinical presentation may be modified, precipitated or caused by intercurrent illness.

TYPE 1 DIABETES

The clinical presentation of type 1 diabetes in younger patients is usually acute with classical osmotic symptoms (Table 2.1).

Symptoms will usually have been present for only a few weeks; weight loss may predominate. In these circumstances, weight loss reflects catabolism of protein and fat resulting from profound insulin deficiency. If the hyperglycaemia is marked, the patient may become severely dehydrated.

Associated symptoms, particularly blurred vision may occur, although these are generally less prominent. Although the islet β-cell destruction of type 1 diabetes is a process that occurs gradually. It is very uncommon to detect type 1 diabetes during the early asymptomatic stages of the condition. Once symptoms appear,

TABLE 2.1 Presenting features of type 1 diabetes

Osmotic symptoms	Associated symptoms
Thirst	Muscular cramps
Polyuria	Blurred vision
Nocturia	Fungal or bacterial infection, usually orogenital
Weight loss	and cutaneous, respectively
Fatigue and lassitude	

diagnosis may sometimes be expedited by awareness of symptoms in other family members with diabetes. Despite the presence of significant osmotic symptoms, patients sometimes do not seek medical advice and may present in DKA (see Table 1.4).

Tip box

Intercurrent illness, such as sepsis, may cause rapid metabolic decompensation in patients with type 1 diabetes.

DKA is a life-threatening medical emergency requiring hospitalization. The diagnosis and management of DKA is considered in more detail in Section 4.

TYPE 2 DIABETES

The majority of patients with type 2 diabetes are diagnosed at a relatively late stage of a long pathological process that develops and progresses over many years.

Tip box

Type 2 diabetes represents a late stage of a complex and progressive pathological process.

The presenting clinical features of type 2 diabetes (Table 2.2) range from none at all to those associated with the dramatic and life-threatening hyperglycaemic emergency of the hyperosmolar non-ketotic syndrome. In many patients with lesser degrees of hyperglycaemia, symptoms may go unnoticed or unrecognized for many years; such undiagnosed diabetes carries the risk of insidious tissue damage.

Tip box

In the UK, African Caribbean people and immigrants from South Asia have the highest rates of diabetes.

Classical osmotic symptoms are may be present in type 2 diabetes – with the notable exception of significant weight loss, which is less common. However, a high index of clinical suspicion must be maintained so that asymptomatic cases are not missed. The absence of weight loss reflects the presence of sufficient secretion of endogenous insulin to prevent catabolism of protein and fat. Most patients with type 2 diabetes are overweight or obese, adding to their

---

TABLE 2.2 Presenting features of type 2 diabetes

None – asymptomatic patients identified by screening

Osmotic symptoms
- Thirst
- Polyuria
- Nocturia
- Blurred vision
- Fatigue/lassitude

Infection
- Recurrent fungal infection (e.g. genital candidiasis)
- Recurrent bacterial infections (e.g. urinary tract)

Macrovascular complications
- Coronary artery disease (angina pectoris, acute myocardial infarction)
- Cerebrovascular disease (transient ischaemic episodes, stroke)
- Peripheral vascular disease (intermittent claudication, rest pain, ischaemic ulceration)

Microvascular complications
- Retinopathy (acute or progressive visual impairment)
- Nephropathy (proteinuria, hypertension, nephrotic syndrome)
- Neuropathy (symptomatic sensory polyneuropathy, foot ulceration, amyotrophy, cranial nerve palsies, peripheral mononeuropathies, entrapment neuropathies)

Associated conditions
- Glaucoma
- Cataracts

---

insulin resistance and hyperinsulinaemia. However lean type 2 diabetes is a definite entity particularly in developing countries.

Patients with diabetes tend to present in four main ways:

- Classical signs and symptoms – osmotic symptoms plus weight loss
- With macrovascular and/or microvascular complications
- Diabetic decompensation – DKA/HONK (hyperosmolar hyperglycaemic state)
- Routine testing at general practitioner (GP) consultations, medical and surgical clinics/insurance medicals.

HISTORY AND INITIAL PHYSICAL EXAMINATION

Having obtained a detailed history, a physical examination should be undertaken (Table 2.3). The consultation should take place in appropriate and comfortable circumstances.

TABLE 2.3 Components of the comprehensive diabetes evaluation

Medical history
- Age and characteristics of onset of diabetes (e.g. DKA, symptomatic laboratory finding)
- Eating patterns, physical activity habits, nutritional status and weight history; growth and development in children and adolescents
- Diabetes education history
- Review pf previous treatment regimens and response to therapy (A1C records)
- Current treatment of diabetes, including medications, meal plan, physical activity patterns, and results of glucose monitoring and patients' use of data
- DKA frequency, severity and cause
- Hypoglycaemic episodes:
  - Hypoglycaemia awareness
  - Any severe hypoglycaemia – frequency and cause
- History of diabetes-related complications:
  - Microvascular: retinopathy, nephropathy, neuropathy (sensory, including history of foot lesions; autonomic, including sexual dysfunction and gastroparesis)
  - Macrovascular: CHD, cerebrovascular disease, PAD
  - Other psychosocial problems dental disease

Physical examination
- Height, weight, BMI
- Blood pressure determination, including orthostatic measurements when indicated
- Fundoscopic examination
- Thyroid palpation
- Skin examination (for acanthosis nigricans and insulin injection sites)
- Comprehensive foot examination:
  - Inspection
  - Palpation of dorsalis pedia and posterior tibial pulses
  - Presence/absence of patellar and Achilles reflexes
  - Determination of proprioception, vibration and monofilament sensation

Laboratory evaluation
- A1C, if results not available within past 2–3 months
- If not performed/available within past year:
  - Fasting lipid profile, including total, LDL and HDL cholesterol and triglycerides
  - Liver function tests
  - Test for urine albumin excretion with spot urine albumin-to-creatinine ratio
  - Serum creatinine and calculated GFR
  - Thyroid-stimulating hormone in type 1 diabetes, dyslipidaemia or women aged over 50 years

Referrals
- Annual dilated eye examination
- Family planning for women of reproductive age
- Registered dietitian for MNT
- DSME

Continued

TABLE 2.3 Components of the comprehensive diabetes evaluation—cont'd

- Dental examination
- Mental health professional, if needed

BMI, body mass index; CHD, coronary heart disease; DKA, diabetic ketoacidosis; DSME, diabetes self-management education; GFR, glomerular filtration rate; HDL, high density lipoprotein; LDL, low density lipoprotein; MNT, medical nutrition therapy; PAD, peripheral arterial disease.
Source: American Diabetes Association (2011). Reproduced with permission.

- The mode of diagnosis and presence of symptoms should be recorded.
- Family history of diabetes should be reviewed.
- For women, enquiry into obstetric (stillbirths, large babies, gestational diabetes) and menstrual history (oligomenorrhoea, especially with features of hyperandrogenism) may be relevant.
- Associated conditions (see Section 1), predisposing and aggravating factors should be identified.
- A detailed history of drug use, smoking habits and alcohol consumption is required along with an enquiry into habitual physical activity and sporting interests.
- Height and weight (plus waist circumference) need to be recorded and body mass index calculated.
- Blood pressure should be measured carefully; lying and standing pressures should be recorded if there is any suggestion of postural hypotension arising from autonomic neuropathy. In diabetes there may be a postural drop with few or no symptoms.
- Evidence of established diabetic complications including neuropathy (including autonomic dysfunction where appropriate) should be sought diligently at diagnosis in patients with type 2 diabetes (see Section 5).
- Unless contraindications exist, notably angle-closure glaucoma, the fundi should be examined through pharmacologically dilated pupils in all patients with type 2 diabetes, as well as in patients with features that are not classical of autoimmune type 1 diabetes.
- Features of other endocrinopathies, signs of marked insulin resistance and specific syndromes of diabetes such as the lipodystrophies are rare.

Physical examination of the patient with newly presenting type 1 diabetes is usually unremarkable, although there may be evidence of recent weight loss and occasionally signs compatible with dehydration. Features of orogenital candidiasis or cutaneous sepsis are not uncommon, but are non-specific. The presence of vitiligo is consistent with the presence of autoimmune disease.

OCULAR COMPLICATIONS

Retinopathy

In patients with type 1 diabetes, the appearance of symptoms provides a fairly reliable indicator of the time of onset of pathological hyperglycaemia. Complications such as retinopathy are therefore usually absent at diagnosis. Visual symptoms such as blurred vision, which results from osmotic changes within the ocular lens, usually resolve within weeks; patients should be advised to defer obtaining prescription eyewear until the diabetes is stabilized.

Patients with type 2 diabetes may present with a spectrum ranging from a normal retina to sight-threatening changes such as haemorrhages, exudates and maculopathy.

Cataract

Cataracts may be present at diagnosis of type 2 diabetes and rarely may develop acutely in type 1 diabetes.

NEPHROPATHY

Proteinuria is the hallmark of diabetic nephropathy. As with the other microvascular complications of diabetes, the development of nephropathy is closely related to the duration of diabetes.

Type 1 diabetes

Tests for microalbuminuria may be positive at diagnosis. This may simply reflect the renal effects of uncontrolled hyperglycaemia and should not automatically be interpreted as evidence of nephropathy requiring specific therapy. The test should be deferred until the diabetes has been stabilized.

Type 2 diabetes

In addition to early nephropathy, the presence of microalbuminuria may reflect a further increase in risk of macrovascular disease (see p. 199). However, because nephropathy can develop during the asymptomatic phase preceding diagnosis, plasma creatinine should

be checked, especially if Albustix-positive (indicative of urinary
protein losses of 500 mg/day or more; see p. 200).

Neuropathy and foot disease

Evidence of these complications should be evaluated
carefully at diagnosis in patients with type 2 diabetes, as detailed
in Section 5.

Macrovascular disease

The close relationship between the components of the insulin
resistance syndrome and type 2 diabetes should prompt the
identification and treatment, (if clinically indicated), of the
associated risk factors for atherosclerosis:

- hypertension
- dyslipidaemia
- microalbuminuria
- renal impairment.

As a minimum, the clinical stigmata of hyperlipidaemia, the
presence of pedal pulses and signs of vascular insufficiency should be
noted. Further investigations including routine bloods (urea and
electrolytes), lipid levels and ECG may be warranted.

SCREENING FOR DIABETES

There has been a significant increase in our understanding of the
pathogenesis of type 1 diabetes. Approximately 10% of patients have
a first-degree relative with type 1 diabetes and therefore subjects at
high risk could be identified using a combination of immune, genetic
and metabolic markers. However, even in high risk groups, screening
is imperfect and the complex methodology is not available other than
for clinical trials.

In the UK Prospective Diabetes Study (UKPDS), the severity of
diabetes-related tissue damage correlated with the glycated
haemoglobin (HbA1c) concentration at diagnosis of type 2 diabetes.
Thus, there is the prospect that earlier intervention in patients
identified by screening of asymptomatic at-risk individuals may
prevent or retard chronic diabetic complications. Type 2 diabetes
satisfies some of the major criteria for a disorder for which screening
would be appropriate. However, there is little evidence to suggest
that population screening is cost effective. It is appropriate to screen
'at risk' groups (see Section 1).

Tip box

Tissue damage at diagnosis of type 2 diabetes reflects the degree and duration of preceding hyperglycaemia.

WHO MAKES THE DIAGNOSIS?

Blood glucose and urine testing are valuable pointer to diabetes. Although glucose oxidase test strips are specific for glucose, glycosuria does not invariably indicate the presence of diabetes; the converse is also true.

In the UK, the diagnosis of diabetes is most commonly made in the GP's surgery. Routine checks, insurance medicals and consultations with opticians or urologists also highlight cases of type 2 diabetes. Diagnosis on the coronary care unit following an acute myocardial infarction is not uncommon. Less commonly, the diagnosis is made when the patient presents with an established complication such as an infected neuropathic foot lesion or symptomatic diabetic retinopathy.

Most often, the diagnosis of diabetes relies on osmotic symptoms plus an increased laboratory blood glucose level, which can be fasting (≥ 7 mmol/L) or random (> 11.1 mmol/L).

Tip box

Measurement of random plasma glucose concentration is often the first-test that prompts further investigation for diagnosing diabetes mellitus.

INITIAL MANAGEMENT

Having confirmed the diagnosis of diabetes, the crucial clinical question is whether insulin treatment is required. In the young patient with acute osmotic symptoms, weight loss and ketonuria, the decision to start insulin is straightforward. Similarly, the overweight or obese middle-aged or elderly patient with minor symptoms will usually be a candidate for a trial of dietary manipulation followed by metformin. In reality very few patients ($< 20\%$) manage with diet alone for the usually advised period of 3 months.

Other oral agents including sulphonylureas, pioglitazone, gliptins etc. can be used from diagnosis, in addition to appropriate dietary measures.

Tip box

In newly diagnosed diabetic patients, the first consideration is whether insulin treatment is required.

Most importantly, the patient should be treated according to clinical need. However, an attempt should be made to place the patient with diabetes within the classification system. Often this assignment to a particular category is not possible with certainty and becomes clear only later. Initial therapy, therefore, does not necessarily confirm the aetiology. The difficulty at diagnosis centres on the degree of endogenous insulin deficiency, the rate of β-cell deterioration, the degree of insulin resistance and the presence of any intercurrent illness. Thus, patients with what proves ultimately to be type 1 diabetes will sometimes be treated with a trial of oral antidiabetic drugs, usually because the clinical and biochemical features were not classical; conversely, patients with type 2 diabetes may need insulin temporarily at diagnosis, especially if there is significant intercurrent illness.

Tip box

Initial treatment with insulin does not necessarily confirm a diagnosis of type 1 diabetes.

It can sometimes be difficult to decide whether a newly presenting, middle-aged, non-obese patient with moderately severe hyperglycaemia has type 2 diabetes that will respond adequately to oral antidiabetic agents or whether the patient would be better treated with insulin from the outset. In this context, it should be remembered that, although relatively uncommon in the elderly, type 1 diabetes might present at any age.

Tip box

Type 1 diabetes may present at any age – even in nonagenarians.

The situation is complicated by increasing awareness of subtypes of diabetes in which insulin deficiency appears to be the predominant feature but which present less dramatically than classical type 1 diabetes. Moreover, even the presence of morbid obesity does not guarantee a diagnosis of type 2 diabetes; occasionally, obese patients present with marked osmotic symptoms and/or ketonuria indicative of insulin dependence.

Tip box

Features of type 1 diabetes may sometimes develop in patients with morbid obesity.

Identification of patients with apparently autoimmune diabetes with a relatively slow onset can be problematic; the prevalence of latent autoimmune diabetes in adults (LADA) is not known but is perhaps under diagnosed (see Section 1). The diagnosis is often made retrospectively (glutamic acid dehydrogenase (GAD) +ve, anti-islet cell +ve) following the rapid failure of treatment with oral antidiabetic agents (see Section 3, p. 97). Useful clinical pointers at diagnosis suggesting that insulin may be required include:

- unintentional weight loss preceding diagnosis
- normal body weight or underweight for height at diagnosis
- presentation with osmotic symptoms of short duration
- marked fasting hyperglycaemia.

Dietary manipulation ± oral agents may sometimes initially produce dramatic improvements. The issue of insulin dependence is particularly difficult in African Caribbean patients who may present with ketosis, even DKA, yet who ultimately prove to have diabetes that is controllable with oral agents or even diet alone.

Personal telephone contact is best to ensure that insulin treatment is initiated with the minimum of delay.

Tip box

Osmotic symptoms, weight loss, raised blood glucose plus ketonuria – liaison with the local hospital diabetes team is important. Insulin treatment should be initiated with the minimum delay in patients with newly diagnosed type 1 diabetes.

KETONURIA

Ketonuria (in concert with hyperglycaemia) usually suggests the presence of a marked degree of insulin deficiency. In these circumstances, ketonuria results from:

- accelerated breakdown of adipocyte triglycerides
- preferential hepatic β-oxidation of the liberated fatty acids to ketone bodies (3-hydroxybutyrate and acetoacetate).

Insulinopenia (absolute or, more commonly, relative) is primarily responsible for the acceleration of ketogenesis. Reduced ketone body clearance by peripheral tissues may also contribute as ketosis develops, and this too is influenced by insulin. Ketonuria in diabetes is sometimes erroneously attributed to fasting or decreased carbohydrate intake. Although ketonuria is a physiological response to fasting in non-diabetic individuals, the crucial distinction in the diabetic patient is the combination of ketonuria in concert with hyperglycaemia.

> **Tip box**
>
> Ketonuria in concert with hyperglycaemia suggests marked insulinopenia.

In non-diabetic individuals, the plasma glucose concentration will be normal, or even marginally reduced, during fasting. In healthy subjects, the mobilization of fatty acids from adipocyte stores is a physiological response mediated by a reduction in endogenous insulin secretion. However, fasting promotes the development of ketosis in patients with type 1 diabetes under circumstances of insulin deficiency. The combination of significant ketonuria together with glycosuria should be interpreted as evidence of a need for prompt measurement of BUN (blood urea nitrogen) and blood glucose, and prompt insulin treatment.

 Significant ketosis is a contraindication to oral antidiabetic therapy – insulin is required.

Conversely, in patients with otherwise typical features of type 1 diabetes, especially weight loss, the absence of ketonuria at diagnosis should not be taken as unequivocal evidence that insulin therapy will not be required.

AUTOIMMUNE AND NON-AUTOIMMUNE TYPE 1 DIABETES

Rarely, young patients with hyperglycaemia but no ketonuria will prove to have an inherited form of diabetes, for instance maturity-onset diabetes of the young (MODY) (see p. 14); such patients often receive insulin therapy from diagnosis, the assumption being that they have type 1 diabetes. A family history with an autosomal dominant inheritance and diagnosis under the age of 25 years are prerequisites for the diagnosis, which may be confirmed in an affected family by genetic testing.

In difficult cases, the presence of serum islet cell, insulin and GAD antibodies may help in the diagnosis of type 1 diabetes (see p. 9).

In addition, although relatively uncommon, non-autoimmune forms of type 1 diabetes are recognized, albeit mainly in people from minority ethnic groups.

PLURIGLANDULAR SYNDROME

The pluriglandular syndrome type II should be borne in mind in patients presenting with features suggesting autoimmune type 1 diabetes. Consideration should be given to checking for other endocrine autoantibodies in the serum, particularly:

- thyroid microsomal and thyroglobulin antibodies
- adrenal antibodies.

Antibody positivity does not predict future autoimmune disease with certainty. However, the prevalence of autoimmune thyroid disease, Addison's disease and other non-endocrine autoimmune disorders such as pernicious anaemia, coeliac disease and premature menopause is increased in patients with type 1 diabetes. Vitiligo is a useful cutaneous marker of autoimmune disease. Periodic checks of target organ function (e.g. thyroid function tests, serum B_{12} level) are indicated even in the absence of clinical features. Coexisting endocrinopathies may adversely affect metabolic stability (see p. 18).

INFLUENCE OF COMORBIDITY

The presence of significant physical or psychological disease may be important modifiers of the presentation and management of diabetes. For example, if malignancy severely limits life expectancy in a patient with diabetes (perhaps precipitated by high-dose dexamethasone), the primary goals of management will be:

- avoidance of osmotic symptoms
- avoidance of major metabolic decompensation; concern about long-term microvascular complications would be lower in the list of priorities.

Insulin may be the most appropriate therapy; considerations such as the likely lack of efficacy of oral agents, concomitant renal and/or hepatic impairment may also preclude alternatives. As a general point, patients with diabetes are more likely to encounter significant comorbidity and may be predisposed to the development of important complications that influence treatment.

Tip box

Diabetic patients are frequently affected by significant comorbidity.

LIFESTYLE MANAGEMENT

Lifestyle advice should be considered as part of the multidisciplinary intervention programme for all diabetic patients. Appropriate management of cardiovascular risk factors such as smoking, physical inactivity and poor diet is important for the prevention of macrovascular disease. Microvascular complications may also be affected by adverse lifestyle factors (e.g. smoking). However, helping patients to modify certain behaviours should take account of other factors such as the patient's:

● willingness to change
● perception of their diabetes
● comorbidities that may be related indirectly to their diabetes, such as depression.

Patients should be offered lifestyle interventions that have a proven benefit in terms of both metabolic and psychosocial outcomes. These could include frequent contact with health professionals (including telephone contact). Psychosocial interventions should be varied and include behaviour modifications, motivational interviewing and patient empowerment.

Education interventions for diabetes are complex, varied, should be evidence-based and suit the needs of the individual. Health-care professionals should receive training in patient-centred interventions. The programme should have specific aims and learning objectives, and should support the development of self-management attitudes, beliefs, knowledge and skills for the patient, their family and carers. It should be structured, be resource effective and have supporting materials including pamphlets and other literature.

Trained educators should deliver lifestyle advice, and the programme should be appropriate to the age and the needs of the patients. The programme should also be assessed against key criteria and quality-assured to ensure sustained consistency.

Lack of head-to-head comparative trials makes it impossible to recommend any specific programme(s). Measurement of HbA1c is the most commonly used method for assessing outcome. However, HbA1c is a marker for glycaemic control and not for quality of life.

HEALTHY EATING

Effective management of diabetes cannot be achieved without an appropriate diet. All patients with newly diagnosed diabetes should receive educational advice from a dietitian as soon as possible after diagnosis (Table 2.4). The initial interview with the dietitian should focus on the patient's preferences and habits. This should include enquiry about who takes responsibility for cooking at home, whether prepackaged convenience foods form a substantial part of the diet and the amount of food eaten outside the home, for example by the business traveller. Ethnic and social influences are of obvious importance, such as the high saturated fat content of traditional South Asian cuisine or the teenager's predilection for fast food (Table 2.5).

Healthy eating is of fundamental importance as part of diabetes health-care behaviour and has beneficial effects on weight, metabolic control and general well-being. Salt restriction is recommended for the prevention of hypertension and cardiovascular disease. Because of their high energy content, fats represent a major source of excess calorie consumption, particularly in convenience and junk foods. It is recommended that saturated fats, derived mainly from meat and dairy products, should comprise less than 10% of total energy intake. Use poly- or mono-unsaturated fatty acids (e.g. olive oil, rapeseed oil) in preference, but not in excess. In addition, consumption of trans-unsaturated fatty acids in excessive amounts may increase the risk of cardiovascular disease via alterations in lipoproteins.

TABLE 2.4 Initial dietary advice for newly diagnosed patients with diabetes

1. Quench thirst with water or low-calorie, carbonated drinks
2. Avoid sugar and obviously sugary foods
3. Use artificial sweeteners in beverages
4. Cereal, bread, pasta or potatoes should form the main part of each meal
5. Meat, grilled rather than fried, and cheese should be a small part of each meal
6. Fish and pulses are good alternatives to meat
7. Eat plenty of fresh fruit and vegetables
8. Use cooking fats and spreads low in saturated and trans-fatty acids – olive oil or reduced fat spreads are preferable
9. Moderate your alcohol consumption
10. Avoid adding salt to food at the table if hypertensive

TABLE 2.5 General dietary advice in diabetes

General guidance on healthy eating should be advised initially
- Increase intake of starchy carbohydrate foods
- Increase fruit and vegetable intake
- Reduce fat intake
- Reduce sugar intake
- Reduce salt intake
- Safe and sensible consumption of alcohol

Aims of dietary advice
- To provide knowledge of healthy eating
- To encourage lifestyle changes in order to reduce obesity and ensure optimal weight
- To maintain blood glucose and lipid levels as near normal as possible
- To reduce the acute complications of diabetes (i.e. hypoglycaemia/ hyperglycaemia)

Objectives of dietary advice
- To tailor dietary advice to suit individual needs, taking account of eating habits, physique, occupation, culture and religious beliefs
- To provide realistic advice
- To provide dietary education to allow patients to understand their diabetes and to achieve independence in management

Dietary goals
- Ensure an adequate and balanced nutritional intake
- Aim to provide 50% energy intake from carbohydrate by increasing intakes of complex carbohydrate/fibre-rich foods
- Limit rapidly absorbed carbohydrate intake
- Ensure that complex carbohydrate foods (starchy foods) are eaten at each meal/snack
- Encourage regular eating habits/meals
- Reduce fat intakes to <30% of energy intake
- Monitor body weight, encouraging weight maintenance and weight reduction when necessary
- Avoid hypoglycaemia

Tip box

People with type 2 diabetes should be given dietary choices for achieving weight loss that may also improve glycaemic control. Options include simple caloric restriction, reducing fat intake, consumption of carbohydrates with lower rather than high glycaemic index, and restricting the total amount of dietary carbohydrate.

NUTRITION THERAPY

Individualized and detailed dietary advice requires the input of trained dietitians. However, the general principles that underpin the diet for most diabetic patient differs little in terms of macronutrient composition from the advice that is currently promulgated as a healthy diet for the population in general. Much more relevant to success in an individual patient is a realistic approach bolstered by adequate practical training for the patient (and relatives) and an ability to communicate the objectives effectively and sympathetically. At the outset, simple, easy-to-follow guidelines are appropriate (see Table 2.3).

Tip box

Nutrition therapy is the cornerstone of the management of all forms of diabetes.

Advised changes in diet are notoriously difficult for the patient to implement. This is especially so for the middle-aged or elderly patient with type 2 diabetes, 75% of whom are overweight or obese. Dietary modifications often run contrary to a lifetime's habits and preferences, which have usually been reinforced by powerful social and cultural influences.

Obese individuals often significantly underestimate their daily calorie consumption. The oft-heard protests from patients about their supposedly miniscule daily food intake has to be gently but firmly repudiated if progress is to be made; recognition of the problem by the patient is usually a step forward. The difficulty lies in not alienating the patient in the process; a judgemental approach is unlikely to be successful. Increased levels of habitual physical exercise should also be encouraged.

The amount of carbohydrate ingested is usually the primary determinant of postprandial response, but the type of carbohydrate also affects this response. Intrinsic variables that influence the effect of carbohydrate-containing foods on blood glucose response include the specific type of food ingested, type of starch (amylase versus amylopectin), style of preparation (cooking method and time, amount of heat or moisture used), ripeness and degree of processing.

The glycaemic index of foods was developed to compare the postprandial responses to constant amounts of different carbohydrate-containing foods. The glycaemic index of a food is the increase above fasting in the blood glucose area over a 2-h period after ingestion of a constant amount of that food (usually a 5-g carbohydrate portion) divided by the response to a reference food (usually glucose or white bread). Multiplying the glycaemic index of the constituent foods by the amounts of carbohydrate in each food and then totalling the values for all foods calculates the glycaemic loads of food, meals and diets. Foods with a low glycaemic index include oats, barley, bulgur, beans, lentils, legumes, pasta, pumpernickel (coarse rye) bread, apples, oranges, milk, yoghurt and ice cream. Fibre, fructose, lactose and fat are dietary constituents that tend to lower the glycaemic response.

Tip box

Several randomized clinical trials have suggested that diets with a low glycaemic index reduce glycaemia in diabetic subjects.

- Fibre – as for the general population, people with diabetes are encouraged to choose a variety of fibre-containing foods such as legumes, fibre-rich cereals (≥ 5 g fibre per serving), fruits, vegetables and whole-grain products because they provide vitamins, minerals and other substances important for good health.
- Palatability – limited food choices and gastrointestinal side-effects are potential barriers to achieving such high fibre intakes.
- Sweeteners – substantial evidence from clinical studies demonstrates that dietary sucrose does not increase glycaemia more than isocaloric amounts of starch.

CARBOHYDRATE IN DIABETES MANAGEMENT

Recommendations:

- A dietary pattern that includes carbohydrate from fruits, vegetables, whole grains, legumes and low-fat milk is encouraged for good health.
- Monitoring carbohydrate, whether by carbohydrate counting, exchanges or experienced-based estimation, remains a key strategy in achieving good glycaemic control.
- The use of glycaemic index and load may provide a modest additional benefit over that observed when total carbohydrate is considered alone.
- Sucrose-containing foods can be substituted for other carbohydrates in the meal plan or, if added to the meal plan, covered with insulin or other glucose-lowering medications. Care should be taken to avoid excess energy intake.
- Sugar alcohols and non-nutritive sweeteners are safe when consumed within the daily intake levels established by the Food and Drug Administration (FDA).

Food and nutritional interventions that reduce postprandial blood glucose excursions are important in this regard, as dietary carbohydrate is the major determinant of postprandial glucose levels. Low-carbohydrate diets might seem to be a logical approach to lowering postprandial glucose. However, foods that contain carbohydrate are important sources of energy, fibre, vitamins and minerals, and are important in dietary palatability.

A number of practices are controversial:

- Unrealistic targets – for some patients the prescription of diets with hopelessly unrealistic targets such as a '1000-kcal daily reducing diet' is a recipe for failure, disillusionment and loss of faith in the dietitian.
- Special foodstuffs – the purchase of products such as cakes aimed specifically at diabetic patients should be discouraged. These are often more expensive, contain calories in the form of sorbitol or fructose, and may cause diarrhoea.

DIETARY RECOMMENDATIONS FOR PEOPLE WITH DIABETES

Weight loss in overweight and obese individuals improves insulin sensitivity and glucose tolerance. Aim for weight maintenance and modest weight loss (5–10 kg in 1 year), which can improve health outcomes.

Weight loss via dietary intervention and therefore hypocaloric intake requires modifications to the type, quantity and/or frequency of food and drink consumed. A weight loss of approximately 0.5 kg per week results from a loss of adipose tissue that entails an energy deficit of 3500 kcal per week. This requires a daily energy deficit of a least 500 kcal per day. To ensure this deficit it is standard practice to aim for a 600-kcal deficit.

Most patients are able to lose weight actively for about 3–6 months, and so studies reporting weight losses at 12 months reflect a mixture of both weight loss and weight maintenance.

CALORIE RESTRICTION

Daily energy requirements may be calculated from the patient's height, age and physical activity using published tables. Adipose tissue contains about 7000 kcal/kg. Sustained weight loss in the obese will occur at a rate of around 0.5 kg/week with a reduction in daily calorie intake of 500 kcal (1.2 MJ). This represents a reduction of around 20% for most patients.

Tip box

A daily reduction of 500 kcal will produce weight loss averaging 0.5 kg per week.

More rapid rates of weight loss will include structural protein (i.e. muscle) as well as fat; this is undesirable because resting energy expenditure, which is determined largely by fat-free mass, will decline as an adaptive response. Resting energy expenditure, which normally accounts for the majority of daily calorie consumption, represents the energy requirements for essential metabolic processes maintaining cell membrane potentials and body temperature. The observation that, on average, the obese have higher resting energy expenditures than the non-obese means that maintenance of body weight requires a proportionately greater calorie intake. Physical exercise, in conjunction with calorie restriction, will help preserve fat-free tissues, thereby maintaining resting energy expenditure; this combination offers advantages over calorie reduction alone.

LOW AND VERY LOW CALORIE DIETS

Low calorie diets (LCD, 800–1800 kcal/day) and very low calorie diets (VLCD, < 800 kcal/day) are associated with modest weight loss (5–6%) at 12 months' follow up. Although VLCD are associated with greater weight loss in the short term (3–4 months), this difference is not sustained at 12 months. These patients require close medical and dietary supervision.

FOOD COMPOSITION

High dropout rate and poor compliance with carbohydrate- and energy-restricted diets demonstrated in trial settings suggests that these diets are not widely applicable or acceptable to patients. However, both low carbohydrate (< 30 g/day) and low fat (< 30% of total daily energy) diets are associated with modest weight loss at 12 months. Low carbohydrate/high protein (LC/HP) diets are more effective than low fat/high carbohydrate (LF/HC) diets at 6 months, but the difference between strategies is usually not significant at 12 months. Reduced calorie diets result in clinically meaningful weight loss regardless of the macronutrients they emphasize.

COMMERCIAL DIETS

A variety of commercial weight reduction programmes are associated with a modest reduction in body weight and a reduction in several cardiac risk factors in overweight and obese premenopausal women at 12 months. At 12 months' follow-up, most commercial diets resulted in a clinically useful weight loss of around 10% in participants who had kept to their original diet, and this was associated with a reduction in hypertension, dyslipidaemia and fasting hyperglycaemia.

MEDITERRANEAN DIET

There is no consistent definition for the Mediterranean diet and therefore it is impossible to comment on.

RECOMMENDATIONS

- Dietary interventions that produce a 600-kcal per day deficit result in sustainable modest weight loss. Where VLCD are indicated for rapid weight loss, patients should be under medical supervision.
- When discussing dietary change with patients, health-care professionals should emphasize achievable and sustainable healthy eating.

In patients with type 2 diabetes, short-term supplementation with omega-3 polyunsaturated fatty acids (PUFA) causes a reduction in triglycerides (TG) but a rise in low density lipoprotein (LDL) cholesterol. It is therefore not generally recommended in people with type 2 diabetes. Vitamin E supplementation is also not recommended in people with type 2 diabetes.

ENCOURAGING DIETARY CHANGE IN CLINICAL PRACTICE

The use of a behavioural approach to dietary interventions in patients with diabetes leads to clinically significant benefit in terms of weight loss, HbA1c, lipids and self-care behaviour for up to 2 years after the initial intervention.

Intensive therapy or contact in patients with diabetes also leads to clinically beneficial effects on weight and glycaemic control during the period of intervention. More education and contact appears to improve outcomes. Prepackaged meal programmes show significant clinical benefit in terms of weight, blood pressure, glycaemic control and lipids during the study period but are impractical outside the trial setting.

Tip box

Clinical interventions aimed at dietary change are more likely to be successful if a psychological approach based on a theoretical model is included.

Weight management in type 2 diabetes

Weight reduction, ideally towards normality but tempered with realistic expectations, is regarded as the cornerstone of managing type 2 diabetes. However, even with intensive personal dietetic support in the setting of a clinical trial, only a minority of patients (approximately 20%) with type 2 diabetes are able to normalize their fasting plasma glucose concentrations. In the UKPDS, weight loss during the initial, intensive, 3-month dietary phase averaged 5 kg; this was associated with a rapid but temporary improvement in fasting plasma glucose concentration.

Weight management is an integral part of diabetes care. Type 2 diabetes is associated with obesity (identified as a BMI >30 kg/m^2). In turn, obesity is associated with a significant negative impact on morbidity and mortality. Weight loss in obese individuals is associated with reductions in mortality, blood pressure, lipid profiles, arthritis-related disability and other outcomes. It is not known what the impact of weight loss is on diabetic retinopathy, nephropathy or neuropathy. The benefits of weight loss on the prevention and remission of both impaired glucose tolerance and established diabetes plus its impact on glycaemic control in people with established diabetes are well established. Weight loss improves insulin sensitivity and glucose tolerance. Weight maintenance and modest weight loss (5–10 kg in 1 year) can significantly improve health outcomes. However, the long-term benefits of weight loss on glycaemic control have not been assessed adequately.

Antioxidants and trace elements

Increased oxidant damage mediated by free radicals has been implicated in the promotion of atheroma. Diets in UK populations may be low in the antioxidant β-carotene and vitamins C and E, and consumption of fresh fruit and vegetables is regarded as a sensible recommendation, albeit founded largely on theoretical considerations at present. There are currently no data supporting routine pharmacological supplementation with antioxidants in diabetes.

Minerals

Salt should be restricted to a maximum of 3 g/day. Diabetic patients have increased exchangeable body sodium levels. In patients with hypertension, particularly if difficult to control, salt intake should be reduced to less than 2.5 g/day Hyporeninaemic hypoaldosteronism, which is a feature of diabetic nephropathy, may warrant dietary restriction of potassium.

Tip box

Dietary salt restriction is beneficial in hypertensive patients.

Body mass index

BMI is an internationally accepted measure and can be used to classify overweight or obesity in adults. BMI takes account of the expected difference in weights of adults of different heights. Values are age-independent and are the same for both sexes.

However, BMI may understate body frames in some ethnic groups. For example, in South Asian Indians a given BMI is associated with greater total percentage fat mass than in the white population. Therefore, lower BMI cut-offs appear appropriate to define obesity-related risk in higher risk groups such as South Asians. South Asian, Chinese and Japanese individuals should be considered overweight at BMI >23 kg/m^2 and obese at BMI >27.5 kg/m^2.

Waist circumference

As BMI is not always an accurate predictor of body fat or fat distribution, particularly in muscular individuals, some caution may be warranted if it is used as the only measure of body fatness in muscular individuals. Waist circumference is at least as good an indicator of total body fat as BMI, and is the best anthropometric predictor of visceral fat.

Men with a waist circumference of 94 cm or more (90 cm or more for Asian men) are at increased risk of obesity-related health problems, and women with a waist circumference of 80 cm or more are at an increased risk of obesity-related health problems.

The World Health Organization (WHO) recommended that an individual's relative risk of type 2 diabetes and cardiovascular disease could be more accurately classified using both BMI and waist circumference. Sex differences are apparent, and waist circumference enhances diabetes prediction beyond that predicted by BMI alone in women but not in men. Waist-to-hip ratio may also be a useful predictor of diabetes and cardiovascular disease risk in adults, but is more difficult to measure than waist circumference.

Tip box

When the BMI is greater than 35 kg/m^2, waist circumference does not add to the absolute measure or risk.

Bioimpedance

There is no clinical evidence to suggest that bioimpedance is a better measure than BMI or waist circumference in the prediction of body fat in adults.

EXERCISE AND PHYSICAL ACTIVITY

DEFINITIONS

Physical activity is defined as any skeletal muscle movement that expends energy beyond resting level (e.g. walking, gardening, stair climbing).

Health-enhancing physical activity is physical activity conducted at a sufficient level to bring about measurable health improvements. This normally equates to a moderate intensity level or above, and can generally be described as activity that slightly raises heart rate, breathing rate and core temperature but in which the patient is still able to hold a conversation.

Exercise is a subset of physical activity that is done with the goal of enhancing or maintaining an aspect of fitness (e.g. aerobic, strength, flexibility, balance).

ASSESSMENT OF PHYSICAL ACTIVITY

Physical activity is a very difficult behaviour to measure because it incorporates mode of activity, duration, frequency and intensity. There is no 'gold standard', and techniques range from heart rate to motion counters and self-reports. Self-report is the easiest format but there is often an over-reporting of minutes spent in activity. It is important in assessing what kind of support a patient needs for increasing or maintaining physical activity. A rate of perceived exertion scale is useful for estimating exercise intensity.

Effects of physical activity and exercise on the management of diabetes

Various guidelines exist for physical activity and exercise in the general population. Greater amounts of activity provide greater health benefits, particularly for weight management. People with type 1 or type 2 diabetes should be encouraged to participate in physical activity or structured exercise to improve cardiovascular risk factors. In patients with type 2 diabetes, physical activity or structured exercise should be encouraged to improve glycaemic control. Structured, supervised exercise programmes and less structured, unsupervised physical activity programmes (of variable activity type and mode of delivery) are effective for improving glycaemic control and cardiovascular risk factors. Exercise intervention significantly decreases plasma triglyceride levels and reduces in visceral adipose tissue.

Adults should also undertake moderate- or high-intensity muscle-strengthening activities that involve all major muscle groups on two or more days per week. Older adults (aged 65 years and older) should avoid inactivity. If regular exercise is not possible owing to limiting chronic conditions, they should be as physically active as their abilities allow. Older adults should also try to do exercises that maintain or improve balance if they are at risk of falling.

In people with type 2 diabetes, physical activity or exercise should be performed at least every second or third day to maintain improvements in glycaemic control. In view of insulin adjustments it may be easier for people with type 1 diabetes to perform physical activity or exercise every day. Aerobic, endurance exercise is usually recommended, although resistance exercise with low weights and high repetitions is also beneficial. A combination of both aerobic and resistance exercise appears to provide greater improvement in glycaemic control than either type of exercise alone.

Tip box

Exercise and physical activity (involving aerobic and/or resistance exercise) should be performed on a regular basis.
  Advice about exercise and physical activity should be individually tailored and diabetes-specific, and should include implications for glucose management and foot care.

ADVICE FOR PATIENTS TAKING INSULIN OR GLUCOSE-LOWERING DRUGS

Exercise with the normal dose of insulin dose and no additional carbohydrate significantly increases the risk of hypoglycaemia during and after exercise. If exercise can be anticipated, a reduction of the normal insulin dose will significantly reduce the risk of hypoglycaemia. The amount of reduction in insulin dose will depend on the time of day, on the insulin and glycaemic levels before exercise, and on the duration and intensity of the exercise being performed. If exercise cannot be anticipated and the insulin has already been taken, extra carbohydrate before exercise reduces the risk of hypoglycaemia.

Injection of insulin into exercising areas and a high temperature increases the absorption of insulin and the risk of hypoglycaemia, and should therefore be avoided. This should be taken into consideration when exercising in hot climates. A further reduction in insulin dose may be required.

> **Tip box**
>
> Individual advice on avoiding hypoglycaemia when exercising by adjustment of carbohydrate intake, reduction of insulin dose and choice of injection site should be given to patients taking insulin.

Patients using glucose-lowering drugs, such as sulphonylureas, may also be at risk of hypoglycaemia during exercise.

DIABETIC COMPLICATIONS AND EXERCISE

A gradual introduction and initial low intensity of physical activity with slow progressions in volume and intensity is recommended for sedentary people with diabetes. Patients with existing complications of diabetes should seek medical review before embarking on exercise programmes. There is a higher risk of myocardial infarction after heavy exertion in sedentary compared with non-sedentary people with type 1 diabetes.

High-intensity exercise may transiently increase albumin excretion rate (AER) in people with or without diabetes. However, there is no known association between exercise participation and development or exacerbation of diabetic complications.

Weight-bearing physical activity and brisk walking programmes in people with type 2 diabetes and peripheral neuropathy (with well fitting shoes/boots) does not increase the risk of foot ulcers.

SMOKING

In the general population tobacco smoking is strongly and dose-dependently associated with all cardiovascular events, including coronary heart disease, stroke, peripheral vascular disease and cardiovascular death. In people with diabetes, smoking is an independent risk factor for cardiovascular disease and the excess risk attributed to smoking is more that additive (Table 2.6). Smoking cessation reduces these risks substantially, with the decrease in risk being dependent on the duration of cessation.

For microvascular disease the evidence is less clear. There is a suggestion that smoking may be a risk factor for retinopathy in type 1 diabetes but not in people with type 2 diabetes.

Those who quit smoking for at least a year experience greater weight gain than their peers who continue to smoke. The amount of weight gained differs according to age, social status and certain

---

TABLE 2.6 Recommendations regarding diabetes and smoking

Assessment of smoking status and history
- Systematic documentation of a history of tobacco use must be obtained from all adolescent and adult individuals with diabetes.

Counselling on smoking prevention and cessation
- All health-care providers should advise individuals with diabetes not to initiate smoking. This advice should be repeated consistently to prevent smoking and other tobacco use among children and adolescents with diabetes under age 21 years.
- Among smokers, cessation counselling must be completed as a routine component of diabetes care.
- Every smoker should be urged to quit in a clear, strong and personalized manner that describes the added risks of smoking and diabetes.
- Every diabetic smoker should be asked if he or she is willing to quit this time.
- If no, initiate brief and motivational discussion regarding need to stop using tobacco, risks of continued use, and encouragement to quit as well as support when ready.
- If yes, assess preference for and initiate either minimal, brief or intensive cessation counselling and offer pharmacological supplements as appropriate.

Effective systems for delivery of smoking cessation
- Training of all diabetes health-care providers in the public health service guidelines regarding smoking should be implemented.
- Follow-up procedures designed to assess and promote quitting status must be arranged for all diabetic smokers.

Source: American Diabetes Association (2011). Reproduced with permission.

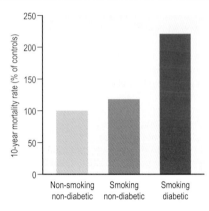

Figure 2.1 Deleterious effect of smoking and disease on 10-year mortality. Death rate is expressed as a percentage of that in age- and sex-matched non-diabetic, non-smoking populations. (Source: Adapted from Bilous and Donnelly (2010). Reproduced with permission.)

behaviours. To prevent weight gain after smoking cessation, individualized interventions, low calorie diets and cognitive behavioural therapy may reduce the associated weight gain without affecting quit rates. Additionally, exercise interventions may be effective in the longer term.

Tip box

Health-care professionals should offer weight management interventions to patients who are planning to stop smoking.

Possible ill effects of smoking include:

- decreased insulin sensitivity
- increased mortality (Fig. 2.1)
- independent risk factor for type 2 diabetes
- atheroma development
- risk factor for complications – retinopathy, nephropathy, necrobiosis lipoidica and cheiroarthropathy (limited joint mobility).

Tip box

All people who smoke should be advised to stop and offered support to help facilitate this in order to minimize cardiovascular and general health risks.

FIRST-LINE INTERVENTIONS

Health-care professionals involved in caring for people with diabetes should advise them not to smoke. Studies in patients with diabetes support the use of intensive management in the form of motivational interviewing or counselling in combination with pharmacological therapies such as bupropion and nicotine replacement. Group behaviour therapy and individual advice is more effective than self-help material. There is no evidence suggesting that counselling strategies to aid smoking cessation or pharmacological intervention in patients with diabetes should differ from those used in the general population.

Tip box

Intensive management plus pharmacological therapies should be offered to all patients with diabetes who wish to stop smoking. Smoking status should continue to be monitored at least annually.

ALCOHOL

Alcoholic beverages are a variable and potentially important component of the diet and may have a bearing on a number of aspects of diabetes (Table 2.7). Alcohol provides energy of 7 kcal/g – almost twice that of carbohydrates and approaching the energy value of fats. Calorie load and risk of hypoglycaemia are the principal concerns.

TABLE 2.7 Potential relevance of excessive alcohol consumption to patients with diabetes

- Calorie burden
  - Obesity
- Hypertension
  - Restriction of alcohol may improve control of hypertension
- Dyslipidaemia
  - Hypertriglyceridaemia
- Hypoglycaemia
  - Exacerbation of insulin or sulphonylurea-induced hypoglycaemia – may occur several hours after consumption
  - Recognition of symptoms of hypoglycaemia may be impaired
- Alcoholic ketoacidosis
  - Even in non-diabetic subjects; rare
- Liver disease
  - Alcoholic steatosis, hepatitis and cirrhosis
- Pancreatitis
  - Risk of secondary diabetes with recurrent or chronic pancreatitis
  - Risk of chronic malabsorption
- Chlorpropamide–alcohol flush syndrome
  - Inhibition of acetaldehyde dehydrogenase
- Neuropathy
  - Exacerbation of chronic diabetic neuropathic syndromes
  - Exacerbation of erectile dysfunction

Tip box

Alcohol can be a significant source of dietary calories.

HEPATIC METABOLISM OF ALCOHOL

The liver metabolizes more than 90% of alcohol. The metabolism of alcohol alters the redox state of the liver. The ratio of reduced to oxidized nicotinamide adenine dinucleotide (NAD) is increased, thereby inhibiting gluconeogenesis.

This inhibition of gluconeogenesis leads to a reduction of endogenous glucose production in the liver, which increases the risk of hypoglycaemia. Hypoglycaemia in diabetic patients may occur at blood alcohol levels not usually associated with intoxication.

As glycogenolysis can sustain hepatic glucose production, the risk of hypoglycaemia is highest when fasting depletes hepatic glycogen stores. Particular caution is required in diabetic patients at high risk of recurrent hypoglycaemia. Conversely, the features of hypoglycaemia are sometimes mistaken as those of alcoholic intoxication; this might lead to serious consequences if the correct metabolic disturbance is not recognized and the appropriate treatment denied. The carrying of a card or wearing of a bracelet that identifies the patient as being diabetic should always be encouraged.

Tip box

The symptoms of hypoglycaemia may be masked by alcohol.

$$\text{Ethanol} + \text{NAD}^+ \xrightarrow[\text{dehydrogenase}]{\text{Alcohol}} \text{Acetaldehyde} + \text{NADH} + \text{H}^+$$

$$\text{Acetaldehyde} + \text{H}_2\text{O} + \text{NAD}^+ \xrightarrow[\text{dehydrogenase}]{\text{Acetaldehyde}} \text{Acetate} + \text{NADH} + \text{H}^+$$

 Alcohol consumption can predispose to hypoglycaemia even in the absence of intoxication.

Alcohol may significantly increase the depth and duration of iatrogenic hypoglycaemia and has been implicated in fatalities. It has also been suggested that alcohol may be an underappreciated risk factor for severe sulphonylurea-induced hypoglycaemia.

Late hypoglycaemia occurring after many hours may necessitate extra carbohydrate or a temporary reduction in insulin dose. There may also be a risk of early reactive hypoglycaemia if mixers with high sugar content stimulate insulin release in patients with sufficient endogenous reserve. It is important that patients appreciate that the symptoms of hypoglycaemia may be masked by alcohol.

> **Hypoglycaemia may occur many hours after alcohol consumption – even the following morning.**

ALCOHOL DEPENDENCE

Alcohol dependence represents a potentially fatal risk to the patient reliant on insulin or treated with sulphonylureas; regular meals should be encouraged. In addition, excess alcohol intake is regarded as a contraindication to metformin therapy because the risk of lactic acidosis may be enhanced by the alterations in redox state. Alcoholic ketoacidosis is an uncommon but serious metabolic disturbance that may develop in diabetic or non-diabetic alcoholics.

RECOMMENDED DAILY CONSUMPTION

The recommended maximum daily consumption of alcohol in the UK is:

- 30 g (3 units) for men
- 20 g (2 units) for women.

Consuming over 40 g/day alcohol increases a man's risk of liver disease, hypertension and some cancers (for which smoking is a confounding factor) and violent death. For women, consuming more than 24 g/day average alcohol increases their risk of developing liver disease and breast cancer.

In the UK, depending on the strength and volume of the measure, 1 unit approximates to a half-pint (375 mL) of beer, a single measure (44 mL) of spirits or a glass (120 mL) of wine. Recommendations to patients should include the following advice:

- Do not substitute alcohol for regular meals or snacks.
- Avoid alcoholic drinks with high sugar content (e.g. sweet wine).

- Avoid lower carbohydrate drinks – they tend to be high in alcohol.
- Avoid alcohol if there is hypertriglyceridaemia, symptomatic neuropathy or refractory hypertension.
- Carry a diabetes identification card in case of emergency.

BENEFICIAL ASPECTS OF ALCOHOL

Alcohol is known to have both beneficial and harmful effects on the biochemical basis of coronary heart disease (CHD) and the psychological consequences of the disease. Observational evidence suggests a protective effect of alcohol consumption for vascular endpoints including death in patients with type 2 diabetes. Moderate quantities of alcohol is associated with favourable effects on cardiovascular risk factors including lower circulating insulin levels, increased high density lipoprotein (HDL)-cholesterol levels and reduced coagulability. Recent observational data from the USA suggest that diabetic patients share the benefits of moderate habitual alcohol consumption on mortality from CHD observed in non-diabetic subjects. Low-to-moderate chronic alcohol intake is associated with lower circulating insulin concentrations and improved insulin sensitivity. There is some evidence from epidemiological studies that the risk of developing type 2 diabetes is inversely associated with alcohol intake; moderate alcohol consumption may decrease the risk of type 2 diabetes. Studies that have stratified alcohol intake describe the familiar 'J' shaped curve relating alcohol consumption and a measure of vascular risk in patients with type 2 diabetes.

MANAGEMENT OF DIABETES

TYPE 1 DIABETES – INITIATING THERAPY

Home-based instruction of the newly diagnosed child or young person appears to be at least as effective as inpatient instruction in terms of glycaemic control, acceptable to the family and/or carers and cost-effective. There is no evidence for a sustained effect of any specific insulin regimen on glycaemic control during the first few months after diagnosis.

Dietary advice as part of a comprehensive management plan is recommended to improve glycaemic control. A dietitian should give specialist dietetic advice with expertise in type 1 diabetes, and all patients should be able to access such training locally and, ideally, at their own diabetes clinic.

GLYCAEMIC TARGETS

There is compelling evidence that good glycaemic control reduces the risk of microvascular and macrovascular complications in people with type 1 diabetes. However, there is no agreed single target for glycaemic control in type 1 patients. Targets recommended by different authorities vary between 6.5% and 7.5%. However, individual preferences, general treatment goals, co-morbidities and other patient factors may require modification of glycaemic goals. In addition, targets also vary within an individual even over a very short period of time, depending on a variety of clinical and non-clinical circumstances.

Tip box

The overall aim is to achieve the lowest possible HbA1c that does not interfere with the patient's quality of life.

INSULIN REGIMENS

Evidence regarding the impact of an intensive insulin regimen upon long-term control is derived principally from the Diabetes Control and Complications Trial (DCCT), which also involved a comprehensive patient support element (diet, exercise plans and monthly visits). Intensive insulin therapy (four injections or more per day, or insulin pump) significantly improved glycaemic control over a sustained period compared with conventional insulin therapy (two injections per day). However, it is difficult to separate the benefits of intensive insulin therapy from the intensive support package.

The choice of insulin regimen and dose depends on several factors: what type of diabetes a person has; their weight; their age; how often they check or intend to check their blood glucose; and, finally, what goals they are trying to achieve.

The principle of insulin replacement is to mimic insulin secretion in a person without diabetes and to achieve the best possible control of blood glucose without causing significant hypoglycaemia. After eating, there is normally a rapid rise in insulin to limit glucose levels after meals. Overnight, low steady levels of insulin (the background or 'basal' insulin level) are sufficient to limit glucose production by the liver.

Appropriate combinations of the above insulins can be tailored to the individual; a certain element of this will be trial and error, but close liaison with the health-care provider usually results in the right regime for that person (Table 3.1). The pre-mixed insulins are a popular starting regimen, and the timing of onset, peak and duration of action will depend on the component parts.

Conventional therapy for type 1 diabetes (twice-daily insulin with support from a multidisciplinary health-care team and regular diabetes and health monitoring) is associated with variable results.

Both basal (e.g. glargine and detemir) and rapid-acting (e.g. lispro, aspart and glulisine) insulin analogues are prescribed widely in the management of type 1 diabetes.

Insulin injection sites

The recommended sites for insulin injection are shown in Figure 3.1. Injection should be given into a pinched-up skin fold using thumb, index and middle finger, taking up the skin and leaving the muscle

TABLE 3.1 Insulin types, names and profiles of insulin action

Type	Name	Onset	Peak	Length of action
Intermediate-acting	Isophane (Insulatard – human or pork, Humulin I)	1 h	6 h	12–18 h
Long-acting	Detemir (Levemir) Glargine (Lantus)	1–2 h	No real peak	12–18 h 18–24 h
Pre-mixed	NovoMix 30, Humalog Mix 25 or 50, Humulin M3	30 min	2–6 h	8–12 h

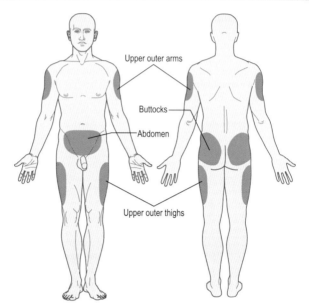

Figure 3.1 Recommended sites for subcutaneous insulin injection.

behind. This will avoid intramuscular injection. Too shallow an injection will be delivered intradermally, and can be painful.

- Insulin absorption is fastest in the abdomen and slowest in the arms and buttocks. Short-acting insulin is best given into the abdomen, and long-acting insulin into the thigh or arm; however, this can be varied according to the most practical site available.
- Most importantly, the injection sites should be 'rotated': if the abdomen is the site used most often then rotating around different points regularly is a good idea. This should avoid lipohypertrophy (an accumulation of fat under the skin), which occurs if the same injection site is used repeatedly. If this occurs, it can be unsightly and increases the variability of insulin absorption.
- If a person rotates from limb to limb, it is good idea to try to stick to a schedule whereby the same area is injected at the same time of day, for example morning injection in the abdomen, teatime injection in the leg.
- Insulin absorption may also be accelerated by exercising that part of the body (e.g. injecting legs and then jogging/running).

Different insulin delivery systems

There are four main devices for insulin injection: needle and syringe; insulin pens (now most commonly used); jet injection devices; and external pumps.

Needle and syringe

This is the traditional method of delivery. The following steps are recommended:

1. Clean the rubber stopper of the bottle with alcohol. If intermediate-acting or long-acting insulin is being used (cloudy insulins), mix by rolling or rotating the bottle.
2. Open the syringe to the number of units that is needed so that there is air to this point in the syringe.
3. Turn the insulin bottle upside down and inject the stopper with the needle.
4. Push the air inside and withdraw the insulin dose required.
5. Give the syringe a few taps with your finger to get the bubbles to the top, and push the bubbles back into the bottle.
6. Pinch up the area of skin to be injected.
7. Insert the needle at a right angle to the skin and push it in; then push down the plunger to administer the insulin.

There are now several aids to needle and syringe delivery: spring-loaded syringe holders; syringe magnifiers to help the visually impaired; syringe-filling devices that click when the insulin has been taken up; and needle guides for when a person cannot see the rubber stop on the bottle where the needle is inserted to take up insulin.

Insulin pens

These pens come with a cartridge already inserted that contains 3.0 mL of the specific insulin and the patient can dial the amount of insulin to be taken. Each unit (or 2 units) is accompanied by a click so that people with visual impairment can hear the number of units; the number will also appear in a window on the pen. The pens allow delivery of 30–70 units; a new needle can be screwed on as necessary. There are several different pens available and it is best to view them and try them out with a diabetes specialist nurse to see which is most suitable.

Jet injection device

These are expensive but good for people who cannot perform the injection for themselves. The device holds a large quantity of insulin to be used for multiple treatments. After dialing up the amount of insulin to be delivered, the device is held against the skin and, on pressing a button, a jet of air forces the insulin through the skin into the tissue underneath. The device is occasionally leaky, with insulin staying above the skin; others report that the injection can be painful.

Traditionally patients are advised to rotate the location of their injection sites; this helps to avoid local reactions to insulin, which are, principally:

- *Allergy.*   Local allergic reactions are uncommon with modern insulin preparations; reactions to diluent or preservatives are sometimes thought to be of relevance; a change of brand may help, but many cases resolve spontaneously. Transient tender nodules developing at the injection site are suggestive; generalized allergic reactions are exceedingly uncommon. Testing kits are available from insulin manufacturers. Major insulin resistance due to high titres of anti-insulin antibodies that cause antigen–antibody complexes is very uncommon; corticosteroids may be useful.
- *Lipohypertrophy.*   Localized areas of lipohypertrophy, although comfortable to inject into, are thought to cause erratic absorption of insulin from the site. The hypertrophy is attributed to the trophic effects of insulin on fat metabolism. Avoidance of the area may lead to regression; liposuction has been used.
- *Lipoatrophy.*   This has become rare since the introduction of highly purified, and more recently human sequence, insulins. It may be improved by the injection of highly purified soluble insulin around the edge of the lesion.

Patients occasionally complain of recurrent minor local bleeding or bruising, which rarely presents any real cause for concern.

Renal failure

Care is required with insulin treatment in patients with progressive renal impairment. Decreased insulin degradation by the failing kidneys, anorexia with decreased caloric intake and reduced renal gluconeogenesis may all contribute. Sometimes substantial reductions in insulin dose may be required.

 Progressive renal failure necessitates reduction in insulin dose.

Some patients with end-stage renal failure on continuous ambulatory peritoneal dialysis (CAPD) inject their insulin into the dialysate bags, thereby delivering insulin intraperitoneally. Insulin requirements vary enormously between patients and are in part dependent on the strength of dialysate used; hypertonic solutions contain high concentrations of glucose.

Disposal of needles

Clipper devices are available for the safe disposal of used syringe needles. Boxes designed to contain used sharps should be disposed of appropriately. Some local authorities offer a needle disposal service.

Altering insulin doses

Patients vary in their capacity and willingness to adjust their own insulin doses. Some will never make an adjustment; the advice of the specialist nurse can be helpful in such cases and close telephone contact is reassuring. Other patients alter doses too frequently according to their latest home capillary readings – this can lead to a 'roller-coaster' effect with glycaemic instability, and is best avoided. Although there are some general principles to be followed, there are no hard-and-fast rules; caution and common sense are guiding principles.

- Alter one insulin dose at a time.
- Alter the appropriate insulin based on knowledge of the pharmacokinetics of the insulin preparations being used. For example, on twice-daily mixtures of short- and medium-acting insulin:
  - Allow a few days to observe the effect of the change; daily fluctuations must be taken into account.
- A relatively small change (2–4 units) is generally safe; larger changes may be indicated in some instances, but care should be taken to avoid inducing hypoglycaemia. Such small alterations are not always appropriate; the magnitude of the increase or decrease should reflect the overall insulin dose. For example, for a patient stabilized on a daily dose of 40 units, a change of 4 units is 10% of the total; for a patient on 100 units, a proportionately similar change would be 10 units. Moreover, when insulin has just been initiated, tiny daily increases in dose may be too cautious. However, experience is required in judging whether larger increases are indicated.
- If recurrent hypoglycaemia occurs at the higher dose, the patient should drop back to the previous dose.

- Remember that increasing the dose of a pre-mixed insulin preparation will increase both the short- and the longer-acting components.
- Be prepared for discrepancies between theory based on insulin pharmacokinetics and the realities of clinical practice.

Unwanted effects of insulin therapy

Weight gain

This is a common consequence of insulin (and sulphonylurea) treatment. In patients with type 1 diabetes, some regain of lost body weight is appropriate; this reflects the physiological anabolic effects of insulin. However, in patients with type 2 diabetes, the initiation of insulin therapy because of inadequate glycaemic control with oral agents is often associated with unwelcome weight gain. Dietary countermeasures may be partially effective, particularly when combined with an exercise programme. Weight gain is not inevitable but it can detract from the sense of achievement for some patients. It tends to plateau after a few months, possibly reflecting the resetting of a physiological homeostatic mechanism.

Insulin oedema

This is a rare complication of insulin therapy. Oedema of the feet and legs develops shortly after the initiation of insulin and resolves with continued therapy. The aetiology is uncertain but insulin-mediated sodium and water retention by the kidney has been postulated.

Transient deterioration of retinopathy

A rapid and sometimes marked transient deterioration in pre-existing retinopathy may follow the institution of improved glycaemic control, for example when insulin is commenced after tablet failure. This appears to be due to a reduction in retinal blood flow that occurs with improved glycaemic control. As a result, already compromised areas of retinal circulation become more ischaemic and further damage may occur.

Insulin neuritis

An uncommon complication is so-called insulin neuritis, wherein acute symptomatic neuropathy, which may be very unpleasant, develops following the institution of insulin treatment. Histological studies in acute painful neuropathies have demonstrated actively regenerating neurons, which are thought to be the origin of the symptoms. Rapid alterations in osmotically active intraneural molecules (e.g. sorbitol) are also thought to be relevant. The prognosis appears to be generally favourable with continued good glycaemic control. Symptomatic treatment may be required until recovery, which may not always be complete; subclinical neuropathy predating the improved control may have been present in some cases.

Postural hypotension

A clinically significant fall in blood pressure shortly after insulin injection is very rare. The vasodilator effects of insulin have been implicated, but the pathophysiology remains uncertain.

Severe insulin resistance

The definition is arbitrary. When daily insulin doses (in excess of 200 units) were needed to control glycaemia, it was considered to reflect severe insulin resistance; this is now largely of historical interest. The concept of insulin resistance is discussed in Section 1.

- *Severe insulin resistance syndromes.* Specific causes of severe insulin resistance, congenital or acquired, are very rare.
- *Brittle diabetes.* Whether this entity exists is regarded as contentious by some. Apparently high insulin requirements with swings in control are a feature of some patients with idiopathic brittle diabetes.
- *Hormonal stress response to intercurrent illness.* Transient insulin resistance may arise in the course of intercurrent illnesses (e.g. sepsis); temporary increases in insulin doses, sometimes necessitating a change to intravenous or multiple subcutaneous doses of short-acting insulin, are required. Insulin may be required during the course of such an illness in patients previously well maintained on oral antidiabetic agents; this will usually be undertaken in the hospital setting. With resolution of the acute episode, reintroduction of oral therapy may be possible.
- *Anti-insulin antibodies.* The role of acquired anti-insulin antibodies, once thought to be an important mechanism of insulin resistance, has faded with modern, less antigenic, insulin preparations.
- *Obesity.* Clinical insulin resistance is confined largely to patients with type 2 diabetes whose obesity and associated insulin resistance limits attainment of glycaemic targets despite large doses of insulin. However, type 1 patients can become obese and develop insulin resistance – possible 'double diabetes'.

Insulin regimens

This is the schedule of insulin that a person will decide upon with their health-care professional, and is based on the type of diabetes, physical needs and lifestyle (in particular eating patterns and

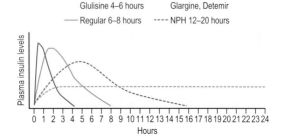

Figure 3.2 Action profiles of injectable insulins. NPH, neutral protamine Hagedorm.

activity). The variables include type of insulin, timing and dose (Fig. 3.2). There are many regimens, but the most common examples are:

● *Insulin added to oral medication.* This combination is worthwhile in those with type 2 diabetes where the fasting blood glucose begins to rise despite maximum oral medication. It most often means a dose of long-acting insulin at bedtime.
● *Twice-daily insulin.* This is either two doses of an intermediate-acting insulin or two doses of a mixed insulin to give more control over postprandial increases in blood glucose (Fig. 3.3). The latter is often used in type 1 diabetes when the individual wants to avoid taking insulin at work/school at lunchtime.
● *Basal-bolus insulin.* This is essentially intensive insulin therapy and is discussed below (Fig. 3.4).

Tip box

If recurrent hypoglycaemia occurs at the higher dose, it should be dropped back to the previous dose. If there is a significant change in diet and weight, this can increase or decrease insulin requirements significantly.

If no change in results is observed, check your insulin (expiry and pen device), plus review your injection site and technique with a health-care professional.

Adverse effects of insulin therapy

Although insulin is no doubt life-saving to many and provides a dramatic improvement in symptoms, to others it is good to be aware of the following adverse effects:

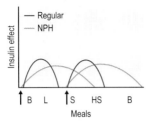

Regular insulin

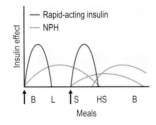

Rapid-acting insulin

Figure 3.3 Twice-daily insulin. B, breakfast; L, lunch; S, supper; HS, hora somni (bedtime); NPH, neutral protamine Hagedorm.

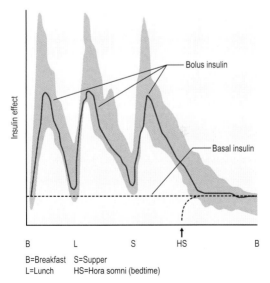

B=Breakfast   S=Supper
L=Lunch   HS=Hora somni (bedtime)

Figure 3.4 Basal-bolus insulin replacement.

- *Hypoglycaemia.* This is the most common disadvantage of insulin therapy and occurs when the amount of insulin taken is too much for the amount of food ingested, exercise undertaken or starting level of blood sugar. It may also occur as a consequence of excess alcohol intake (see Section 4).
- *Weight gain.* When insulin is started, a person will begin to retain fat; this is normal to some extent. People will find they are unable to eat as much as they did previously without putting on weight and therefore they should beware of overeating. Also, eating snacks to avoid hypoglycaemia should be limited as much as possible. It is usually better to reduce the insulin dose rather than eating to justify it.
- *Insulin allergy.* This is now extremely rare due to the use of human insulin.

Rapid-acting insulin analogues

Rapid-acting insulin analogues have a small but statistically significant effect on glycated haemoglobin (HbA1c) that, in the context of long-term glycaemic control, is unlikely to be clinically significant. However, there is a reduction in hypoglycaemia associated with their use, and insulin analogues have been associated with an improvement in treatment satisfaction scores.

Basal insulin analogues

Basal insulin analogues appear to offer no clinically significant improvement in glycaemic control, but are associated with fewer severe hypoglycaemic episodes, particularly nocturnal episodes. Insulin detemir is associated with less weight gain than neutral protamine Hagedorm (NPH) insulin, but many individuals require twice-daily dosing. Basal insulin analogues appear to offer greater patient satisfaction but no clear change in quality of life.

> **Tip box**
>
> Basal insulin analogues should be used in adults with type 1 diabetes who are experiencing severe or nocturnal hypoglycaemia. In type 1 diabetic patients who are not experiencing severe or nocturnal hypoglycaemia, NPH insulin could be considered.

Rapid-acting and basal insulin analogues in children and adolescents

In children and adolescents, the use of rapid-acting and basal insulin analogues offers similar glycaemic control, rates of overall hypoglycaemia, and rates of nocturnal hypoglycaemia to that of regular human insulin. Therefore, children and adolescents should be offered insulin analogues, regular human insulin and NPH preparations, or an appropriate combination of these.

The insulin regimen should be tailored to the individual to achieve the best possible glycaemic control without disabling hypoglycaemia.

> **Tip box**
>
> Intensive insulin therapy should be delivered as part of a comprehensive support package. In general this refers to regular contact between patients and their families/carers and the local multidisciplinary diabetes team delivering specific health-care strategies.

Continuous subcutaneous insulin infusion therapy

Continuous subcutaneous insulin infusion (CSII) or 'insulin pump' therapy allows programmed insulin delivery with multiple basal infusion rates and flexible bolus dosing of insulin with meals. In developed countries its usage is increasing in patients with type 1 diabetes who are expert at carbohydrate counting or have undertaken an appropriate structured education course. Carbohydrate counting is an essential skill to support intensified insulin management in type 1 diabetes, by either multiple daily injections (MDI) or CSII. CSII therapy requires considerable input from the patient along with the diabetes nurse specialists and dietitians, in addition to the purchase of a pump and consumables.

Pumps are often the size of a pager and are worn on a belt or in the clothing, with thin plastic tubing coming from the pump to a needle that penetrates the skin, usually in the abdomen. It is in place 24 hours a day, and this device is as close as one can get to the constant gradual administration of insulin that is taking place in the body.

Some important points to know about pumps

- They do not measure blood sugar and so the pump still needs to be directed by blood sugar measurements with a meter and dose adjustments.
- There are two basic rates of delivery: the *basal rate*, which is a slow, continuous trickle when a person is not eating, and the *bolus rate*, which is a much higher flow rate delivered when a meal is about to be eaten.
- Much guidance is required, especially at the start, from the diabetes specialist nurse and/or doctor, in addition to a dietitian.
- National Institute for Health and Clinical Excellence (NICE) guidelines recommend that pumps be considered in those

where other insulin regimes have 'failed' – where it is not possible to reduce HbA1c to less than 7.5% without causing 'disabling hypoglycaemia'. Pumps should also be considered only for patients who are committed to gaining the considerable expertise and competence that the effective use of a pump requires.

Advantages of pumps
- They are flexible and good for people whose meal times are unpredictable.
- They have built-in safety devices to stop overdosage.
- They generally do improve control, reducing uncomfortable swings in blood sugar, and result in a better HbA1c.

Disadvantages of pumps
- Skin infections can occur as the infusion set is left *in situ* for a few days.
- Ketoacidosis can occur rapidly if the pump disconnects, as short-acting insulin is the only form given.
- Blood glucose must be measured frequently to adjust the pump for best control.
- They are expensive (more than £2500, with annual costs of about £1200).
- Limited availability of pumps supplied from the National Health Service.

Tip box

Concerns have been raised over the lack of independent studies to allow objective comparison of MDI and CSII.

However, in patients with type 1 diabetes, CSII therapy has been associated with an improvement in glycaemic control with reported mean falls in HbA1c of between 0.2% and 0.4% (2.2–4.4 mmol/mol) or greater mean treatment satisfaction scores.

CSII therapy should be considered for patients unable to achieve their glycaemic targets and in patients who experience recurring episodes of severe hypoglycaemia. Pump therapy management requires a local multidisciplinary pump clinic for patients who have undertaken structured education. Patients using CSII therapy should agree targets for improvement in HbA1c and/or reduction in hypoglycaemia with their multidisciplinary diabetes care team. Progress against targets should be monitored and, if appropriate, alternative treatment strategies should be offered.

Tip box

An insulin pump is recommended for those with very low basal insulin requirements (such as infants and very young children) where even small doses of basal insulin analogue may result in hypoglycaemia.

Inhaled insulin

A number of drug companies have developed inhaled insulins. In principle, this was a way of avoiding giving insulin by injection, but the dose of insulin needed is about seven times the amount needed, compared with injection. The accuracy of dosing has proved difficult and, because the insulin is being absorbed through the lungs, there has been some doubt about long-term safety – it would be difficult to know for many years whether inhaling insulin might impair lung function.

One preparation has been recently withdrawn from the market, but inhaled insulins continue to be developed. Currently there are no preparations available for use.

TYPE 2 DIABETES – INITIATING THERAPY

The immediate purpose of lowering blood glucose is to provide relief from symptoms (thirst, polyuria, nocturia and blurred vision). Thereafter, the aim is to prevent microvascular complications: retinopathy, nephropathy and neuropathy.

Hyperglycaemia, along with hypertension and dyslipidaemia, is associated with macrovascular complications (myocardial infarction (MI), stroke and peripheral arterial disease). The effects of glucose-lowering therapies on cardiovascular morbidity and mortality are therefore of major importance (and not just on glucose-lowering).

ORAL HYPOGLYCAEMIC AGENTS

Modifications to diet and lifestyle are seldom sufficient to produce good, long-term, metabolic control in patients with type 2 diabetes. Thus, pharmacological adjuncts are required in the majority of patients early in their management. Historically, orally active agents are usually employed first-line, whereas insulin is reserved for patients in whom tablets prove insufficient.

The choice of drug depends on both clinical and biochemical factors; as with all pharmacological agents, antidiabetic therapy should be initiated only following careful consideration of the possible benefits and risks of treatment for the individual patient.

> **Tip box**
>
> Selection of oral antidiabetic agents should be based on the potential benefits and risks to the patient.

Classification

Oral antidiabetic drugs may usefully be classified by their actions as being either:

- hypoglycaemic agents, or
- antihyperglycaemic agents.

This distinction, which reflects differences in chemistry and hence mode of action, is clinically relevant. Drugs in the latter category do not usually cause hypoglycaemia when used as monotherapy. It should be noted that other drugs, not used primarily as antidiabetic agents, may also lower plasma glucose concentrations (Table 3.2). The latter agents may potentiate the glucose-lowering effects of other drugs.

> **Tip box**
>
> Antihyperglycaemic agents may potentiate the hypoglycaemic actions of other drugs.

Combination oral agent therapy

For patients inadequately controlled by monotherapy, biguanides and sulphonylureas may be usefully combined; the effect may be synergistic (i.e. greater than a simple additive effect). Combination therapy is more likely to be effective in patients with less severe degrees of fasting hyperglycaemia. However, many patients will still not attain adequate glycaemic control. In these circumstances, the addition of a third agent will often result in further improvement.

TABLE 3.2 Hypoglycaemic and antihyperglycaemic drugs used to treat type 2 diabetes

Hypoglycaemic drugs	Antihyperglycaemic drugs
Sulphonylureas	Biguanides
Repaglinide	α-Glucosidase inhibitors
	Thiazolidinediones
	GLP-1 analogues/DPP-4 inhibitors

GLP, glucagon-like peptide; DPP, dipeptidyl peptidase.

> **Tip box**
>
> Metformin and sulphonylureas may be usefully combined in patients with type 2 diabetes.

The time-honoured conventions concerning the clinical use of oral antidiabetic agents have attracted criticism, and the optimal order of selection of therapy for patients with type 2 diabetes remains uncertain. However, the benefits of improved glycaemic control with either oral antidiabetic agents or insulin, particularly on microvascular complications, are clear. However, most clinicians would agree that metformin is the drug of choice for overweight patients.

> **Tip box**
>
> Additional benefit from oral antidiabetic agents is rarely obtained by escalating doses; consider adding an agent from another class, or consider insulin therapy.

Use of insulin in type 2 diabetes

The question of when to either abandon oral agents in favour of insulin or to add in insulin therapy is a particularly difficult one. This is especially so in the case of an obese patient who continues to have inadequate glycaemic control despite strenuous nutritional and lifestyle advice. The morbidly obese patients may require very high insulin doses to achieve satisfactory glycaemic control.

The waning of response to oral agents reflects the gradual attrition of endogenous insulin secretion that characterizes type 2 diabetes. Dietary compliance is also likely to be important in some cases. Non-obese patients masquerading as type 2 patients may have sufficient β-cell reserve at diagnosis to have a satisfactory response to oral agents. A proportion of these middle-aged to elderly patients have autoimmune markers associated with type 1 diabetes. These patients represent a subgroup called latent autoimmune diabetes in adults (LADA; see p. 59).

> **Tip box**
>
> Failure of an adequate therapeutic response to oral antidiabetic agents supports the case for insulin treatment.

Contraindications to oral antidiabetic agents

There are a number of acute or temporary clinical situations where oral antidiabetic agents are contraindicated in patients with type 2 diabetes; insulin therapy should be instituted in these circumstances

TABLE 3.3 Indications for insulin in type 2 diabetes

Clinical indication	Rationale for insulin therapy
Major acute intercurrent illness (e.g. septicaemia, MI)	Deterioration in metabolic control with sulphonylureas and risk of lactic acidosis with biguanides
Pregnancy	Inadequate metabolic control with oral antidiabetic agents; safety concerns about medication other than metformin and glibenclamide
Surgery	Risk of perioperative hypoglycaemia (especially with long-acting sulphonylureas); risk of lactic acidosis with biguanides
Acute major metabolic decompensation (DKA or HONK/HHS)	Absolute or marked relative insulin deficiency in concert with insulin resistance mandates insulin therapy

DKA, diabetic ketoacidosis; HONK, hyperosmolar non-ketotic coma; HHS, hyperosmolar hyperglycaemic state; MI, myocardial infarction.

(Table 3.3). After resolution or recovery, a satisfactory therapeutic response may be attained following the reintroduction of oral agents.

BIGUANIDES

Although the data for clinically relevant outcomes with metformin are limited, they are stronger than for any other oral agent for the treatment for type 2 diabetes. Metformin (dimethylbiguanide) should be considered as the first-line oral treatment option for overweight patients (body mass index (BMI) > 25 kg/m^2; Asians > 23 kg/m^2) with type 2 diabetes.

Metformin has been the only biguanide available in the UK since the late 1970s. It was introduced into the USA only in 1995.

The metabolic actions of metformin are complex and remain incompletely understood. It can be used either as monotherapy or in combination with other therapies such as sulphonylureas – where the effect on glycaemia is greater than that observed with either drug alone. It is also used as an adjunct to insulin therapy. Metformin's mode of action, pharmacokinetics and its adverse effects are distinct from those of the sulphonylureas.

Mode of action

In contrast to the sulphonylureas, metformin does not increase insulin secretion. Metformin suppresses gluconeogenesis, thereby reducing hepatic glucose output, which is the principal determinant of fasting plasma glucose levels. In addition, metformin appears to improve insulin action and serves to limit postprandial plasma glucose excursions by promoting tissue glucose uptake with oxidation or storage as glycogen. These effects appear to be due mainly to intracellular actions of the drug distal to the interaction between insulin and its membrane receptor.

Effects on fatty acid metabolism may also contribute to the improvement in glycaemia through decreased activity of the glucose–fatty acid (Randle) cycle in muscle and liver; these substrates compete for uptake and oxidation (see Section 1, p. 45). Through increasing insulin sensitivity, metformin has effects on some of the components of the metabolic syndrome. In addition, the beneficial effects of metformin therapy in overweight patients previously demonstrated are not explained solely by improvement in glycaemia. In particular, metformin appears to have a cardioprotective role in overweight type 2 patients.

In summary, metformin decreases hepatic glucose production and may improve peripheral glucose disposal while suppressing appetite and promoting weight reduction. Activation of the energy-regulating enzyme AMP-kinase in liver and muscle is a principal mode of action.

> **Tip box**
> Metformin has beneficial effects on some components of the metabolic syndrome.

Pharmacokinetics

Metformin is absorbed predominantly from the small intestine, attaining high local concentrations. The bioavailability of an oral dose is 50–60%; the mean plasma half-life is between 2 and 3 hours, necessitating 2–3 daily doses. Metformin is not bound to plasma proteins and is therefore not subject to displacement by other drugs such as sulphonylureas. No hepatic metabolism occurs, with virtually the entire drug dosage being excreted unchanged in the urine by the renal tubules.

Adverse effects

Metformin is a safe and well tolerated drug.

Gastrointestinal disturbances

Symptoms include nausea, anorexia, abdominal discomfort and diarrhoea. The absolute risk increase of diarrhoea is approximately 7% and the symptoms resolve rapidly on withdrawal. A minority of patients are unable to tolerate these effects. Metformin is available as a slow-release (SR) preparation that is associated with fewer side-effects. Introduction of metformin at a low dose (500 mg daily for the first week) can help to reduce the frequency and severity of gastrointestinal symptoms, which may be transient and self-limiting – 'Start low, go slow'. Other side-effects are rare; although reduced serum concentrations of vitamin B_{12} and folate are well documented, anaemia is virtually never encountered and in practice the clinical risk can be ignored.

Lactate metabolism

The principal contraindication is renal impairment, as this leads to accumulation of the drug. Metformin is contraindicated in patients with an estimated glomerular filtration rate (eGFR) of 30 units or less. Renal function should be checked at least annually.

Metformin therapy does not lead to an increase in lactic acid levels and there is no evidence that it increases the risk of developing lactic acidosis (see p. 161). However, metformin should be avoided in clinical conditions in which lactate production is increased (e.g. cardiopulmonary disease) or hepatic clearance impaired (e.g. alcohol abuse).

 Renal impairment is the principal contraindication to metformin therapy.

Hypoglycaemia

When used as monotherapy, metformin is associated with a low risk of hypoglycaemia. However, metformin does potentiate the hypoglycaemic risks of oral hypoglycaemic agents such as sulphonylureas.

GLYCAEMIC CONTROL

Metformin, sulphonylureas, insulin, meglitinides and α-glucosidase inhibitors all have similar effects on HbA1c. In non-obese patients, metformin monotherapy reduces postprandial glycaemia, hypercholesterolaemia and hyperinsulinaemia.

SULPHONYLUREAS

Sulphonylureas increase endogenous release of insulin from pancreatic β-cells. The drugs available are classed according to their date of release: first generation (acetohexamide, chlorpropamide, tolbutamide, tolazamide), second generation (glipizide, gliclazide, glibenclamide (glyburide), gliquidone, glyclopyramide) and third generation (glimepiride). The first-generation agents are now rarely used.

Sulphonylureas should be considered as oral agents especially in patients who are not overweight, who are intolerant of, or have contraindications to, metformin.

Mode of action

Sulphonylureas bind to an ATP-dependent K^+ (KATP) channel on the cell membrane of pancreatic β-cells inhibiting the tonic, hyperpolarizing efflux of potassium. This causes the electric potential over the membrane to become more positive. This depolarization opens voltage-gated Ca^{2+} channels. The rise in intracellular calcium leads to increased fusion of insulin granulae with the cell membrane, and therefore increased secretion of (pro)insulin.

There is some evidence that sulphonylureas also sensitize β-cells to glucose, that they limit glucose production in the liver, that they decrease lipolysis (breakdown and release of fatty acids by adipose tissue) and decrease clearance of insulin by the liver.

Hypoglycaemia/weight gain/adverse effects

Patients taking sulphonylureas have a higher rate of major hypoglycaemia (defined as requiring third-party help or medical intervention) than patients on diet alone. Weight gain is also significantly greater. A recent population-based study showed that 1 person in every 100 treated with a sulphonylurea each year experienced an episode of major hypoglycaemia, compared with 1 in every 2000 treated with metformin and 1 in every 10 treated with insulin. Weight gain of approximately 5 kg was observed in the sulphonylurea arm versus the placebo arm.

Cardiovascular morbidity

There have been concerns regarding the cardiovascular safety of sulphonylureas dating from the early 1970s. In 1970, the University Group Diabetes Program (UGDP) reported a detrimental effect of the sulphonylurea, tolbutamide, on cardiovascular disease (CVD).

TABLE 3.4 Plasma half-lives, duration of action and metabolism of the sulphonylureas

	Half-life (h)	Duration of action (h)	Active/inactive metabolites
First-generation agents			
Tolbutamine	4–8	6–12	No
Tolazamide	4–7	12–24	Yes
Chlorpropamide	24–48	24–72	Yes
Second-generation agents			
Glipizide	1–5	<24	No
Gliclazide	6–15	<24	No
Glibenclamide	10–16	<24	Both
Glimepiride	5–8	~24	Both
Gliquidone	12–24	<24	Yes

It was reported that CVD mortality was higher in patients given tolbutamide than in those given insulin (12.7% versus 6.2%, respectively). In a further large retrospective cohort study, there was a 24–61% excess risk for all-cause mortality with sulphonylureas in comparison with metformin. However, other studies, including the UKPDS, have not confirmed this.

MEGLITINIDE ANALOGUES

Meglitinides act on the same β-cell receptor as sulphonylureas, but have a different chemical structure. They have not been assessed for their long-term effectiveness in decreasing microvascular or macrovascular risk, and are more expensive than other glucose-lowering agents. Weight gain is more common and hypoglycaemia is more frequent in those treated with meglitinides compared with metformin.

Repaglinide

The carbamoylmethyl benzoic acid derivative, repaglinide, is a rapid-acting insulin secretagogue (meglitinide being the non-sulphonylurea portion of the glibenclamide molecule). Repaglinide binds to a distinct portion of the ATP-dependent K^+ channel in the β-cell membrane. However, unlike sulphonylureas, repaglinide does not stimulate exocytosis of insulin.

NATEGLINIDE

This is a phenylalanine derivative that also produces rapid and brief secretion of insulin when administered with meals. In the UK, a limited licence restricts its use to combination therapy with metformin.

Pharmacokinetics

Repaglinide is rapidly absorbed, has a short plasma half-life (less than 60 min), is hepatically metabolized and is excreted principally (90%) in the bile. It is designed for use only when a meal is consumed; if a meal is skipped, no drug is taken. The tablet should ideally be taken 30 min before the meal. This mealtime dosing allows for more flexibility than is possible with once- or twice-daily sulphonylureas, which have much longer duration of action (Table 3.4). Thus, repaglinide can be viewed as a prandial glucose regulator.

Clinical efficacy

Repaglinide achieves reductions in fasting glucose levels, postprandial glucose levels and reductions in HbA1c concentrations similar to those of metformin, sulphonylureas, insulin and α-glucosidase inhibitors. As with sulphonylureas, selection of patients is important; there should be sufficient β-cell reserve to allow effective stimulation of endogenously synthesized insulin. Combining repaglinide with metformin results in control that is superior to the control obtained with either agent used alone.

> **Tip box**
> Repaglinide allows flexible dosing with meals for patients with type 2 diabetes.

Safety and tolerability

Repaglinide is generally well tolerated. Side-effects include hypoglycaemia and weight gain. Contraindications are similar to those for sulphonylureas. Repaglinide appears to be a relatively safe choice in mild-to-moderate renal impairment. However, cautious dose titration is recommended.

α-GLUCOSIDASE INHIBITORS

α-Glucosidase inhibitors are oral glucose-lowering agents that specifically inhibit α-glucosidases in the brush border of the small intestine. These enzymes are essential for the release of glucose from more complex carbohydrates. As a result they inhibit postprandial glucose peaks, thereby leading to decreased post-load insulin levels, especially in comparison with sulphonylureas. Acarbose, miglitol and voglibose are the α-glucosidase inhibitors available commercially, and as monotherapy reduce HbA1c by approximately 0.8% (8.7 mmol/mol) compared with placebo.

Compared with placebo, α-glucosidase inhibitors have minimal effects on body weight. As predicted from their mechanism of action, hypoglycaemic adverse effects do not occur. Abdominal discomfort (flatulence, diarrhoea and stomachache) are the most frequently occurring adverse effects inhibitors and are dose-related.

THIAZOLIDINEDIONES

Mode of action

Thiazolidinediones (pioglitazone and rosiglitazone) increase whole-body insulin sensitivity by activating nuclear receptors and promoting esterification and storage of circulating free fatty acids in subcutaneous adipose tissue.

The thiazolidinediones lower glucose by two main mechanisms:

- increased glucose disposal in peripheral tissues (the principal effect)
- decreased hepatic glucose production.

These actions are mediated via effects of the drugs with a specific nuclear receptor – the peroxisome proliferator-activated receptor (PPAR)-γ. Activation of this receptor increases the transcription of certain insulin-sensitive genes, influencing adipocyte differentiation and function. Binding of thiazolidinediones to this complex induces a conformational change that ultimately alters the expression of genes involved in the regulation of lipid metabolism, including:

- lipoprotein lipase
- fatty acid transporter protein
- fatty acyl-CoA synthetase
- malic enzyme
- glucokinase.

Effects on glucose transporter (GLUT)-4 and adipocyte leptin expression have also been reported. The combined effect is to increase the uptake of non-esterified fatty acids and increase lipogenesis within adipocytes. However, the precise mechanisms through which these drugs improve insulin sensitivity in glucose metabolism remains to be determined.

Effects on the glucose–fatty acid cycle is an attractive possibility; amelioration of insulin resistance via reduction in adipocyte-derived or possibly through tumour necrosis factor-α is another. Combining a thiazolidinedione (TZD) with a sulphonylurea or metformin is beneficial and enhances the glucose-lowering effect.

Glycaemic control

Thiazolidinediones require the presence of a sufficient amount of insulin in order to exert a therapeutic effect. Pioglitazone can be added to metformin and sulphonylurea therapy, or substituted for either in cases of intolerance. When combined with insulin therapy in insulin-treated obese patients, insulin doses may be reduced substantially with a concomitant improvement in glycaemic control.

Pioglitazone is effective at lowering HbA1c as monotherapy, and in dual or triple therapy when combined with metformin, sulphonylureas or insulin. However, there is no convincing evidence that pioglitazone monotherapy has benefits over metformin or sulphonylurea monotherapy.

Cardiovascular effects

A meta-analysis of 84 published and 10 unpublished trials of pioglitazone compared with placebo or other therapy, and excluding the Prospective Pioglitazone Clinical Trial in Macrovascular Events (PROactive trial), reported a reduction of all-cause mortality with pioglitazone, but no significant effect on non-fatal coronary events. A further meta-analysis with 16 390 patients found a reduction in the primary composite endpoint (death, MI or stroke) with pioglitazone versus control. However, the PROactive trial suggested a reduction in fatal and non-fatal MI in the subgroup with previous MI. In patients with previous stroke, subgroup analysis showed that pioglitazone reduced fatal or non-fatal stroke, whereas there was no effect on stroke risk in patients with any history of previous stroke.

Studies on congestive heart failure (CHF) found an increased risk of CHF in TZD therapy in comparison with placebo or other medications, with an overall relative risk of 1.72. The PROactive study found that, although more patients treated with pioglitazone had a serious heart failure event compared with placebo ($P = 0.007$), mortality due to heart failure was similar to that with placebo. Pioglitazone does not have a negative inotropic effect on the heart. The cardiac failure appears, mostly, to be due to the increased plasma volume induced by TZD treatment.

Pioglitazone should not be used in patients with heart failure.

Weight gain

Increases of several kilograms in body weight have been reported in clinical trials. This appears to be due to the insulin-sensitizing and lipogenic effects of TZD therapy; improved glycaemic control may also reduce urinary glucose losses. Thiazolidinediones appear preferentially to increase subcutaneous fat deposits, whereas visceral adiposity is reduced.

Hypoglycaemia

Thiazolidinediones are classed as antihyperglycaemic rather than oral hypoglycaemic agents. The risk of hypoglycaemia exists when the drugs are combined with agents such as sulphonylureas or insulin; careful monitoring of blood glucose is required and doses of other agents doses may have to be reduced, sometimes substantially.

Fractures

Pioglitazone treatment is associated with an increased risk of peripheral fracture in both women and men.

INCRETINS

It has been known for many years that glucose administered orally gives rise to much higher insulin levels than glucose given intravenously despite similar or even higher plasma glucose levels. This increase is due to the release of intestinal humoral substances. Incretins are a group of gastrointestinal hormones that cause this increase in the amount of insulin released from the β-cells of the islets of Langerhans. This increase occurs before blood glucose levels are increased. These intestinal humoral substances also slow the rate of absorption of nutrients into the bloodstream by reducing gastric emptying, and in many patients directly reduce food intake by central effects on satiety. They also inhibit glucagon release from the α-cells of the islets of Langerhans. The two main candidate molecules that fulfil criteria for the incretin effect are glucagon-like peptide (GLP)-1 and glucose-dependent insulinotropic peptide (GIP). Both GLP-1 and GIP are inactivated rapidly by the enzyme dipeptidyl peptidase (DPP)-4. Type 2 patients have a blunted incretin response, and infusion studies have shown that GIP is ineffective in type 2 diabetes (Fig. 3.5).

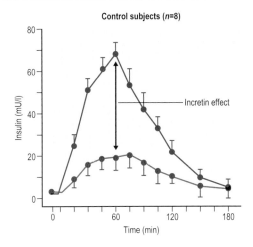

Control subjects (n=8)

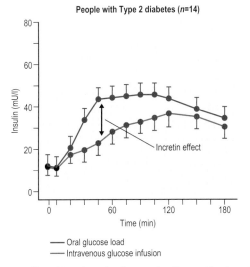

People with Type 2 diabetes (n=14)

— Oral glucose load
— Intravenous glucose infusion

Figure 3.5 Effect of incretin on insulin secretion (Source: Nauck et al. (1996). © Springer. Redrawn with permission.)

GLUCAGON-LIKE PEPTIDE-1 AGONISTS

GLP-1 is produced in the intestinal α-cells in the small intestine. It is one of the key 'incretin' hormones – a group of rapidly metabolized peptides secreted from the gut in response to food that amplify secretion of insulin from pancreatic β-cells and inhibit inappropriate glucagon secretion. GLP-1 also slows gastric emptying, resulting in slowed absorption of glucose following meals, and reduce appetite. GLP-1 agonists mimic endogenous GLP-1 activity, but are resistant to breakdown by the DPP-4 enzyme, resulting in more prolonged action.

Glycaemic control

Two GLP-1 agonists are currently available:

● Both need to be administered subcutaneously.
● Exenatide, which requires twice-daily injection, has a half-life of 4 h.
● Liraglutide, which requires once-daily injection, has a half-life of 11–13 h.

Both exenatide 10 µg (twice daily) and liraglutide 1.2/1.8 mg (once daily) added to oral glucose-lowering agents (metformin and sulphonylureas) reduce mean HbA1c by over 1%.

Hypoglycaemia/weight gain/adverse effects

GLP-1 agonists are generally well tolerated. The most frequent adverse events are gastrointestinal, especially nausea, which is generally reported as mild to moderate and settles in 8–10 weeks. If the patient is warned about this potential side-effect, the medication is usually well tolerated. Severe hypoglycaemia is rare and occurs only when sulphonylureas are co-prescribed. Mild to moderate hypoglycaemia occurs in approximately 10% of patients.

GLP-1 agonist treatment often results in weight loss. Weight loss was reported in study participants in the range of 1.6–3.1 kg. Hence, weight loss is a possible advantage of GLP-1 agonist therapy compared with insulin therapy and other oral glucose-lowering drugs, such as sulphonylureas and thiazolidinediones.

GLP-1 agonists may be used to improve glycaemic control in obese adults (BMI ≥ 35 kg/m^2) with type 2 diabetes who are already prescribed metformin and/or sulphonylureas. A GLP-1 agonist may be added as a third-line agent in those who do not reach target glycaemia on dual therapy with metformin and sulphonylureas (as an alternative to adding insulin therapy).

There have been suggestions that GLP-1 agonists are associated with increased risk of pancreatitis. However, there is insufficient evidence to determine whether these agents increase the background rates of acute pancreatitis in patients with diabetes.

DIPEPTIDYL PEPTIDASE-4 INHIBITORS (GLIPTINS)

DPP-4 inhibitors are oral agents that inhibit activity of the enzyme DPP-4 and hence prolong the actions of endogenous GLP-1. Three DPP-4 inhibitors are currently available: sitagliptin, vildagliptin and saxagliptin.

Glycaemic control

Compared with placebo, sitagliptin, vildagliptin, alogliptin, linagliptin, and saxagliptin have all been shown to be effective at lowering HbA1c by nearly 0.7 to 1%.

Hypoglycaemia/weight gain/adverse effects

DPP-4 is a membrane-associated peptidase that is expressed widely in tissues such as liver, lung, intestine and kidney. It is also known as CD26 and is distributed on T-cells, β-cells and natural killer cells. DPP-4 inhibitors, in the trials undertaken, have been well tolerated. However, they have so many roles that careful monitoring is necessary.

No severe hypoglycaemia was reported in study participants taking DPP-4 inhibitors alone. In combination with metformin, rates of hypoglycaemia were 6–10-fold lower with gliptins than with sulphonylureas. Gliptins are weight-neutral.

Published studies for sitagliptin and vildagliptin have medium-term follow-up (maximum 2 years); therefore, the long-term effects of these drugs on microvascular complications, cardiovascular disease and mortality are unknown. There is a statistically significant increase in all-cause infection following treatment with sitagliptin, but not with vildagliptin or saxagliptin.

SODIUM–GLUCOSE CO-TRANSPORTER INHIBITORS: FLOZINS

Phlorizin is a naturally occurring phenol glycoside first isolated from the bark of an apple tree in 1835. Early studies in animals showed that oral ingestion of phlorizin caused renal glycosuria and weight loss without hyperglycaemia; these findings were later confirmed in humans. The therapeutic potential of phlorizine is limited by poor oral bioavailability because of its tendency to be hydrolysed in the gut to its aglycone, phloretin. Because the majority of filtered glucose is reabsorbed in the early proximal convoluted tubule, and because non-selective sodium-glucose co-transporter (SGLT) inhibitors may also block GLUT-1, research has focused specifically on SGLT2 as a molecular target to increase urinary glucose excretion. Chemically, most SGLT2 inhibitors are glycosides derived from the prototype, phlorozin.

There are now several SGLT2 inhibitors in early clinical development, among which the leading compounds are sergiflozin and dapagliflozin. These novel SGLT2 inhibitors are pro-drugs that require conversion to the active 'A' form for activity against SGLT2 receptors. SGLT2 inhibitors potentially have the advantage of lowering plasma glucose levels irrespective of the underlying pathology of hyperglycaemia, and therefore may be useful in both type 1 and type 2 diabetes. They should also combine easily with both other oral and injectable treatments for diabetes.

Evidence for the safety of renal glycosuria on long-term kidney function comes from individuals with familial renal glycosuria. The prolonged excretion of urine with high sugar concentrations is classically reputed to be a risk factor for the development of genitourinary infections. So far, an approximate doubling of episodes of vulvovaginitis and balanitis has been reported, although it is less clear whether urinary tract infections are also increased in frequency or severity. Clinic development will also have to include testing SGLT2 inhibitors in diabetic patients with impaired renal function and/or microalbuminuria, who are at risk of further renal and cardiovascular disease.

Other potential adverse affects of SGLT2 inhibitors relate to the non-selective inhibition of GLUT pathways outside the kidneys. For example, non-specific inhibition of SGLT by phlorozin affects glucose uptake in the brain and inhibits the activation of the ventromedial hypothalamic responses to hyperglycaemia. Phlorozin has also been reported to inhibit alveolar fluid absorption in the lungs. Therefore, SGLT2 specificity is important for new agents entering clinical development.

GLYCAEMIC MONITORING

BLOOD GLUCOSE MONITORING

Many different strips and dedicated meters are available and will continue to progress and improve. Some meters simply measure the blood glucose, whereas others can store a lot of additional information such as exercise and extra carbohydrate intake. Stored information can be downloaded and graphs created. Adequate training and a system of quality control are vital. Even when trained health professionals use such systems, misleading results are possible, particularly in the lower range of blood glucose results. The diagnosis of diabetes cannot be made on the basis of a meter reading.

Practical limitations to self-testing include:

- inadequate manual dexterity (e.g. deforming rheumatoid arthritis or advanced neuropathy; post-stroke)
- intellectual inability or incapacity
- visual handicap.

When to test?

In type 1 diabetes, single readings are of relatively limited value, except to confirm or, sometimes importantly, to exclude the possibility of acute hypoglycaemia (see p. 126). More useful is a 'profile' of tests performed at different times of the day, usually in close relation to meals, typically:

- before breakfast
- before lunch
- before evening meal
- before retiring to bed.

In addition, a test at 0200–0300 hours, although inconvenient, may be important for patients in whom nocturnal hypoglycaemia (which may be asymptomatic) is suspected. Tests before and after exercise can be used to guide reductions in insulin dose or need for additional carbohydrate (see p. 74).

In patients in whom particularly 'tight' glycaemic control is required (e.g. pregnancy in diabetes) patients are often asked to test 2–3 hours postprandially.

Self-monitoring of blood glucose (SMBG) is a commonly used strategy for both type 1 and type 2 diabetes. It is a fundamental and established component of self-management in people with type 1 diabetes. The frequency and accuracy of testing vary considerably between patients; records vary from non-existent to meticulously charted profiles from dedicated (and sometimes obsessional) individuals. Fabricated results are well recognized. Discomfort and inconvenience are the main factors that discourage regular testing in many patients; expense is another consideration for patients in some countries. Self-monitoring guides adjustment of insulin or other medication for patients and health professionals as part of a comprehensive package of diabetes care, encourages self-empowerment and promotes better self-management behaviours. Frequent blood glucose monitoring is associated with an improvement in glycaemia.

Occasionally self-monitoring may fail to improve diabetes control and has been associated with negative psychological outcomes. Other methods of self-monitoring include self-monitoring of urine glucose (SMUG) and measurement of blood or urine ketones. Continuous monitoring of interstitial glucose (CMG) is an alternative for people with type 1 diabetes who have persistent problems with glycaemic control.

Tip box

The importance of SMBG whilst driving should be reinforced in people with type 1 diabetes.

SELF-MONITORING OF BLOOD GLUCOSE IN PEOPLE WITH TYPE 1 DIABETES

Continuous glucose monitoring

Although SMBG is a vital part of the management of glycaemia in people with type 1 diabetes, many patients do not routinely monitor glucose levels either postprandially or overnight, which may leave undetected episodes of hyperglycaemia and hypoglycaemia, respectively. Systems using continuous monitoring of glucose are generally considered for use only by patients who experience particular difficulties in maintaining normal glucose levels or who have been transferred to continuous subcutaneous insulin infusion therapy.

SELF-MONITORING IN PEOPLE WITH TYPE 2 DIABETES

The evidence for the benefit of SMBG in people with type 2 diabetes is conflicting. The impact of SMBG on management of glycaemic control is positive but small for patients not on insulin: the benefit in glycaemic control is greatest for those using insulin. However, it is difficult to use the evidence base to define which groups of patients with type 2 diabetes will gain most benefit from SBGM. Extrapolation from the evidence would suggest that specific subgroups of patients might benefit. These include those who are at increased risk of hypoglycaemia or its consequences, and those who are supported by health professionals in acting on glucose readings to change health behaviours, including appropriate alterations in insulin dosage.

Motivated patients with type 2 diabetes who are using sulphonylureas may benefit from routine use of SMBG to reduce risk of hypoglycaemia. SMBG may be considered in the following groups of people with type 2 diabetes who are not using insulin:

- those at increased risk of hypoglycaemia
- those experiencing acute illness
- those undergoing significant changes in pharmacotherapy of fasting, for example during Ramadan
- those with unstable or poor glycaemic control (HbA1c >8.0% (64 mmol/mol))
- those who are pregnant or planning pregnancy.

Tip box

SMGB is recommended for patients with type 1 or type 2 diabetes who are using insulin and have been educated in appropriate alterations of insulin dosage.

Fingerprick devices

Sterile, disposable, single-use lancets may be used in conjunction with simple, hand-held, mechanical devices by which a fingerprick sample is obtained with a minimum of discomfort. This aids compliance and helps to ensure that an adequate sample is obtained. The depth of the puncture can be adjusted. Used lancets must be disposed of appropriately.

Tip box

Routine self-monitoring of blood glucose in people with type 2 diabetes who are using oral glucose-lowering drugs (with the exception of sulphonylureas) is not recommended.

Urine glucose monitoring in patients with type 2 diabetes

Some old studies suggest that urine testing is equivalent to blood testing, but these studies were generally carried out in an era when HbA1c levels were higher than would now be considered acceptable, limiting the applicability of these data to current practice. There is no evidence describing an impact of urine monitoring on rates of hospital admission, rates of diabetic ketoacidosis (DKA), or mortality.

> **Tip box**
>
> Routine self-monitoring of urine glucose is not recommended in patients with type 2 diabetes.

Blood and urine ketone monitoring

Ketone monitoring using urine, or more recently blood, is generally accepted practice in the management of type 1 diabetes. Detection of ketones can assist with insulin adjustments during illness or sustained hyperglycaemia to prevent or detect DKA.

Blood ketone measurement is a more accurate predictor of ketosis/acidosis than urine ketone measurement. Blood ketone monitoring with increased health-care professional support is preferable to urine ketone monitoring in young adults with type 1 diabetes.

> **Tip box**
>
> There is insufficient evidence to advise on the routine measurement of ketones in patients with type 1 or type 2 diabetes.

PRINCIPLES OF EDUCATION IN DIABETES

EDUCATION IN ADULTS WITH DIABETES

It is recommended that structured patient education should be available to all people with diabetes and their carers at the time of initial diagnosis, and then as required on an ongoing basis, based on a formal, regular assessment of need.

There is insufficient evidence currently available to recommend a specific type of education or provide guidance on the setting for, or frequency of, sessions. There is good evidence, at least in the short term, that diabetes education improves clinical outcomes and quality of life. The model has moved from primarily didactic presentations to more empowerment-based models.

NICE clinical guideline CG66 on type 2 diabetes (2010, update) recommends that a patient education programme is selected that meets the criteria laid down by the Department of Health and Diabetes UK report on structured patient education in diabetes. Although these guidelines were written with type 2 in mind, the principles for type 1 diabetes should be no different.

The programme should:

- have a person-centred, structured curriculum that is theory-driven and evidence-based, resource-effective, has supporting materials, and is written down

- be delivered by trained educators who have an understanding of education theory appropriate to the age and needs of the programme learners, and are trained and competent in the delivery of the principles and content of the programme they are offering, including the use of different teaching media
- provide the necessary resources to support the educators, and that the educators are properly trained and given time to develop and maintain their skills
- have specific aims and learning objectives and should support development of self-management attitudes, beliefs, knowledge and skills for the learner, their family and carers
- be reliable, valid, relevant and comprehensive
- be flexible enough to suit the needs of the individual, for example including the assessment of individual learning needs, and to cope with diversity, for example meeting the cultural, linguistic, cognitive and literacy needs in the locality
- offer group education as the preferred option, but with an alternative of equal standard for a person unable or unwilling to participate in group education
- be familiar to all members of the diabetes health-care team and integrated with the rest of the care pathway, and that people with diabetes and their carers have the opportunity to contribute to the design and provision of local programmes
- be quality-assured and reviewed by trained, competent, independent assessors who assess it against key criteria to ensure sustained consistency
- have its outcomes audited regularly.

Multidisciplinary teams providing education should include, as a minimum, a diabetes specialist nurse (or a practice nurse with experience in diabetes) who has knowledge of the principles of patient education, and a dietitian. Although not formally assessed in this appraisal, input from other disciplines, such as podiatry, has potential value. The composition of the team and the way that members interact may vary between programmes, but team functioning should be tailored to the needs of different groups of people with diabetes.

Education is considered to be a fundamental part of diabetes care. People with diabetes, whether they are using insulin or other means of achieving glycaemic control, have to assume responsibility for the day-to-day control of their condition. It is therefore critical that they understand the condition and know how to treat it, whether this is through an appreciation of the basis of insulin replacement therapy and its optimal use, or through lifestyle management, including nutrition and physical activity.

The aim of education for people with diabetes is to improve their knowledge and skills, enabling them to take control of their own condition and to integrate self-management into their daily lives. The ultimate goal of education is improvement in the following areas:

- control of vascular risk factors, including blood glucose, blood lipids and blood pressure
- management of diabetes-associated complications, if and when they develop
- quality of life.

Education in adults with type 1 diabetes

Structured education based on principles of adult learning (including patient empowerment and experiential learning) is associated with improved psychosocial well-being, reduced anxiety and overall improvement in quality of life in people with type 1 diabetes. Adults with type 1 diabetes experiencing problems with hypoglycaemia or who fail to achieve glycaemic targets should have access to structured education programmes.

In recent years the DAFNE (Dose Adjustment for Normal Eating) education programme has been introduced for adults with type 1 diabetes. Patients taking part in the DAFNE programme obtained an average 1% improvement in HbA1c, overall improvement in quality of life and improved dietary freedom. No effect was noted in frequency of severe hypoglycaemia or patient-perceived hypoglycaemia.

Other packages such as BITES (Brief Intervention in Type 1 Diabetes – Education for Self-efficacy) and BERTIE (Bournemouth Type 1 Intensive Education) have been introduced as part of the education package for adults with type 1 diabetes. Patients participating in these programmes have found varying or no improvement in terms of satisfaction, HbA1c, rates of hypoglycaemia, blood pressure, lipids, weight, BMI or use of insulin.

A number of structured education programmes have also been developed specifically for patients who have significant problems with hypoglycaemia. These include Hypoglycaemia Anticipation, Awareness and Treatment Training (HAATT), HyPOS and Blood Glucose Awareness Training (BGAT). Improvements in hypoglycaemia rates and hypoglycaemia awareness seen in these programmes are not associated with a deterioration in overall glycaemic control.

EDUCATION FOR CHILDREN AND ADOLESCENTS WITH TYPE 1 DIABETES

Structured education based on developing problem-solving skills has a positive effect on a number of behavioural outcomes (including frequency of SMBG, better compliance with sick-day rules, increased levels of exercise, dietary intake and improved medication adherence) and overall quality of life.

There appears to be no difference as to whether group or individual (one-to-one) structured education is associated with better outcomes.

> **Tip box**
>
> Children and adolescents should have access to programmes of structured education that has a basis in enhancing problem-solving skills.

EDUCATION IN PATIENTS WITH TYPE 2 DIABETES

Structured education based on principles of adult learning (including patient empowerment and experiential learning) is associated with improved psychosocial well-being, reduced anxiety, and overall improvement in quality of life in patients with type 2 diabetes. The best known type 2 education package is the DESMOND (Diabetes Education and Self-Management for Ongoing and Newly Diagnosed). This programme did not lead to improvement in HbA1c after 12 months but was associated with around 1 kg greater weight loss, 5% less cigarette smoking, a greater understanding of diabetes and a lower prevalence of depression.

Most education interventions are associated with some HbA1c improvement, particularly in the short term – the magnitude of change is usually in the range of 0.3% (3 mmol/mol) to 1.0% (11 mmol/mol) improvement. The programmes may lead to patients reducing their diabetes medication, improving their knowledge outcomes, increasing the number of days exercising and an improvement in patient empowerment.

ORGANIZATION OF DIABETES CARE

DIABETES CENTRES

Patients (and their families) require education backed up by readily available expert assistance from a multidisciplinary diabetes care team. Arrangements for care vary markedly between countries with differing health-care systems. Purpose-built, hospital-based diabetes centres have proved to be popular in the UK and elsewhere. Such centres fulfil a multitude of functions:

- diagnosis and assessment of new patients
- long-term follow-up (usually for selected groups where adequate arrangements exist for the provision or sharing of follow-up with primary care teams; see below)
- continuing education of patients and staff
- education for other groups (e.g. community-based nurses)
- screening for chronic complications (see Section 5)
- specialist foot care
- provision of specialist medical care for special groups (e.g. pre-pregnancy and during pregnancy, young patients)
- assessment and treatment of erectile dysfunction (see p. 188)
- provision of telephone advice.

The aim is to provide these services in an accessible and comfortable environment. The active participation of patients, both as individuals and collectively, is to be encouraged; more generally, the concept of self-care is important in the management of a chronic disorder such as diabetes for which the patient, suitably educated and supported, is ultimately largely responsible. Diabetes care may be regarded as a cooperative process between the patient and the health-care system. Thus, although patients rightly deserve minimum standards of care (e.g. the European Patients' Charter), it is also recognized that they have certain obligations to ensure that appropriate care is delivered by acquiring knowledge to enable self-care on a day-to-day basis and to maintain regular contact with the health-care team.

Tip box

The philosophy of self-management for patients with diabetes should be actively encouraged.

Specialized care

Special clinics (sometimes outside normal office hours) for adolescents and young adults are held in many centres. Care of special groups of patients such as children and pregnant women may be located either in the diabetes resource centre or in another hospital department, according to local circumstances.

Staff

Staffing of the diabetes centre will typically include:

- consultant diabetologist – specialist training in diabetes; team leader
- specialist diabetes nurse – most health districts in the UK have at least one, and often more. Responsibilities include education and provision of day-to-day practical direction and support for patients, both in hospital and in the community, organization of staff training, development and implementation of local policies, commissioning of new equipment, introduction and evaluation of new treatments and technologies, research and audit. The diabetes specialist nurse should be well versed in counselling and education skills. Nurses may elect to concentrate on special groups such as children.
- dietitian
- podiatrist

In addition, the services of other specialists will also be required as necessary:

- nephrologist
- obstetrician
- vascular surgeon
- ophthalmic surgeon
- cardiologist
- psychologist.

Shared clinics, for instance between a diabetologist and a nephrologist or an obstetrician, are popular and may help to reduce the number of visits while facilitating the sharing of relevant information.

INPATIENT CARE

The problems surrounding inpatient care for people with diabetes have been long established. There are a number of concerns; these include disempowerment, distress, a lack of staff knowledge including in the management of acute diabetes complications, issues with food and food and medication timing, medicines mismanagement, and a lack of information provision. It is vital that these issues are addressed to ensure people with diabetes receive high-quality care.

Diabetic patients account for a disproportionate amount of hospital inpatient activity. Hospital admission is now rarely required for initiation of insulin therapy, but is necessary for the management of acute metabolic emergencies (see Section 4). Hospitalization is also frequently required for the management of serious acute microvascular and macrovascular complications, notably foot ulceration (see p. 188). Other common conditions such as unstable coronary heart disease and cardiac failure usually necessitate emergency or elective admission.

Surgery is required more often by diabetic patients (see above); close liaison between the surgical and diabetes services is obviously desirable. Written protocols for the management of diabetes during surgery or MI (see p. 207), DKA (see p. 148) or labour (see p. 250) should be agreed upon, implemented, audited and refined. This should be a continual process aiming not just to maintain but also to raise standards of care.

Diabetes UK recently published standards of care in hospital. The principles should be of a level that ensures:

- pre-assessment planning for elective admissions is undertaken and implemented
- every person with diabetes has an assessment and care plan for their hospital stay that is regularly updated as appropriate
- coordination and administration of medications and food in a timely manner
- access to food and snacks appropriate for maintaining good diabetes management
- protocols are in place for the timely prevention and management of hypoglycaemia and hyperglycaemia, including self-management of these complications where appropriate
- people are supported to optimize blood glucose control during their hospital stay
- information about the inpatient stay is provided to people with diabetes
- people with diabetes have access to the specialist diabetes team and education
- effective multidisciplinary communication between staff
- a discharge and follow-up plan is developed for each individual.

SUPPORTED SELF-MANAGEMENT OF DIABETES

People with diabetes wishing to self-manage:

- should be supported to do so where appropriate
- should have access to their self-monitoring equipment
- should have access to education, including information about how to access a structured education programme.

In order to support the delivery of the above, there needs to be:

- the implementation of diabetes training for all medical and nursing staff to ensure health-care professionals are equipped with the necessary competencies
- the development and implementation of protocols and/or systems to cover: communication, ongoing referral, surgery, prevention, and the timely and effective management of acute complications
- the implementation of audit and the commissioning of models of care shown to be effective.

DIABETES INPATIENT SPECIALIST NURSE (DISN)

Patients with diabetes should have evaluation of their glycaemic control and support in the management of their diabetes from a diabetes nurse specialist in an effort to reduce length of stay.

The inception of the diabetes inpatient specialist nurse (DISN) has led to an improvement in the management of inpatients with diabetes along with a significant reduction in inpatient bed-days. The role of the DISN has been to:

- act as a resource for expert advice and training for nursing staff, medical staff and other health-care professionals
- provide a highly specialized diabetes management and education service to patients referred within secondary care
- lead and contribute to strategic issues relating to diabetes care
- carry out audit and research work in connection with all aspects of diabetes care and participate in quality assurance programmes
- communicate with all areas, both professional and voluntary
- work as part of the diabetes team to provide a multidisciplinary service input with extended knowledge and skills in diabetes management.

DIABETES IN PRIMARY CARE

The long-term management of diabetic patients in the UK is increasingly being supervised in whole or in part in primary care; this is regarded as particularly appropriate for patients with type 2 diabetes who have satisfactory glycaemic control and no significant diabetic complications. Problems with metabolic control or the detection of complications should prompt consideration of specialist advice. Various models of care have been described, for example:

- miniclinics – performed in general practice but based on hospital clinics

- integrated care systems – wherein patient management is shared between the primary and secondary sectors to a greater or lesser degree.

Local circumstances will influence the arrangements within a particular health district. This approach requires close cooperation between hospital-based and primary provision to ensure high standards of care. Ready access to the hospital service and diabetes specialist nurses is necessary. An effective patient register and recall system are crucial components of successful diabetes care within a general practice setting. Regular audit of process and outcome is required; this pertains to hospital-based clinics as well as primary care clinics.

Tip box

A dynamic and regular process of audit is necessary to identify deficiencies and ensure improvements in practice.

Some studies have shown that prompted management of diabetes in primary care can result in good rates of attendance and satisfactory performance of blood pressure measurement and retinal examination. Conversely, unstructured care can lead to losses to follow-up, inferior glycaemic control and increased mortality rates.

Tip box

A prompted recall system is regarded as a prerequisite for successful care of diabetes in primary care.

OUT-OF-HOURS SUPPORT

Experience of dedicated diabetes hotlines shows that parents of younger children and patients with a short duration of diabetes are more likely to use this service. However, there is no evidence suggesting that a dedicated diabetes helpline prevents acute complications and hospital admissions.

TRANSITION FROM PAEDIATRIC TO ADULT SERVICES

Young people with diabetes often move from the paediatric services to the adult health-care system at a time when diabetes control is known to deteriorate. There is consensus that the needs of adolescents and young people need to be managed actively during this transition period. Transition models have evolved according to local circumstances and beliefs, and their complexity makes comparison very difficult. There is little evidence available on the different adolescent transition models and their benefits, and there is no evidence to recommend a particular transition model.

- Patients and their families favour a structured transition from paediatric to adult services together with adequate information along the way.
- A structured transition process appears to improve clinic attendance and reduces loss to follow-up in the adult services.

Paediatric and adult services should work together to develop structured transition arrangements that serve the needs of the local population.

MANAGEMENT OF DIABETES AT SCHOOL

Educational and health services should work together to ensure that children with diabetes have the same quality of care within the school day as outside it. There is no reason, if appropriate planning, education and training of school personnel are in place, why diabetic schoolchildren cannot full participate in the school experience.

Intensification of diabetes management requires increased monitoring and insulin use and, as this significantly improves glycaemic control, appropriate facilities should be available to all children while at school, including the treatment of hypoglycaemia.

ACUTE METABOLIC COMPLICATIONS

HYPOGLYCAEMIA

TYPE 1 DIABETES

Hypoglycaemia is the most-feared complication of therapy in insulin-treated patients. Unfortunately, iatrogenic hypoglycaemia is a common and serious hazard of treatment. It has a substantial clinical impact in terms of mortality, morbidity and quality of life. The risk of hypoglycaemia increases as glycaemic control is improved and in intensive insulin therapy it is the principal factor limiting the attainment of lower glycaemic targets.

Tip box

The risk of severe hypoglycaemia is inversely related to glycaemic control.

Iatrogenic hypoglycaemia usually results from a mismatch between:

- supply of glucose for metabolic requirements (e.g. as a result of a missed meal)
- rate of utilization (e.g. an increase due to physical exercise)
- a relative excess of insulin leading to a fall in the circulating glucose concentration.

In the Diabetes Control and Complication Trial, the overall risk of severe hypoglycaemia was increased approximately 3-fold in the intensively treated group. This was observed despite strenuous efforts to exclude patients who were thought to be at high risk of hypoglycaemia. The relation between rate of severe hypoglycaemia and mean glycated haemoglobin (HbA1c) level was inverse and curvilinear. Factors predisposing to severe hypoglycaemia are presented in Table 4.1. However, in a significant proportion of hypoglycaemic episodes, a clear predisposing factor cannot be identified even with very careful scrutiny of the circumstances.

TABLE 4.1 Risk factors for severe hypoglycaemia

- History of severe hypoglycaemia
- History of symptomatic unawareness of hypoglycaemia
- Impaired counter-regulatory hormone responses
- Intensive insulin therapy
- Glycated haemoglobin within the non-diabetic range
- Long-duration type 1 diabetes
- Alcohol consumption

Tip box

Asymptomatic hypoglycaemia is a contraindication to intensive insulin therapy.

In patients with type 1 diabetes, insulin levels reflect the absorption of exogenous insulin and do not fall as the plasma glucose levels fall.

Other causes of hypoglycaemia in insulin-treated patients are presented in Table 4.2. Their effects in individual patients are variable.

The symptoms and signs of acute hypoglycaemia may be divided into two main categories:

● Autonomic (adrenergic) – arising from activation of the sympathoadrenal system (Table 4.3). During hypoglycaemia, the body normally releases adrenaline (epinephrine) and related substances. This serves two purposes:
  1. the β-effect of adrenaline is responsible for the typical symptoms of hypoglycaemia (tremor, sweating, palpitations, etc.) warning the patient that hypoglycaemia is present
  2. the β-effect of adrenaline also stimulates the liver to release glucose (gluconeogenesis and glycogenolysis).

TABLE 4.2 Causes of recurrent hypoglycaemia in insulin-treated patients

Changes in insulin pharmacokinetics

- Change of anatomical injection site
- Development of renal impairment
- Effect of ambient temperature
- Effect of exercise on insulin absorption
- Change of insulin, e.g. human to quick-acting analogue (take analogue with meal rather than 30–40 min before)

Altered insulin sensitivity

- Acute resolution of insulin resistance postpartum
- Hypopituitarism or Addison's disease
- Hypothyroidism
- Weight loss or calorie/carbohydrate restriction
- Resolution of drug-induced insulin resistance, e.g. withdrawal of steroid therapy

Others

- Recovery of partial endogenous insulin secretion (honeymoon period)
- Malabsorption syndrome, e.g. coeliac disease
- Gastroparesis due to autonomic neuropathy
- Severe liver disease
- Eating disorders (anorexia/bulimia)

TABLE 4.3 Autonomic, neuroglycopenic and non-specific symptoms and signs in acute hypoglycaemia

Autonomic (adrenergic)

- Tremor
- Sweating
- Anxiety
- Pallor
- Nausea
- Tachycardia
- Palpitations
- Shivering
- Increased pulse pressure

Neuroglycopenia

- Impaired concentration
- Confusion
- Irrational, uncharacteristic or inappropriate behaviour
- Difficulty in speaking
- Non-cooperation or aggression
- Drowsiness progressing to coma
- Focal neurological signs including transient hemiplegia
- Focal or generalized convulsions
- Permanent neurological damage if prolonged, severe hypoglycaemia

Non-specific

- Hunger
- Weakness
- Blurred vision

- Neuroglycopenic – resulting from inadequate cerebral glucose delivery (Table 4.3). Specific symptoms vary by age, duration of diabetes, severity of the hypoglycaemia and the speed of the decline. The symptoms in a particular individual may be similar from episode to episode, but are not necessarily so and may be influenced by the speed at which glucose levels are dropping, as well as the previous incidence of hypoglycaemia.

Under experimental conditions, adrenergic activation occurs at a higher plasma glucose concentration than the level at which cerebral function becomes impaired (2.7 mmol/L). Thus, the patient is often alerted to the falling plasma glucose concentration by adrenergic activation and is usually able to take corrective action.

Hypoglycaemia and the brain

Cerebral function is critically dependent on an adequate supply of glucose from the circulation. Glucose is transported into the brain across the blood–brain barrier by a facilitative glucose transporter protein, GLUT-1. Studies in humans indicate that the rate of glucose transport into the brain can be modified by changes in plasma glucose levels. In particular, antecedent hypoglycaemia causes upregulation of glucose transport, so that more glucose is transported across the blood–brain barrier during subsequent episodes of hypoglycaemia. This adaptive response has important clinical implications.

Cognitive impairment progresses ultimately to loss of consciousness as plasma glucose falls. Seizures and transient focal neurological deficits may occur.

Tip box

Recurrent severe hypoglycaemia may cause intellectual impairment.

The most serious consequence of acute hypoglycaemia is cerebral dysfunction with the risk of:

- injury (to self or others). As a result of neuroglycopenia, the patient may become irrational and aggressive. Prompt assistance from another party may then be required to avert loss of consciousness and more serious sequelae.
- Generalized epileptic seizures.
- Coma.

Clinically, hypoglycaemia may be usefully graded as follows:

Grade 1   Biochemical hypoglycaemia in the absence of symptoms.
Grade 2   Mild symptomatic – treated successfully by the patient.
Grade 3   Severe – assistance required from another person.
Grade 4   Very severe – may cause coma or convulsions.

Hypoglycaemia – counter-regulation

The physiological response to acute hypoglycaemia comprises:

- suppression of endogenous insulin secretion.
- activation of a hierarchy of counter-regulatory responses (Fig. 4.1).

Counter-regulatory hormone responses

As plasma glucose concentration progressively falls, hormones that antagonize the actions of insulin are secreted in the following sequence:

- catecholamines – adrenaline and noradrenaline (epinephrine and norepinephrine)

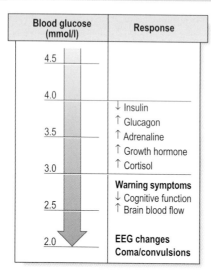

Figure 4.1 Hierarchy of hormonal responses to acute hypoglycaemia. NB: Thresholds are modifiable by factors such as antecedent hypoglycaemia.

- glucagon
- cortisol
- growth hormone.

Secretion of catecholamines occurs in the setting of generalized sympathetic nervous system activation. Glucagon and catecholamines are the principal hormones that protect against acute hypoglycaemia. These hormones stimulate glycogenolysis and gluconeogenesis, thereby increasing hepatic glucose production; enhanced hormone-stimulated lipolysis also contributes to recovery from hypoglycaemia through stimulatory effects on gluconeogenesis. If the response of either glucagon or catecholamines is inadequate, the other will usually compensate. However, deficiency of both will result in severe hypoglycaemia.

Cortisol and growth hormone play a less important role during acute hypoglycaemia, being more important in the later recovery of glucose levels. However, deficiencies of these hormones, for example cortisol deficiency in autoimmune Addison's disease (which is more common in patients with type 1 diabetes), can lead directly to or exacerbate hypoglycaemia. Hypopituitarism may have a similar effect.

Failure of counter-regulatory hormone responses predisposes to severe recurrent hypoglycaemia.

Hypoglycaemia unawareness

Hypoglycaemic unawareness is particularly common in patients:

- with long-standing type 1 diabetes
- who attempt to maintain glucose levels close to the normal range.

In addition, certain drugs and alcohol may impair a patient's perception of these symptoms. β-Blockers are designed to blunt the β-effect of adrenaline and related substances. Hence, if hypoglycaemia occurs in someone who is using this type of drug, he or she may have reduced adrenergic warning symptoms such as tremor and palpitations. β-Blockers may also reduce adrenaline's effect of stimulating the liver to make glucose, and therefore may lead to the hypoglycaemia being slightly more severe and/or more protracted. β-Blockers are not contraindicated in diabetes, but patients should be aware of these possible problems.

During hypoglycaemia, the body normally releases adrenaline and related substances. The reduction in the β-effect of adrenaline reduces the typical symptoms of hypoglycaemia and blunts liver glycogenolysis and gluconeogenesis. As a result the patient may not be aware that their glucose level is low and the liver produces less glucose.

Attenuation of the adrenaline response is usually due to the glycaemic threshold for the response being shifted to a lower plasma glucose concentration. This can be aggravated by previous episodes of hypoglycaemia.

'Hypoglycaemia begets hypoglycaemia' – antecedent hypoglycaemia alters the glycaemic threshold for counter-regulatory hormone secretion – the brain becomes 'used to' the low glucose concentration. Clinical studies have shown that intensive insulin therapy leads to symptoms that develop at lower plasma glucose levels. Neuronal glucose transporters increase in number in response to repeated hypoglycaemia. As a result, the hypoglycaemic threshold for the brain to signal adrenaline release falls. Consequently, the patient has less time between the onset of symptoms and the development of severe neuroglycopenia.

Tip box

Although the loss of warning symptoms has been described as a form of acquired autonomic dysfunction, it is generally accepted that classical diabetic autonomic neuropathy *per se* is not usually responsible for loss of hypoglycaemia awareness.

Recurrent hypoglycaemia, even if asymptomatic, is therefore a contraindication to intensive insulin therapy in patients with type 1 diabetes. Hypoglycaemic unawareness will sometimes disappear when the frequency of hypoglycaemic episodes has declined, but this is not always the case. With care and expert supervision, this may not necessarily compromise overall glycaemic control as judged by glycated haemoglobin concentrations.

Tip box

Severe hypoglycaemia carries risks of coma, convulsions, injury and sometimes death.

As adrenaline release is a function of the autonomic nervous system, the presence of autonomic neuropathy causes the adrenaline release in response to hypoglycaemia to be lost or blunted. However, it is accepted that classical autonomic neuropathy is not usually responsible for loss of hypoglycaemic awareness.

Advice about driving. Patients with loss of warning symptoms of hypoglycaemia should not continue driving motor vehicles. Hypoglycaemia while driving can have serious consequences. This should be conveyed to the patient and the advice recorded in the patient's case notes. Fatalities have occurred occasionally involving innocent bystanders. In the UK, patients should also be reminded that it is their legal responsibility to inform the driving licensing authority – the UK Driver and Vehicle Licensing Authority (DVLA). If the patient has a history of moderate or severe hypoglycaemic episodes, a hospital specialist's report is usually requested by the DVLA. The patient should be advised to do regular blood glucose tests before driving (which they should record) and to carry simple carbohydrate in the car.

 Patients with loss of warning symptoms of hypoglycaemia must not drive motor vehicles.

Nocturnal hypoglycaemia

Hypoglycaemia in type 1 diabetes is particularly common during the night and often goes undetected. Prevention of severe nocturnal hypoglycaemic events remains one of the most challenging goals in the treatment of diabetes. With the prevention of severe hypoglycaemia, it is likely that more people would be able to move toward optimal glycaemic control. Insulin-induced hypoglycaemia is also implicated in occasional sudden death in young patients. Prolonged severe hypoglycaemia, often exacerbated by excessive alcohol consumption, may produce cerebral oedema and permanent brain damage. The risk of hypoglycaemia bars insulin-treated diabetics from certain occupations.

 Nocturnal hypoglycaemia is often asymptomatic in insulin-treated patients.

The frequent occurrence of nocturnal hypoglycaemia – which may affect more than 50% of patients and often goes unrecognized – may be an important cause of hypoglycaemia unawareness. In addition, the physiological responses to insulin-induced hypoglycaemia are impaired during stages 3–4 (slow wave) of sleep.

Conventional strategies to minimize nocturnal hypoglycaemia include:

- reducing the dose of evening intermediate insulin
- moving the time of the evening injection of intermediate insulin to 2200 hours
- eating a snack containing 10–20 g carbohydrate before bed
- avoiding excess alcohol consumption.

Tip box

In patients on an intensified basal-bolus insulin regimen, insulin analogues are recommended in adults with type 1 diabetes who are experiencing severe or nocturnal hypoglycaemia.

Nocturnal hypoglycaemia often due to poor dietary compliance, and excess alcohol intake has been implicated in the sudden death of some young patients (so-called 'dead in bed' syndrome). The cause remains unproven, but catecholamine-mediated falls in plasma potassium concentration leading to cardiac arrhythmias have been implicated.

Treatment of insulin-induced hypoglycaemia

Grade 1–2 hypoglycaemia
The blood glucose level can usually be raised to normal within minutes with 15–20 g carbohydrate – overtreatment should be avoided if at all possible. Insulin-treated patients are advised to carry

dextrose tablets or Lucozade at all times. At the onset of symptoms, patients should take:

- 2–4 dextrose tablets
- 2 teaspoonfuls of sugar (10 g), honey or jam (ideally in water), or
- a small glass of carbonated sugar-containing soft drink.

If there is no improvement within 5–10 min, the treatment should be repeated. If the next meal is not imminent, a snack (e.g. biscuit, sandwich, piece of fruit) should be eaten to maintain blood glucose. Over-treatment should be avoided if possible.

Grade 3–4 hypoglycaemia

Friends, colleagues or relatives may recognize the development of hypoglycaemia before patients themselves. A subtle change in appearance or behaviour may prompt a third party to encourage oral carbohydrate consumption. Unfortunately, cognitive dysfunction may lead to a negative or even hostile response. If the level of consciousness falls, it often becomes hazardous to try forcibly to administer carbohydrate by mouth. Alternatives include:

- *Buccal glucose gel*. Proprietary thick glucose gels (e.g. Glucogel, formerly known as Hypostop) or honey (with variable efficacy) can be smeared on the buccal mucosa.
- *Glucagon*. Parenteral glucagon (1 mg = 1 unit) can be given by intravenous, subcutaneous or, most reliably and conveniently, intramuscular injection. Glucagon is a hormone that rapidly counters the metabolic effects of insulin in the liver, causing glycogenolysis and release of glucose into the blood. Glucagon can raise the glucose by 3–6 mmol/L within minutes of administration.

Tip box

Glucagon is unsuitable and ineffective in starved patients, particularly in patients with a history of alcohol abuse.

Glucagon comes in a glucagon emergency rescue kit, which includes tiny vials containing 1 mg, the standard adult dose. The glucagon in the vial is a lyophilized pellet: it must be reconstituted with 1 ml sterile water, which is included in the 'kit'. Relatives or friends can learn how to reconstitute and administer glucagon, and this should bolster confidence when dealing with a patient prone to recurrent, severe hypoglycaemia. If glucagon is ineffective within 10–15 min, intravenous dextrose should be administered.

Tip box

Intramuscular glucagon may be administered by relatives or friends to hypoglycaemic patients.

- *Intravenous glucose.* Administer 25 mL 50% dextrose (or 100 mL 20% dextrose) into a large vein. If a person is unconscious, has had seizures, or has an altered mental status and cannot receive oral glucose gel or tablets, emergency personnel should establish a peripheral or central intravenous line and administer a solution containing dextrose and saline. Dextrose 25% and 50% are heavily necrotic owing to their hyperosmolarity, and should be given only through a patent intravenous line – any infiltration can cause tissue necrosis. Thrombophlebitis is also a well-recognized complication of intravenous delivery.

  Hypertonic (50%) dextrose must be administered into a large vein in order to avoid extravasation.

Recovery from hypoglycaemia may be delayed if:

- the episode of hypoglycaemia has been prolonged or severe
- an alternative/additional cause for impairment of consciousness (e.g. stroke, drug overdose) coexists
- the patient is postictal (seizure caused by hypoglycaemia).

If the development of cerebral oedema is suspected, computed tomography of the brain should be undertaken and the adjunctive treatment considered: intravenous dexamethasone (4–6 mg 6-hourly) or mannitol. However, evidence for the efficacy of these drugs, or for other measures such as controlled hyperventilation, is poor.

Insulin overdose

Occasionally, patients present having deliberately administered an excessive dose of insulin with the intent of self-harm. It is usually possible to treat the resulting hypoglycaemia with a continuous infusion of 5% or 10% dextrose. Psychiatric assessment is required after recovery. Occasionally, severe, prolonged hypoglycaemia may result in permanent cognitive damage, personality change or chronic behavioural difficulties. The potential for neuronal damage resulting from severe recurrent hypoglycaemia is a particular concern in young children.

Insulin species/type and risk of hypoglycaemia

In the UK, there was intense debate about the effect of insulin species in relation to warning symptoms of hypoglycaemia. The issue arose from complaints from a small number of patients that, on changing from animal to human sequence insulin, symptoms were reduced in intensity predisposing to recurrent hypoglycaemia. This loss of hypoglycaemic awareness cannot be explained on the basis of differences in pharmacokinetics or the presence of high titres of anti-insulin antibodies.

Alternative causes of hypoglycaemia must always be excluded. However, it has been accepted that the patient's views should be respected; a request to change insulin type should be treated sympathetically.

Behavioural problems specific to type 1 diabetes

Idiopathic 'brittle diabetes'

This term is well known to most professionals involved with the care of diabetes. Disruptive episodes of hypoglycaemia may alternate with recurrent ketoacidosis leading to repeated hospitalization. This leads to an enormous amount of attention on the individual concerned. The patients are typically females in their teens with psychosocial difficulties. The symptoms are often associated with menstrual irregularities.

No convincing evidence has emerged in favour of an intrinsic difference in the metabolism of these individuals. There is anecdotal evidence of astonishing degrees of deliberate manipulation that has been known to mislead many well-meaning and experienced professionals. The long-term outlook is poor for these patients; some die from acute metabolic emergencies or suicide. Attempts can be made to alter this self-destructive behaviour pattern, but the problem often remains resistant to reasoned support.

Considerable difficulties in glycaemic control can occur as a result of a number of problems including delayed gastric emptying (gastroparesis) (see p. 18), drug interactions (e.g. β-blockers, steroids) and problems with insulin absorption.

Factitious remission of type 1 diabetes

There are rare reports of factitious 'remission' of type 1 diabetes. In this situation, patients claim that insulin requirements have fallen dramatically and spontaneously. Uncommon organic causes of increased insulin sensitivity (e.g. hypothyroidism, adrenal insufficiency) must be excluded.

Hypoglycaemia by proxy

This is a particularly disturbing but rare situation in which a patient (usually a child) is subjected to deliberate hypoglycaemia by parents or carers; fatalities have been recorded.

TYPE 2 DIABETES

Most of the research into hypoglycaemia has looked at hypoglycaemia in the insulin-deficient type 1 diabetic population. The occurrence of hypoglycaemia in the treatment of type 2 diabetes is well recognized, but is more protean in nature, having different risk factors and clinical features according to the nature of the antihyperglycaemic therapy, the extent of the insulin secretory deficit and the duration of diabetes.

The most common cause of hypoglycaemia in type 2 diabetes, resulting in significant physical and psychological morbidity, is iatrogenic, occurring with the use of insulin secretagogues (particularly sulphonylureas) and insulin therapy. These may overwhelm the normal defences that should protect against a significant fall in plasma glucose concentration, primarily by preventing a fall in circulating insulin. Risk of severe hypoglycaemia is further increased by any defects in the other systems for maintaining glucose concentrations. For example, defects in glucagon responses to hypoglycaemia develop in type 2 diabetes along with defects in the other stress responses. Specific therapies may worsen these defects; for example, sulphonylurea therapy sustains intrapancreatic insulin levels during hypoglycaemia, which may further impair glucagon responses.

Risk factors for individual episodes of hypoglycaemia in patients with type 2 diabetes include behavioural, physiological and therapeutic factors. The most common behavioural factor that precipitates individual episodes of severe hypoglycaemia is missed or irregular meals. Other lifestyle factors include alcohol, exercise and incorrect use of glucose-lowering medication (dose/timing).

Therapeutic/physiological factors associated with increased risk include older age, duration of diabetes, presence of co-morbidities, renal impairment, loss of residual insulin secretion, defective counter-regulation and loss of awareness of hypoglycaemia. The use of other medications may also increase risk.

Patient age also affects subjective awareness of hypoglycaemia. In the elderly, neuroglycopenic symptoms specifically related to articulation and coordination, which include unsteadiness, blurred or double vision, lack of coordination and slurred speech, are more common. There are experimental data to show that the adrenergic symptoms of hypoglycaemia decline with increasing age, whereas the tendency for cognitive dysfunction in hypoglycaemia increases.

Time of day is also important – even in the absence of pharmacological therapy, the lowest plasma glucose level of the day is just before the evening meal and unsuspected hypoglycaemia can occur at this time once drug therapy is started. Intensification of treatment targets will increase the risk of severe hypoglycaemia, although this effect will depend on the nature of the treatment used and the degree of insulin deficiency in the patient.

In addition, in type 2 diabetes hypoglycaemia has also been suggested as a private experience that is often not discussed with health-care providers. Hypoglycaemia may be a much greater burden for patients than health professionals are aware. Type 2 patients reported in a recent UK survey that they often received very little information and guidance from health professionals regarding adverse effects of their glucose-lowering regimens.

In patients on lifestyle adjustment and/or insulin-sensitizing treatments, the risk of hypoglycaemia is negligible. Based on patient reporting, the UK Prospective Diabetes Study (UKPDS) 73 showed rates of 0.1% and 0.3% for lifestyle and metformin, respectively, in patients receiving diet alone or monotherapy for 6 years from diagnosis. The recent Diabetes Outcome Progression Trial (ADOPT) reported rates of around 10% in patients on insulin sensitizers (metformin or a thiazolidinedione) over the 5 years of treatment (again all self-reported). Severe episodes were reported in very few patients (0.1%) on either treatment. Patients are more at risk of hypoglycaemia when an insulin sensitizer is combined with insulin or insulin secretagogues.

With the increasing drive for more strict glucose control in type 2 diabetes and new therapies that may carry different risks for hypoglycaemia from established therapies, a review of the risks of hypoglycaemia in type 2 diabetes is appropriate.

Tip box

Severe sulphonylurea-induced hypoglycaemia is a medical emergency, requires admission to hospital and has a high case-fatality rate.

Risk factors for severe sulphonylurea-induced hypoglycaemia

Hypoglycaemia rates with the third-generation sulphonylureas (e.g. glimepiride), second-generation sulphonylureas (glipizide and gliclazide) and the metiglinides (e.g. repaglinide and nateglinide) appear to be lower than those with glibenclamide and chlorpropamide. This is thought to be related partly to duration of action, but there may be other contributory factors. For example, agents predominantly excreted via the kidney (e.g. glibenclamide) should be avoided in renal impairment and in the elderly. There is also some evidence for differential effects on insulin sensitivity.

The risk of hypoglycaemia in patients taking an α-glucosidase inhibitor or thiazolidinedione appears to be low, but this risk is increased significantly if these drugs are taken along with a sulphonylurea.

Mild symptomatic hypoglycaemia is not reported to have any serious clinical effects, apart from the potential for inducing defects in counter-regulatory responses and impaired awareness to subsequent hypoglycaemia. Nevertheless, people with diabetes are fearful of hypoglycaemia and even clinically trivial events may be sufficient to inhibit concordance with therapy.

> **Tip box**
>
> Although, all sulphonylureas have the potential to cause severe hypoglycaemia, long-acting sulphonylureas, such as chlorpropamide and glibenclamide, are particularly liable to cause severe hypoglycaemia.

Rates of hypoglycaemia with insulin vary according to the regimen and the stage of evolution of the person's diabetes. In the UKPDS, patients who were newly diagnosed at the start of the study and randomized to insulin therapy reported 'any' hypoglycaemia rates of around 33% at year 1 and around 43% at year 10. Corresponding rates for severe episodes (defined as episodes requiring third-party help or medical intervention) were approximately 1.2% and 2.2%, respectively. In contrast, there is also some evidence to suggest that the frequency and severity of hypoglycaemia reduces with time as β-cell function deteriorates.

Newly emerging therapies based around enhancement of incretin action result in improved glycaemic control through a variety of mechanisms. The incretin, glucagon-like peptide (GLP)-1, released from the small intestine after eating, enhances insulin responses to glucose, as well as suppressing glucagon postprandially. The glucose-lowering effect of GLP-1 analogues and gliptins are glucose-dependent and therefore the hypoglycaemic risk of these agents appears much less.

Management

Recurrent symptoms suggestive of hypoglycaemia should prompt a reduction in dose or withdrawal of the medication responsible. Patients with severe sulphonylurea-induced hypoglycaemia should be admitted promptly to hospital; relapse following initial resuscitation with oral or intravenous glucose may necessitate prolonged infusions of dextrose. Delivery of an intravenous bolus of dextrose – a potent insulin secretagogue – will stimulate further insulin release, especially in patients with relatively well-preserved β-cell function. This predictable consequence of treatment, combined with the long duration of action of drugs such as chlorpropamide and glibenclamide, explains the tendency for hypoglycaemia to recur.

Tip box

Relapse after resuscitation is common in severe sulphonylurea-induced hypoglycaemia.

Treatment of hypoglycaemia in type 2 diabetes

- Intravenous dextrose. This remains the mainstay of therapy; it is well recognized that continuous infusions of 5% or 10% dextrose may be required for several days.
- Glucagon. This is less likely to work in type 2 diabetes as hepatic glycogen stores are usually very low when the patient presents with hypoglycaemia. In addition, glucagon also stimulates endogenous insulin release.

The antihypertensive agent, diazoxide, and the somatostatin analogue, octreotide, offer a more direct approach by inhibiting stimulated endogenous insulin secretion; these drugs have been used successfully as adjuncts to intravenous dextrose. However, neither is licensed for this indication in the UK.

- Diazoxide. This drug antagonizes the actions of sulphonylureas by opening adenosine triphosphate (ATP)-sensitive potassium channels in the membranes of islet β-cells. However, the drug is associated with adverse cardiovascular effects, including tachycardia and orthostatic hypotension, which may be hazardous particularly in elderly patients with a compromised vasculature or impaired baroreceptor reflexes.
- Octreotide. This has been shown to be an effective and well-tolerated agent for the prevention of sulphonylurea-induced hypoglycaemia under controlled experimental conditions. However, clinical experience for this indication remains very limited.
- Mannitol and dexamethasone have been recommended for cerebral oedema; however, the evidence base remains poor.

As high plasma insulin levels increase the transport of potassium into cells, serum potassium levels should always be monitored and intravenous supplements administered if hypokalaemia develops.

DIABETIC KETOACIDOSIS

Diabetic ketoacidosis (DKA) is a potentially life-threatening complication in type 1 diabetic patients. DKA results from an absolute shortage of insulin; in response, the body switches to burning fatty acids and producing acidic ketone bodies, which cause most of the symptoms and complications.

DKA may be the first symptom of previously undiagnosed diabetes, but it may also occur in known diabetics for a variety of reasons, such as poor compliance with insulin therapy or intercurrent illness. Vomiting, dehydration, deep gasping breathing, confusion and occasionally coma are typical symptoms. DKA is diagnosed with blood and urine tests; it is distinguished from other, rarer forms of ketoacidosis by the presence of high blood sugar levels.

DKA can affect patients in any age group. In some published series, female patients predominate. A small subgroup, predominantly females under the age of 20 years, may present with multiple episodes. Many episodes of DKA are avoidable with appropriate early action.

DEFINITION

The cardinal biochemical features of DKA are:

- hyperketonaemia – glucose and ketones in urine; fingerprick blood ketones > 3.0 mmol/L
- metabolic acidosis – pH < 7.3; bicarbonate < 15 mmol/L
- hyperglycaemia – plasma glucose > 11 mmol/L.

MORTALITY

DKA was first described in 1886 and, until the introduction of insulin therapy in the 1920s, it was almost universally fatal. Despite adequate and timely treatment, DKA still carries a mortality rate of approximately 3–4%, but varies between centres. Although a number of DKA-related deaths are the inevitable consequence of associated conditions such as overwhelming infection or myocardial infarction, others are still potentially preventable; delays in presentation or diagnosis and errors in management remain important factors.

MECHANISM

DKA arises because of absolute lack of insulin in the body. The lack of insulin and corresponding excess of glucagon leads to increased release of glucose by the liver from glycogen through gluconeogenesis. High glucose levels spill over into the urine, taking water and solutes (such as sodium and potassium) along with it in a process known as osmotic diuresis. Renal gluconeogenesis is also enhanced in the presence of acidosis. Glucose disposal by peripheral tissues such as muscle and adipose tissue is reduced by deficiency of insulin while raised plasma levels of catabolic hormones and fatty acids induce tissue insulin resistance. This whole process can lead to significant dehydration.

The absence of insulin leads to the release of free fatty acids from adipose tissue. Fatty acids are the principal substrate for hepatic ketogenesis and are converted to coenzyme A (CoA) derivatives prior to transportation into the mitochondria by an active transport system (the carnitine shuttle). In DKA, the hormonal imbalance strongly favours entry of fatty acids into the mitochondria and the preferential formation of ketone bodies:

- acetoacetate
- 3-hydroxybutyrate.

Within the mitochondria, fatty acyl-CoA undergoes β-oxidation resulting in the formation of acetyl-CoA, which is then oxidized completely in the tricarboxylic acid cycle, utilized in lipid synthesis, or partially oxidized to ketone bodies. Acetone is formed by the spontaneous decarboxylation of acetoacetate. Although acetone concentration is increased in ketoacidosis, it does not contribute to the metabolic acidosis. Acetone is highly fat-soluble and is excreted slowly via the lungs.

In the absence of insulin-mediated glucose delivery, β-hydroxybutyrate can serve as an energy source for the brain, and is possibly a protective mechanism in case of starvation. The ketone bodies have a low pH and therefore cause a metabolic acidosis. The body initially buffers this with the bicarbonate buffering system, but this is quickly overwhelmed and other mechanisms such as hyperventilation compensate for the acidosis, to lower the blood carbon dioxide levels. This hyperventilation, in its extreme form, may be observed as 'Kussmaul respiration'. In addition, ketones participate in osmotic diuresis and lead to further electrolyte losses.

Ketone body disposal

With the exception of the liver, most tissues have the capacity to utilize ketone bodies. Oxidation of ketone anions during treatment neutralizes the acidosis by the generation of equimolar amounts of bicarbonate ions. Excretion of ketone bodies via the kidney and lung is also important. However, urinary ketone excretion exacerbates the loss of cations such as sodium and potassium.

In various situations, such as infection, insulin demands rise but are often not matched because the patient fails to increase their insulin dose. Blood sugars rise, dehydration ensues, and resistance to the normal effects of insulin increases further by way of a vicious circle.

As a result of the above mechanisms, the average adult patient with DKA has a total body water shortage of about 6 L (or 100 mL/kg). In addition, there are substantial losses of sodium, potassium, chloride, phosphate, magnesium and calcium.

CAUSE

DKA occurs most frequently in those who already have diabetes, although it may be the first presentation in someone who was not previously known to be diabetic. There is often a particular underlying problem that has led to the DKA episode. This may be intercurrent illness (pneumonia, influenza, gastroenteritis, a urinary tract infection), pregnancy, inadequate insulin administration (e.g. defective insulin pen device), myocardial infarction, stroke or the use of recreational drugs. Young patients with recurrent episodes of DKA may have an underlying eating disorder, or may be using insufficient insulin for fear that it will cause weight gain. In 30–40% of cases, no cause for the DKA episode is found.

PREVENTION

Attacks of DKA can be prevented in known diabetic patients by adherence to 'sick day rules'; these are clear-cut instructions to patients how to treat themselves when unwell. Instructions include advice on:

- how much extra insulin to take when glucose levels appear uncontrolled
- an easily digestible diet rich in carbohydrates and salt
- means to suppress fever and treat infection
- recommendations when to call for medical/nursing help.

SIGNS AND SYMPTOMS

The symptoms of an episode of diabetic ketoacidosis usually evolve over the period of about 24 hours. Predominant symptoms are nausea and vomiting, pronounced thirst, excessive urine production and, particularly in the young, abdominal pain that may be severe. Those who measure their glucose levels themselves may notice hyperglycaemia. In severe DKA, breathing becomes laboured and of a deep, gasping character – Kussmaul respiration. Coffee ground vomiting (vomiting of altered blood) occurs in a minority of patients; this tends to originate from erosion of the oesophagus. In severe DKA, there may be confusion, lethargy, stupor or even coma.

On physical examination there is usually clinical evidence of dehydration, such as a dry mouth and decreased skin turgor. If the dehydration is profound enough to cause a decrease in the circulating blood volume, tachycardia and low blood pressure may be observed. Often, a 'ketotic' odour is present, which can be described as 'fruity' and is often compared to the smell of pear drops. If Kussmaul respiration is present, this is reflected in an increased respiratory rate. The abdomen may be tender to the point that an acute abdomen may be suspected, such as acute pancreatitis, appendicitis or gastrointestinal perforation.

Eruptive xanthomata and lipaemia retinalis are recognized complications that respond to treatment of the ketoacidosis. Serum transaminases and creatine phosphokinase may be non-specifically raised in DKA.

DIAGNOSIS

Investigations

Diabetic ketoacidosis may be diagnosed when the combination of hyperglycaemia, acidosis and ketones on urinalysis is demonstrated (Table 4.4). Arterial blood gas measurement is usually performed to confirm the acidosis. Subsequent measurements taken to monitor progress may be taken from a vein, as there is little difference between the arterial and the venous pH.

In addition to the above, blood samples are usually taken to measure urea and creatinine (markers of renal function, which may be impaired in DKA as a result of dehydration) plus electrolytes. Furthermore, markers of infection (complete blood count, C-reactive protein (CRP)) and acute pancreatitis (amylase and lipase) may be measured. Given the need to exclude infection, chest radiography and urinalysis are usually performed. However,

TABLE 4.4 Initial management of a patient with suspected diabetic ketoacidosis

History

Initially, brief and relevant, including:
- Previous episodes of DKA
- Potential precipitating causes
- Co-morbid conditions

Physical examination

Rapid but thorough assessment for:
- Signs of dehydration
- Level of consciousness
- Metabolic acidosis (Kussmaul respiration)
- Systemic hypotension
- Hypothermia
- Gastric stasis
- Precipitating conditions (e.g. pneumonia, pyelonephritis)

Biochemical assessment

Confirm diagnosis by bedside measurement of:
- Blood glucose (by glucose–oxidase reagent test strip)
- Urinary ketones (Ketostix)

Venous blood is withdrawn for laboratory measurement of:
- Glucose
- Urea (BUN)
- Electrolytes (sodium, potassium $\pm$ chloride)
- Complete blood count
- Blood cultures

An arterial blood sample (corrected for hypothermia) is taken for:
- pH
- Bicarbonate
- P_{CO_2}
- P_{O_2} (if shocked)

Repeat laboratory measurement of blood glucose, electrolytes, urea, gases at 2 and 6 h

Other investigations

As indicated by the circumstances:
- Chest X-ray
- Microbial culture of urine, sputum
- ECG
- Sickle cell test

BUN, blood urea nitrogen; DKA, diabetic ketoacidosis; ECG, electrocardiography; P_{CO_2}, partial pressure of carbon dioxide; P_{O_2}, partial pressure of oxygen.

DKA is associated with the release of various cytokines that lead to increased markers of inflammation (increased white cell count and CRP) even in the absence of infection.

If, as a result of confusion, recurrent vomiting or other symptoms, cerebral oedema is suspected, computed tomography of brain should be performed to assess its severity and to exclude other problems such as stroke.

● *Thromboembolism* – if the patient is elderly or very dehydrated, subcutaneous low molecular weight heparin should be considered.

Criteria

DKA is distinguished from other hyperglycaemic diabetic emergencies by the presence of large amounts of ketones in blood and urine, and marked metabolic acidosis. Hyperosmolar non-ketotic state (HONK) or hyperglycaemic hyperosmolar syndrome (HHS) is much more common in type 2 diabetes and features increased plasma osmolarity (above 350 mosmol/kg) due to profound dehydration and concentration of the blood. Mild acidosis and ketonaemia may occur in HONK, but not to the extent observed in DKA. There is a degree of overlap between DKA and HONK, as in DKA the osmolarity may also be increased. In most situations it is relatively easy to classify a case as either DKA or HONK.

Ketoacidosis is not always the result of diabetes. It may also result from alcohol excess and from starvation; in both states the glucose level is normal or low. Metabolic acidosis may occur in diabetic patients for other reasons, such as poisoning with ethylene glycol or paraldehyde.

A 2006 American Diabetes Association statement (for adults) categorized DKA into one of three stages of severity:

● *Mild:* blood pH mildly decreased to between 7.25 and 7.30 (normal 7.35–7.45); serum bicarbonate decreased to 15–18 mmol/L (normal above 20 mmol/L); the patient is alert
● *Moderate:* pH 7.00–7.25, bicarbonate 10–15 mmol/L; mild drowsiness may be present
● *Severe:* pH below 7.00, bicarbonate below 10 mmol/L; stupor or coma may occur.

Metabolic acidosis has a number of potential serious pathological effects:

● exert a negative inotropic effect on cardiac muscle
● exacerbate systemic hypotension via peripheral vasodilatation
● increase the risk of ventricular arrhythmias
● induce respiratory depression with pH < 7.0
● exacerbate insulin resistance.

DKA usually presents with an anion gap acidosis (anion gap typically 25–35 mmol/L). A wide variety of acid–base disturbances

---

TABLE 4.5 Causes of anion gap acidosis

- Ketoacidosis
  - Diabetic ketoacidosis
  - Alcoholic ketoacidosis
- Lactic acidosis
- Chronic renal failure
- Drug toxicity
  - Methanol (metabolized to formic acid)
  - Ethylene glycol (metabolized to oxalic acid)
  - Salicylate poisoning (severe)

---

have been reported. Some causes are listed shown in Table 4.5. The anion gap is increased when plasma:

$$[\text{sodium}] - ([\text{chloride}] + [\text{bicarbonate}]) > 15 \, \text{mmol/L}$$

Potassium is not included because the plasma level of this ion may be altered significantly by acid–base disturbances. Proteins, phosphate, sulphate and lactate ions account for the normal anion gap of about 10–15 mmol/L. When the anion gap is increased, measurement of the plasma concentration of specific anions (e.g. ketone bodies, lactate) may confirm the aetiology of the acidosis.

MANAGEMENT

Hyperglycaemia

Delays in initiating therapy may be disastrous and the diagnosis should be considered in any unconscious or hyperventilating patient.

The main aims in the treatment of diabetic ketoacidosis are replacing the lost fluids and electrolytes while suppressing the high blood sugars and ketone production with insulin (Table 4.6). Admission to an intensive care unit or similar high-dependency area for close observation may be necessary.

- A urinary catheter should be inserted if the patient is oliguric.
- Patients with hyperkalaemia should have a cardiac monitor in order to monitor for peaked T waves.
- Patients who are drowsy or have a reduced conscious level should have a nasogastric tube inserted to avoid aspiration.

Fluid replacement

Despite a proportionally greater loss of body water, plasma sodium concentrations are usually normal or low (Table 4.7). However, in DKA, plasma electrolyte concentrations may be falsely depressed by

TABLE 4.6 Guidelines for the management of severe diabetic ketoacidosis in adults

Fluids and electrolytes

Volumes:
- 1 L/h × 3, thereafter adjusted according to requirements

Fluids:
- Isotonic ('normal') saline (150 mmol/L) is routine
- Hypotonic ('half-normal') saline (75 mmol/L) if serum sodium exceeds 150 mmol/L (no more than 1–2 L – consider 5% dextrose with increased insulin if marked hypernatraemia)
- 5% dextrose 1 L 4–6-hourly when blood glucose has fallen to 15 mmol/L (severely dehydrated patients may require simultaneous saline infusion)
- Sodium bicarbonate (100 mL) as 1.26% solution* (or 8.4% solution if large vein cannulated) if pH <7.0 (with extra potassium – see text)

Potassium:
- No potassium in first 1 L unless initial plasma potassium level <3.5 mmol/L
- Thereafter, add following dosages to each 1 L of fluid, If plasma K^+:
  - <4.0 mmol/L, add 40 mmol KCl (severe hypokalaemia may require more aggressive KCl replacement)
  - 3.5–5.5 mmol/L, add 20 mmol KCl
  - >5.5 mmol/L, add no KCl

Insulin

By continuous intravenous infusion:
- A bolus of 20 units intravenously may be given while an insulin infusion is being prepared
- Give 6 units/h initially until blood glucose level has fallen to 15 mmol/L. Thereafter, adjust rate (1–4 units/h usually) during dextrose infusion to maintain blood glucose concentration at 5–10 mmol/L until patient is eating again

Other points

- Search for and treat precipitating cause (e.g. infection, myocardial infarction)
- Hypotension usually responds to adequate fluid replacement
- CVP monitoring in elderly patients or if cardiac disease present
- Pass nasogastric tube if conscious level impaired to avoid aspiration of gastric contents
- Urinary catheter if conscious level impaired or no urine passed within 4 h of start of therapy
- Continuous ECG monitoring may warn of hyperkalaemia or hypokalaemia (plasma potassium should be measured at 0, 2 and 6 h – or more often as indicated)
- Adult respiratory distress syndrome (ARDS) – mechanical ventilation (100% oxygen, IPPV); avoid fluid overload
- Mannitol (up to 1 g/kg intravenously) if cerebral oedema suspected. Dexamethasone as alternative (induces insulin resistance). Consider cranial CT to exclude other pathology (e.g. cerebral haemorrhage, venous sinus thrombosis)

Continued

TABLE 4.6 Guidelines for the management of severe diabetic ketoacidosis in adults—cont'd

- Treat specific thromboembolic complications if they occur
- Meticulously updated clinical and biochemical record using a purpose-designed flow chart

*1.26% sodium bicarbonate ($NaHCO_3$) = 12.6 g $NaHCO_3$, 150 mmol each of Na^+ and HCO_3^-/L.
CT, computed tomography; CVP, central venous pressure; DKA, diabetic ketoacidosis; ECG, electrocardiography; IPPV, intermittent positive-pressure ventilation.

TABLE 4.7 Average electrolyte deficits in adults with diabetic ketoacidosis

Electrolyte	Deficit (mmol)
Sodium	500
Chloride	350
Potassium	300–1000
Calcium	50–100
Phosphate	50–100
Magnesium	25–50

grossly raised plasma lipid concentrations. Plasma should therefore be inspected for turbidity.

The amount of fluid depends on the estimated degree of dehydration (Table 4.8). If dehydration is so severe as to cause hypovolaemic shock or a depressed level of consciousness, rapid infusion of saline is recommended to restore circulating volume.

TABLE 4.8 Assessment of hydration (over-estimation of dehydration is dangerous)

Degree of dehydration	Clinical signs
Mild, 3%	Only just clinically detectable
Moderate, 5%	Dry mucous membranes, reduced skin turgor
Severe, 8%	As above, plus sunken eyes, poor capillary return
+ Shock	May be severely ill with poor perfusion, thready rapid pulse (reduced blood pressure is not likely and is a very late sign)

TABLE 4.9 Initial fluid replacement

Fluid	Rate (mL/h)	Time (h)
0.9% sodium chloride 1 L	1000	1
0.9% sodium chloride 1 L with potassium chloride	500	2
0.9% sodium chloride 1 L with potassium chloride	500	2
0.9% sodium chloride 1 L with potassium chloride	250	4
0.9% sodium chloride 1 L with potassium chloride	250	4
0.9% sodium chloride 1 L with potassium chloride	250	4
0.9% sodium chloride 1 L with potassium chloride	125	8
Total	7 L	25

When the circulating volume has been restored, this should be followed by gradual correction of interstitial and intracellular fluid deficits. Overenthusiastic fluid replacement may lead to respiratory distress syndrome and/or cerebral oedema.

● Use sodium chloride 0.9% (see example, Table 4.9) – infusion rates will vary between patients; remember the risk of possible cardiac failure in elderly patients.
● If hypotension (systolic blood pressure < 100 mmHg) or signs of poor organ perfusion are present, consider use of colloid if increased rate of sodium chloride 0.9% does not restore circulating volume.
● Measure U&Es, venous bicarbonate and laboratory glucose at the end of hour 2 and hour 4.

Tip box

Considerable care is required in elderly patients or those with cardiac disease; monitoring of CVP or pulmonary wedge pressure is strongly recommended in these circumstances.

Insulin

The aims of insulin treatment in DKA are:

● inhibition of lipolysis (and hence ketogenesis)
● inhibition of hepatic glucose production
● enhanced disposal of glucose and ketone bodies by peripheral tissues.

Some guidelines recommend a bolus of insulin of 0.1 unit insulin per kilogram of body weight. This may be administered immediately after the potassium level is known. Insulin administration can lead to dangerously low potassium levels (see below). In order to reduce the theoretical risk of cerebral oedema, some guidelines recommend delaying the initiation of insulin until 1 h after fluids have been started.

In adults, insulin can be given at rate of around 6 units per hour to reduce the blood sugar level and suppress ketone production. Guidelines differ as to what dose to use when blood sugar levels start falling; some recommend reducing the dose of insulin (to 3 units/h) once the glucose concentration falls below 14.0 mmol/L. Below this blood glucose level it is often useful to start a glucose/K/insulin infusion.

Blood glucose concentrations tend to fall more slowly during treatment in patients with higher levels of catabolic hormones caused by infection or other serious illnesses.

- *Transfer to subcutaneous insulin.* The first subcutaneous injection should comprise or include an appropriate dose of short-acting insulin. Precise recommendations are difficult to make. The subcutaneous insulin should continue to be administered for 30–60 min before the intravenous infusion is terminated to allow time for absorption of insulin from the subcutaneous depot, thereby avoiding transient insulinopenia.
- *Intramuscular insulin.* If intravenous insulin administration is impracticable for any reason, an intramuscular regimen can be used as a safe alternative. This begins with a bolus of 20 units short-acting insulin, followed by 6 units/h into the deltoid until blood glucose level has reached 15 mmol/L. Insufficient rehydration may cause erratic absorption of intramuscular injections, resulting in apparent insulin resistance.

Potassium

Potassium levels can fluctuate severely during the treatment of DKA, because insulin decreases potassium levels in the blood by redistributing it into cells. DKA leads to considerable total body potassium deficit (300–1000 mmol/L). As a result of acidosis, insulin deficiency and renal impairment plasma potassium levels are usually normal or high at presentation. However, potassium concentration will fall during treatment. Target potassium concentration is 4.0–5.0 mmol/L.

Tip box

Plasma potassium concentration is an unreliable indicator of whole-body potassium status.

TABLE 4.10 Suggested potassium replacement	
Plasma potassium (mmol/L)	Potassium added (mmol)/L fluid)
<3.5	40*
3.5–5.5	20
>5.5	0

*Severe hypokalaemia may require more aggressive replacement. Must be given in 1 L fluid; avoid infusion rates of potassium >20 mmol/h.

There should be no potassium in the first litre unless known to be <3.5 mmol/L. Thereafter, add dosages below to each 1 L of fluid, as shown in Table 4.10.

Tip box

Check plasma potassium on admission, after 2 hours and then 4-hourly until the rate of fluid infusion is 8-hourly or slower.

Hypokalaemia increases the risk of dangerous irregularities in the heart rate.

 Severe hypokalaemia complicating treatment of DKA is potentially fatal and is usually avoidable.

Bicarbonate

The administration of sodium bicarbonate solution rapidly to improve the blood pH remains controversial. There is little evidence to indicate that it improves outcome beyond standard therapy.

Administration of bicarbonate into the extracellular space is associated with a number of potentially serious adverse effects, particularly hypokalaemia, and may actually exacerbate intracellular acidosis. Bicarbonate ions (which cannot diffuse across cell membranes) combine with H^+ ions extracellularly, producing carbonic acid which dissociates into water and carbon dioxide. The latter readily enters cells where the reverse reaction occurs, generating H^+ (and bicarbonate ions) intracellularly.

Paradoxical acidosis of cerebrospinal fluid (the clinical significance of which is disputed), adverse effects on the oxyhaemoglobin dissociation curve and overshoot alkalosis are other unwanted effects. Concern has also been expressed about the potential for accelerating ketogenesis (and lactate generation) by increasing pH with bicarbonate. The fall in blood ketone body and lactate concentrations is delayed by sodium bicarbonate infusion.

The use of bicarbonate is therefore discouraged, although some guidelines recommend it for extreme acidosis (pH < 6.9), and smaller amounts for severe acidosis (pH 6.9–7.0).

Phosphate

There is always some depletion of phosphate, a predominantly intracellular ion. Plasma levels may be very low. There is no evidence that replacement has any clinical benefit and phosphate administration may lead to hypocalcaemia.

> **Care must be taken to avoid iatrogenic hypocalcaemia if phosphate replacements are administered.**

CEREBRAL OEDEMA

Cerebral oedema, which is the most dangerous complication of DKA, is probably the result of a number of factors (Table 4.11). Some authorities maintain that it is the result of over-vigorous fluid replacement, but the complication may develop before treatment has been commenced. It is more likely to occur in those with more severe DKA, in children, and in the first episode of DKA. Likely factors in the development of cerebral oedema are dehydration, acidosis, increased level of inflammation and coagulation. Together these factors lead to decreased blood flow to parts of the brain, which may then swell once fluid replacement is commenced. The swelling of brain tissue leads to raised intracranial pressure, which is reflected in a rising blood pressure and a falling heart rate, and ultimately herniation, where the swollen brain compresses vital structures in the brain stem, leading to death.

Cerebral oedema, if associated with coma, necessitates admission to intensive care, artificial ventilation and close observation. The administration of fluids should be slowed. The ideal treatment of cerebral oedema in DKA is not established, but intravenous mannitol and hypertonic saline (3%) are often used (as in some other forms of cerebral oedema) in an attempt to reduce the swelling.

TABLE 4.11 Complications of diabetic ketoacidosis

Complication	Clinical findings
Cerebral oedema	This is unpredictable, occurs more frequently in younger children and newly diagnosed diabetics, and has a mortality rate of around 25%. Producing a slow correction of the metabolic abnormalities reduces the risk
Hypokalaemia	This is preventable with careful monitoring and management
Aspiration pneumonia	Use a nasogastric tube in semiconscious or unconscious patients
Gastric stasis	A succussion splash may be evident on abdominal examination
Adult respiratory distress syndrome	ARDS has been reported in patients with DKA, usually in patients under 50 years of age. Clinical features include dyspnoea, tachypnoea, central cyanosis and non-specific chest signs. Arterial hypoxia is characteristic and chest X-ray reveals bilateral pulmonary infiltrates. Management involves respiratory support with IPPV and avoidance of fluid overload
Thromboembolism	Thromboembolic complications can cause mortality in DKA as a consequence of: • dehydration • increased blood viscosity • increased coagulability DIC has also been reported as a rare complication. The role of routine anticoagulation has not been clearly established in DKA and in the absence of other risk factors is not generally recommended
Rhinocerebral mucormycosis	Rarely, an aggressive opportunistic fungal infection develops in patients with DKA or other metabolic acidoses. The lesion arises in the paranasal sinuses and rapidly invades adjacent tissues (nose, sinuses, orbit and brain). Treatment comprises correction of acidosis, surgical excision of affected tissue and parenteral antifungal agents. The course is often fulminant and the condition carries a high mortality rate
Rhabdomyolysis	Increased plasma myoglobin and creatine kinase concentrations may occur in DKA. However, clinically important renal complications of rhabdomyolysis are uncommon. Acute renal failure caused by rhabdomyolysis may be somewhat more common in the diabetic hyperosmolar non-ketotic syndrome but is nonetheless a rare complication

DIC, disseminated intravascular coagulation; DKA, diabetic ketoacidosis; IPPV, intermittent positive pressure ventilation.

RESOLUTION

Resolution of DKA is defined as general improvement in the symptoms, such as the ability to tolerate oral nutrition and fluids, normalization of blood acidity (pH > 7.3) and absence of ketones in blood (< 1 mmol/L). Once this has been achieved, insulin may be switched to the usual subcutaneously administered regimen, 1 h after which the intravenous administration can be discontinued.

> **Tip box**
>
> An episode of DKA should prompt a thorough review of the precipitating events; re-education may be indicated.

In patients with suspected ketosis-prone type 2 diabetes, determination of antibodies against glutamic acid decarboxylase (GAD) and islet cells may aid in the decision whether to continue insulin administration long-term (if antibodies are detected), or whether to attempt treatment with oral medication as in type 2 diabetes.

The commonest causes of failure to respond to treatment for DKA are mechanical problems. These include the pump being inadvertently switched off, set at the wrong rate, or blockage of the delivery line. It is sound practice to cross-check (and record on the flow chart) the prescribed rate of insulin delivery against the volume infused each hour during treatment.

During treatment of DKA, there is increased conversion of 3-hydroxybutyrate to acetoacetate. Nitroprusside-based urine tests may therefore raise concerns that ketosis is either not resolving or is even worsening. A rising plasma bicarbonate concentration will allay such fears.

COUNSELLING AND FOLLOW-UP

DKA is a life-threatening condition. It therefore demands a thorough exploration of the circumstances leading to the admission. There is often a need for re-education of the patient (and sometimes of health-care professionals). Re-emphasis of the 'sick day rules' may be required – in particular the importance of continuing insulin therapy. The problem of recurrent DKA in adolescents is often more problematic. The elderly patient with type 1 diabetes, particularly if intellectually impaired, or otherwise infirm or socially isolated, is also at risk of recurrent episodes.

All patients with DKA should be referred to the diabetes team on the day after admission.

The patient should not be discharged until biochemically normal, eating normally and established on subcutaneous insulin.

DIABETIC HYPEROSMOLAR NON-KETOTIC SYNDROME – HYPEROSMOLAR HYPERGLYCAEMIC SYNDROME

Diabetic HONK syndrome is a characterized by:

- marked hyperglycaemia (plasma glucose often in excess of 50 mmol/L)
- profound dehydration with pre-renal uraemia
- depression of the level of consciousness; coma is well recognized.

It occurs in type 2 diabetes, is much less common than DKA, and is associated with a much higher mortality rate. The high mortality rate in part reflects the high incidence of serious associated disorders and complications. The preferred term used by the American Diabetes Association is hyperosmolar hyperglycaemic state (HHS).

PATHOPHYSIOLOGY

HONK is usually precipitated by an infection or another acute illness. A relative insulin deficiency leads to a serum glucose level that is usually higher than 33 mmol/L and a resulting serum osmolarity that is greater than 350 mosmol/L. Due to an osmotic diuresis patients develop polyuria, which, in turn, leads to volume depletion, haemoconcentration and a further increase in blood glucose level. Unlike DKA, ketosis is absent. It is suggested that the hyperosmolar state and the presence of some plasma insulin suppresses lipolysis.

CLINICAL PRESENTATION

Patients with HONK are usually middle-aged or elderly. Black patients are more frequently represented in big series of hyperosmolar non-ketotic decompensation relative to their contribution to episodes of DKA. Up to two-thirds of cases occur in patients with previously undiagnosed type 2 diabetes.

Characteristic symptoms are:

- polyuria
- intense thirst
- gradual clouding of consciousness.

In the absence of vomiting, which is a prominent symptom of DKA, many patients drink large volumes of carbonated, glucose-containing drinks that only exacerbate thirst and hyperglycaemia. The symptoms may develop over several weeks. Coma and severe dehydration with arterial hypotension are common, and reversible focal neurological signs or motor seizures may occur. Many patients are in a moribund state when admitted to hospital.

The increasing haemoconcentration and volume depletion may result in:

- hyperviscosity and increased risk of thrombosis
- disordered mental functioning
- neurological signs, including focal signs such as sensory or motor impairments or focal seizures or motor abnormalities, such as flaccidity, depressed reflexes, tremors or fasciculations.

DIAGNOSIS

The insidious nature of the condition often leads to delays in diagnosis. The hyperosmolar non-ketotic syndrome must be considered in the differential diagnosis of any patient presenting with otherwise unexplained impairment of consciousness or focal neurological signs, dehydration or shock.

- *Urinalysis.* This will reveal heavy glycosuria and a negative or perhaps 'trace' reaction with Ketostix.
- *Blood chemistry.* The diagnosis is confirmed by a markedly raised plasma glucose concentration. Pre-renal uraemia, a raised haematocrit and a mild leukocytosis are common. Depression of consciousness generally occurs when plasma osmolality exceeds around 340 mosmol/L. Although there is considerable interindividual variation, alternative causes of an impaired level of consciousness should be considered in patients whose osmolality is less marked (Table 4.12).

TABLE 4.12 Plasma osmolality

Plasma osmolality (the osmotic pressure exerted by a fluid across a membrane) can be measured in the laboratory (e.g. by freezing point depression) and estimated using the formula:

$$\text{Plasma osmolality (mosmol/L)} = 2 \times (\text{plasma Na}^+ + \text{plasma K}^+) \\ + \text{plasma glucose} + \text{plasma urea}$$

(where Na^+, K^+, glucose and urea are in mmol/L)
The values for Na^+ and K^+ are doubled to allow for their associated Cl^- anions.

Although total body sodium is reduced, plasma sodium concentration at presentation may be low, normal or high, depending on the degree of concomitant water deficit. The degree of dehydration is generally greater than in DKA. As in DKA, hypertriglyceridaemia and hyperglycaemia may falsely depress the sodium concentration.

Tip box

Plasma sodium concentrations may be depressed by hyperglycaemia or hypertriglyceridaemia.

Although renal impairment may lead to some retention of H^+ ions, and hypotension may produce a degree of lactic acidaemia, plasma bicarbonate is usually above 15 mmol/L. Non-traumatic rhabdomyolysis may occasionally be severe enough to precipitate acute renal failure.

TREATMENT

Successful management of HONK depends on good general care of the unconscious patient and prompt recognition and treatment of underlying causes.

- *Initial therapy.* Intravenous rehydration, electrolyte replacement and insulin therapy are usually similar to that recommended for DKA. Controversy surrounds the choice of isotonic or hypotonic saline for initial rehydration. It is recommended that isotonic saline (150 mmol/L) is used in preference to hypotonic saline (75 mmol/L) unless plasma sodium exceeds 150 mmol/L. A rise in plasma sodium is frequently observed as blood glucose falls with treatment, and water moves back into the intracellular compartment. The rise in sodium may also be partially explained by the reciprocal relationship that exists between plasma glucose and sodium concentrations.
- *Thromboembolic complications.* Despite the high frequency of thromboembolic complications in patients with HONK, the role of routine anticoagulation remains uncertain. Neurological signs usually reverse when hyperglycaemia is controlled; epilepsy also responds to insulin and rehydration, but often not to specific antiepileptic drugs in the presence of hyperosmolality.
- *Subsequent antidiabetic treatment.* Insulin treatment is usually required for the first few months. However, these patients generally secrete significant quantities of endogenous insulin,

allowing successful long-term treatment with oral hypoglycaemic agents. Possible precipitating factors (e.g. thiazide diuretics, glucose drinks) should be carefully avoided in the future.

LACTIC ACIDOSIS

Lactic acidosis is a condition characterized by low pH in body tissues and the blood accompanied by the build-up of lactate, and is considered a distinct form of metabolic acidosis. The condition typically occurs when cells receive too little oxygen (hypoxia), for example during vigorous exercise. In this situation, impaired cellular respiration leads to lower pH levels. Simultaneously, cells are forced to metabolize glucose anaerobically, which leads to lactate formation. Therefore, raised lactate levels are indicative of tissue hypoxia, hypoperfusion and possible damage. Normal fasting blood lactate concentrations range from approximately 0.5 to 1.5 mmol/L. Lactic acidosis is characterized by lactate levels >5 mmol/L and serum pH <7.35.

PATHOPHYSIOLOGY

Most cells in the body normally metabolize glucose to form water and carbon dioxide. First, glucose is broken down to pyruvate through glycolysis. Then, mitochondria oxidize the pyruvate into water and carbon dioxide by means of the Krebs cycle and oxidative phosphorylation, which requires oxygen. The net result is ATP, the energy carrier used by the cell to drive useful work such as muscle contraction. When the energy in ATP is utilized during cell work, protons are produced. The mitochondria normally incorporate these protons back into ATP, thus preventing build-up of protons and maintaining neutral pH.

If the oxygen supply is inadequate, the mitochondria are unable to continue ATP synthesis at a rate sufficient to supply the cell with the required ATP. In this situation, glycolysis is increased to provide additional ATP, and the excess pyruvate produced is converted into lactate and released from the cell into the bloodstream, where it accumulates over time. Although increased glycolysis helps compensate for less ATP from oxidative phosphorylation, it cannot bind the protons resulting from ATP hydrolysis. Therefore, the proton concentration rises and causes an acidosis.

Lactate production is initially buffered intracellularly; for example, the lactate-producing enzyme lactate dehydrogenase binds one proton per pyruvate molecule converted. When such buffer systems become saturated, cells will transport lactate into the blood stream. Hypoxia causes both build-up of lactate and acidification, and lactate is therefore a good 'marker' of hypoxia, but lactate itself is not the cause of the low pH.

The signs of lactic acidosis are deep and rapid breathing, vomiting, and abdominal pain – symptoms that may easily be mistaken for other problems.

CLASSIFICATION

The *Cohen–Woods classification* categorizes causes of lactic acidosis as follows:

- Type A: decreased perfusion or oxygenation
- Type B:
  - B1 – underlying diseases (sometimes causing type A)
  - B2 – medication or intoxication
  - B3 – inborn error of metabolism.

CAUSES

There are several different causes of lactic acidosis including:

- Genetic conditions:
  - diabetes mellitus and deafness
  - glycogen storage disease
  - fructose 1,6-diphosphatase deficiency
  - pyruvate dehydrogenase deficiency
- Drugs:
  - phenformin
  - isoniazid toxicity
  - potassium cyanide (cyanide poisoning)
- Other:
  - muscular exercise
  - diabetic ketoacidosis
  - hypoxia and hypoperfusion
  - haemorrhage, sepsis and shock
  - regional hypoperfusion (bowel ischaemia, marked cellulitis)
  - ethanol toxicity
  - hepatic disease
  - non-Hodgkin's and Burkitt's lymphoma.

Hyperlactataemia in DKA

Significant hyperlactataemia is found in 10–15% of patients with DKA and usually responds to routine treatment of the ketoacidosis. Blood lactate concentration increases when treatment is instituted. Insulin suppresses gluconeogenesis, thus reducing hepatic extraction of lactate from the blood, while facilitating peripheral glucose uptake. The rise in lactate is usually transient.

Biguanides and lactic acidosis

The incidence of lactic acidosis in diabetic patients has declined dramatically since the withdrawal of the biguanide phenformin in many countries, including the UK and USA during the 1970s. Phenformin was thought to bind to the inner mitochondrial membrane and interfere with oxidative metabolism. The incidence of lactic acidosis associated with phenformin was relatively high and unfortunately metformin has lived in phenformin's shadow. Metformin is very unlikely to cause lactic acidosis, but if a patient develops lactic acidosis on metformin the prognosis is extremely poor.

TREATMENT AND PROGNOSIS

The generally poor prognosis associated with severe lactic acidosis is determined largely by the severity of the underlying condition. An exception is lactic acidosis secondary to generalized epileptic convulsions; this is self-limiting and requires no specific treatment.

Tip box

Transient lactic acidosis following convulsions does not require bicarbonate therapy.

Despite controversy surrounding the theoretical and clinical benefits of alkali therapy, intravenous bicarbonate remains the mainstay of supportive treatment for cases of severe lactic acidosis. In most cases the best advice is to obtain expert help.

- *Intravenous bicarbonate.* The role of bicarbonate is contentious. In one double-blind, placebo-controlled trial of intravenous administration of sodium bicarbonate, no improvement in cardiac haemodynamics occurred, although significant improvement in the arterial partial pressure of carbon dioxide ($Paco_2$) occurred. Animal models of lactic acidosis have shown that intravenous administration of bicarbonate may increase lactate production (particularly by the splanchnic bed), decrease portal vein flow, lower intracellular pH in muscle and liver, lower arterial pH, and worsen the cardiac output.

The use of bicarbonate in patients with severe metabolic acidosis and arterial pH <7.15 should probably be reserved to maintain the pH >7.15 until the underlying process is corrected. Massive quantities may be required to raise arterial pH; simultaneous dialysis has been recommended to avoid sodium overload.

● *Sodium dichloroacetate.* Dichloroacetate is the most potent stimulus of pyruvate dehydrogenase, the rate-limiting enzyme for the aerobic oxidation of glucose, pyruvate and lactate. Dichloroacetate may inhibit glycolysis and, thereby, lactate production. Dichloroacetate also exerts a positive inotropic effect that has been attributed to improvement in myocardial glucose use and high-energy phosphate production. Data from animal studies and one placebo-controlled double-blind clinical trial showed that dichloroacetate was superior to placebo in improving the acid–base status of the patients; however, the magnitude of change was small and did not alter haemodynamics or survival.

Dialysis

Dialysis may be a useful mode of therapy when severe lactic acidosis exists in conjunction with renal failure or congestive heart failure. Dialysis allows bicarbonate infusion without precipitating or worsening fluid overload. Therefore, dialysis corrects acidosis by restoring the buffer pool. Haemodialysis or continuous haemofiltration used in conjunction with alkali infusion may be tolerated in a patient with cardiovascular instability. However, the overall benefit of such therapy to a patient's outcome is not known.

Haemodialysis may also be beneficial in removing metformin when accumulation of this drug is associated with lactic acidosis.

CHRONIC COMPLICATIONS

OCULAR COMPLICATIONS

Clinically significant ocular complications associated with diabetes include:

- transient visual disturbances secondary to osmotic changes (or briefer episodes secondary to hypoglycaemia)
- retinopathy – the predominant cause of blindness in type 1 diabetes
- cataracts – develop earlier in diabetic patients
- glaucoma – primary or secondary to diabetic retinopathy
- iritis – associated with autoimmune type 1 diabetes.

DIABETIC RETINOPATHY

Diabetic retinal disease is the commonest cause of visual impairment in patients with type 1 diabetes. Diabetic retinopathy is more than likely to occur in patients who have poorly controlled diabetes and its prevalence increases with the duration of diabetes. Fifty per cent of patients with type 1 diabetes will have some form of retinopathy after 10 years. Approximately 5–10% of patients with type 2 diabetes will present with retinopathy (with a small number having sight-threatening retinopathy).

The following risk factors have been shown to determine the development and progression of diabetic retinal disease:

- poor glycaemic control
- raised BP (BP)
- duration of diabetes
- microalbuminuria and proteinuria
- raised triglycerides
- anaemia
- pregnancy
- smoking
- serum cholesterol (for macular exudates and oedema).

Clinically significant macular oedema and hard exudate formation but not proliferative retinopathy or retinopathy progression appears to be associated with total, high density lipoprotein (HDL) and low density lipoprotein (LDL) cholesterol levels.

Patients with multiple risk factors should be considered at particularly high risk of developing diabetic retinal disease.

Pathology

Microvascular leakage and non-perfusion are the main aetiopathogenic processes. The tight junction of the endothelial cells constitutes the inner blood retinal barrier. Pericytes wrapped round the capillaries are thought to be responsible for the structural integrity of the blood vessel. In diabetic patients there is a reduction in pericytes and endothelial cells leading to a breakdown of this barrier.

Microaneurysms are the first clinically detectable lesions and represent a dilated part of the perivenular capillaries; they occur due to a reduction in the number of endothelial cells and pericytes. They appear as tiny round dots and can occur anywhere in the retina.

Intraretinal haemorrhages can also be dot or blot in shape if they lie in the deeper compact layers of the retina, or flame-shaped if they lie in the nerve fibre layer (obeying the arrangement of the nerve fibres).

Hard exudates appear yellow and waxy with relatively distinct margins and represent intraretinal deposition of serum lipids. They usually border normal and oedematous retina, are found in the posterior pole, and can often be seen in a circinate pattern around a cluster of microaneurysms.

Retinal oedema represents leaky capillaries and is often difficult to delineate with direct ophthalmoscopy. It should always be suspected in the presence of hard exudates. Visual acuity declines if the retinal oedema involves the fovea.

Pre-proliferative diabetic retinopathy

Pre-proliferative diabetic retinopathy develops in eyes that initially may show only simple background retinopathy, and is caused by retinal ischaemia.

Pre-proliferative diabetic retinopathy is characterized by:

- vascular changes consisting of venous changes in the form of 'beading', 'looping' and 'sausage-like' segmentation. The arterioles may also be narrowed and even obliterated, resembling a branch retinal artery occlusion.
- cotton-wool spots, caused by capillary occlusion in the retinal nerve fibre layer. Interruption of axoplasmic flow caused by the ischaemia, and subsequent build-up of transported material within the nerve axons, is responsible for the white appearance of these lesions.
- dark blot haemorrhages, which represent haemorrhagic retinal infarcts.
- intraretinal microvascular anomalies (IRMAs), representing either dilated pre-existing vessels or early intraretinal new vessels. They are found within an area of capillary non-perfusion.

Pre-proliferative changes suggest increasing retinal ischaemia and precede proliferative retinopathy. They indicate worsening retinopathy and a likely need for laser photocoagulation. The presence of ischaemic maculopathy should be assessed as it could lead to irreversible loss of vision.

Classification of diabetic retinopathy

Conventionally involvement of retina in patients with diabetes has been classified as background, pre-proliferative retinopathy and proliferative retinopathy. Macula may be involved (maculopathy) with any of the above forms of retinopathy (Table 5.1).

Another commonly used grading system is the Early Treatment Diabetic Retinopathy Study (ETDRS) system (Table 5.2).

TABLE 5.1 Grading system used for screening for diabetic retinopathy (UK National Guidelines)

RETINOPATHY (R)

Level R0: No visible retinopathy

Level R1: Background diabetic retinopathy (BDR) – mild
The presence of at least one of any of the following features anywhere:
- Dot haemorrhages
- Microaneurysms
- Hard exudates
- Cotton-wool spots
- Blot haemorrhages
- Superficial/flame-shaped haemorrhages

Level R2: Background diabetic retinopathy (BDR) – observable
- Four or more blot haemorrhages in one hemi-field only (inferior and superior hemi-fields delineated by a line passing through the centre of the fovea and optic disc)

Level R3: Background diabetic retinopathy (BDR) – referable
Any of the following features:
- Four or more blot haemorrhages in both inferior and superior hemi-fields
- Venous beading
- IRMA

Level R4: Proliferative diabetic retinopathy (PDR) – referable
Any of the following features:
- Active new vessels
- Vitreous haemorrhage

Level R5: Blind or phthisical eye

Level R6: Not adequately visualized
- Retina not sufficiently visible for assessment – technical failure

---

Continued

TABLE 5.1 Grading system used for screening for diabetic retinopathy (UK National Guidelines)—cont'd

MACULOPATHY (M)

Level M0: No maculopathy

No features ≤2 disc diameters from the centre of the fovea sufficient to qualify for M1 or M2 as defined below.

Level M1: Lesions as specified below within a radius of >1 but ≤2 disc diameters from the centre of the fovea

Level M2: Lesions as specified below within a radius of ≤1 disc diameter of the centre of the fovea

- Blot haemorrhages
- Hard exudates

PHOTOCOAGULATION (P)

Laser photocoagulation scars present

OTHER LESIONS (OL)

Other non-diabetic lesions present:

- Pigmented lesion (naevus)
- Age-related macular degeneration
- Drusen maculopathy
- Myelinated nerve fibres
- Asteroid hyalosis
- Retinal vein thrombosis

IRMA, intraretinal microvascular anomaly.

Screening

Diabetic retinopathy can progress significantly without the patient being aware of any problems. The primary aim of screening is the detection of potentially sight-threatening retinopathy in asymptomatic people so that treatment, where required, can be performed before visual impairment occurs.

Retinal screening is defined as the ongoing assessment of fundi with no diabetic retinopathy or non-sight-threatening diabetic retinopathy. Once sight-threatening eye disease develops, treatment is usually required. Diabetic retinopathy screening does not remove the need for a regular general eye examination to monitor changes in refraction and to detect other eye disease.

In patients with type 1 diabetes it takes 5–6 years for retinopathy to progress. In type 1 patients aged 11 years or older, it can take 1–2 years for retinopathy to progress. A population-based study demonstrated the prevalence of retinopathy to be 14.5% for any retinopathy and 2.3% for proliferative and pre-proliferative

TABLE 5.2 The Early Treatment Diabetic Retinopathy Study (ETDRS) system

Grade	Features
NPDR	
None	Normal retina
Early	Microaneurysms only
Mild	Microaneurysms plus: • retinal haemorrhages and/or • hard exudates ($>1DD$ from fovea)
Moderate	Mild; NPDR plus: • haemorrhage and/or cotton-wool spots (<5) and/or • venous beading/looping or IRMA in one quadrant
Severe	Moderate NPDR plus 4/2/1 rule: • microaneurysm/haemorrhages in four quadrants, or • venous beading/looping in two or more quadrants, or • IRMA in one quadrant
Very severe	Any two or more of the 'severe categories'
PDR	
PDR without HRC	NVE or NVD $<$ ½DD
PDR with HRC	NVE or NVD $>$ ½DD plus preretinal and/or vitreous haemorrhages

DD, disc diameter; HRC, high-risk changes; IRMA, intraretinal microvascular anomaly; NPDR, non-proliferative diabetic retinopathy; NVD, new vessels on the disc; NVE, new vessels elsewhere in the retina; PDR, proliferative diabetic retinopathy.

retinopathy in children and adolescents with insulin-dependent diabetes mellitus diagnosed before the age of 15 years and who were older than 9 years at the time of examination. Pre-proliferative retinopathy has been identified as early as 3.5 years after diagnosis in patients postpuberty, and within 2 months of onset of puberty.

Direct ophthalmoscopy
The direct ophthalmoscope is the instrument of choice for fundus examination by medical students and physicians. It allows for a magnified, monocular image of the retina and optic disc.

Non-mydriatic camera
A non-mydriatic camera does not usually require the patient's eyes to be dilated; however, a much greater success rate can be achieved if tropicamide or similar mydriatic eye drops are used. Non-mydriatic

cameras operate by using an infrared-sensitive video camera image to position and focus the image of the retina. As no visible light is used, the patient's pupil will not constrict, and a photograph can then be taken using the built-in flash. The flash duration is so short that the exposure is made before the pupil can react.

The Scottish Diabetic Retinal Screening programme uses the Topcon TRC-NW6, which incorporates one central and eight fixed peripheral internal fixation points. Using each of these fixation points will cover 85° of the retina. The central fixation point allows a repeatable photograph of the posterior pole.

Grading and quality assurance

Retinal photographs should be graded using digital images by an appropriately trained grader to facilitate quality assurance.

Automated grading can operate as the initial screener to exclude a majority of images with 'no retinopathy' before manual grading. The specificity of automated grading is lower than for manual grading, for equivalent sensitivity. Automated grading may be used for distinguishing no retinopathy from any retinopathy in a screening programme providing validated software is used. It has a similar sensitivity for detecting referable retinopathy, but may be less sensitive at detecting diabetic maculopathy (Table 5.3).

Either one-field 45–50° retinal photography or multiple-field photography can be used for screening purposes.

General principles of management of diabetic retinopathy

Glycaemic control

Tight glycaemic control reduces the risk of onset and progression of diabetic eye disease in type 1 and 2 diabetes. The Diabetes Control and Complications Study (DCCT) demonstrated that intensive glycaemic control reduces the risk of onset of diabetic retinopathy, progression of pre-existing retinopathy, and the need for laser for patients with type 1 diabetes. The UK Prospective Diabetes Study

---

TABLE 5.3 Systematic screening for diabetic retinal disease

- Patients with type 1 diabetes should be screened from age 12 years
- Patients with type 2 diabetes should be screened from diagnosis
- Patients with diabetes with no diabetic retinopathy could be screened every 2 years – all others should be screened at least annually
- Visual acuity measurements often help in the interpretation of maculopathy

(UKPDS) demonstrated similar reduction in the risk of onset and progression in diabetic retinopathy in patients with type 2 diabetes.

Control of blood pressure

The UKPDS demonstrated that the risk of progression of diabetic retinopathy was decreased with tight control of BP (with either captopril or atenolol) and led to an almost 35% relative reduction in the need for retinal photocoagulation. Data from the UKPDS suggests that BP lowering rather than use of a specific agent may be responsible for the benefits. The EURODIAB Controlled Trial of Lisinopril in Insulin-dependent Diabetes (EUCLID) study (using lisinopril) and the Diabetic Retinopathy Candesartan Trials (DIRECT) demonstrated delay in the progression of retinopathy using drugs that act on the renin–angiotensin–aldosterone axis.

Management of dyslipidaemia

The Early Treatment Diabetic Retinal Screening (ETDRS) and DCCT revealed that raised serum cholesterol concentration was related to the development and progression of diabetic maculopathy. Recent studies suggest that aggressive lipid lowering is beneficial in prevention of progression of maculopathy.

Multifactorial risk reduction

The Steno-2 trial and other studies have shown the benefit of multiple interventions, which included behavioural therapy (dietary intervention, exercise and smoking cessation) and pharmacological intervention (reduction of BP, improvement in glycaemic control and lipid modification).

Reducing glycated haemoglobin (HbA1c) by 1.5% (16.4 mmol/mol) and, if possible, to 7% (53 mmol/mol) in type 1 and 2 diabetes plus reducing BP to 144/82 mmHg significantly reduces the incidence and progression of sight-threatening diabetic eye disease. There is no evidence to suggest that lowering BP to a level below 130/75 mmHg has a deleterious impact on retinopathy progression. Therefore, reducing BP and HbA1c below these targets is likely to reduce the risk of eye disease further. Microvascular endpoints (including retinopathy) are decreased:

- by 37% with each 1% (11 mmol/mol) reduction in HbA1c
- by 13% for each 10-mmHg reduction in systolic BP.

Rapid improvement of glycaemic control can result in short-term worsening of diabetic retinal disease, although the long-term outcomes remain beneficial. This is often seen in the rapid improvement of glycaemic control in the first trimester of pregnancy.

However, pregnancy is in itself is considered an independent risk factor for the progression of diabetic retinopathy.

Laser photocoagulation, if required, should be completed before any rapid improvements in glycaemic control are achieved.

Proliferative diabetic retinopathy

Proliferative diabetic retinopathy (PDR) affects about 5–10% of the diabetic population and is more common in type 1 diabetes.

Neovascularization is the hallmark of PDR. New vessels are commonly seen along the retinal arcades, but can occur at the optic disc or elsewhere in the retina. As a general rule, the retina distal to the neovascularization should be considered as ischaemic, and it has been estimated that more than one-quarter of the retina has to be non-perfused before neovascularization occurs. Ischaemia upregulates the vascular endothelial growth factor (VEGF) that stimulates neovascularization. New vessels start as endothelial proliferations, and pass through the internal limiting membrane to lie in the potential plane between the retina and the posterior vitreous face. PDR can result in visual deterioration from ischaemia, haemorrhage and tractional retinal detachment involving the macula (Table 5.4).

Diabetic maculopathy

Involvement of the macula with exudative or ischaemic changes has a potential to involve the fovea, thus threatening vision. Exudative maculopathy may be amenable to treatment but ischaemic changes are not.

TABLE 5.4 Guidelines for referral for specialist assessment of diabetic retinopathy

Clinical problem	Urgency (within)
Sudden loss of vision	1 day
Evidence of retinal detachment	1 day
New vessel formation (on the disc or elsewhere)	1 week
Vitreous or pre-retinal haemorrhage	1 week
Rubeosis iridis	1 week
Hard exudates within 1DD of the fovea or clinically significant macular oedema	4 weeks
Unexplained drop in visual acuity	4 weeks
Unexplained retinal findings	4 weeks
Severe or very severe non-proliferative retinopathy is present	4 weeks

Diabetic maculopathy can present in the following patterns:

- *Focal* – focal leakage, characterized usually by the presence of a cluster of microaneurysms surrounded by retinal thickening and a complete or incomplete ring of hard exudates
- *Diffuse* – diffuse retinal thickening and exudation from capillaries often involving the fovea. Cystoid changes suggest chronicity of the condition
- Ischaemic – diagnosed ideally by fluorescein angiography, representing an enlarged or irregular foveal avascular zone. Clinically it may lack features; however, the hallmarks are reduced visual acuity, deep blot haemorrhages and IRMAs.

Laser photocoagulation

The efficacy of photocoagulation has been demonstrated in the Diabetic Retinopathy Study (DRS) and ETDRS studies. It is believed that the regression of neovascularization is due to the destruction of ischaemic and hypoxic retina with the reduction in angiogenic factors.

Panretinal photocoagulation is now the main modality of treatment for proliferative diabetic retinopathy and severe non-proliferative diabetic retinopathy (NPDR). Clinically significant macular oedema (CSMO) can be treated with focal or grid photocoagulation.

Panretinal laser involves the application of 500 μm of Argon laser photocoagulation spots, each separated by an interval of a similar spot size to the mid-peripheral retina. A row of laser burns are initially placed approximately three disc diameters temporal to the fovea to avoid getting closer to the fovea. About 1500 burns are usually required (in two to three sessions). Severe cases may require further photocoagulation. The aim is to cover the ischaemic areas and regression of new vessels occurs in almost 80% of cases. Fundus fluorescein angiography (FFA) should be undertaken initially to delineate the ischaemic areas, or should be done to ensure coverage of ischaemic areas with laser if good regression of neovascularization is not achieved even with initial retinal photocoagulation.

Laser treatment can be associated with pain, transient visual loss, loss of visual field (inevitable) and, sometimes, reduced visual acuity and choroidal damage.

In very aggressive cases of PDR, an intravitreal injection of an anti-VEGF can give a valuable window period until the laser photocoagulation takes effect which can take up to 2 weeks.

Macular laser

Laser photocoagulation is considered primarily for clinically significant macular oedema. This can be applied focally to leaking microaneurysms or in a grid pattern over the macula in case of diffuse macular oedema. The spot sizes used vary from 50–100 μm and power just sufficient to cause a minimal blanch. Use of higher power can result in reduction of visual acuity. Utmost care should be taken to avoid the foveal avascular zone. Ideally macular laser should be undertaken only after angiographic assessment.

Other modalities of locally managing macular oedema are with intravitreal injections of triamcinolone acetonide or anti-VEGF. The effects of these injections, however, are usually only short-lived.

Vitrectomy

Early vitrectomy is of proven value for improving long-term vision in patients with type 1 diabetes and persistent vitreous haemorrhage. Its value in type 2 diabetes is less certain. Patients with type 1 or type 2 diabetes who have severe fibrovascular proliferation threatening the macula with or without retinal detachment also have better visual acuity after vitrectomy.

- Patients with type 1 diabetes and persistent vitreous haemorrhage should be referred for early vitrectomy.
- Vitrectomy should be performed in patients with tractional retinal detachment threatening the macula and should be considered in patients with severe fibrovascular proliferation.
- Patients with type 2 diabetes and vitreous haemorrhage that is too severe to allow photocoagulation should be referred for consideration of a vitrectomy.

Cataract extractions in patients with diabetes

Visual outcome following cataract surgery in patients with diabetes is closely linked to age and severity of retinopathy present before surgery. Although postoperative progression of pre-existing proliferative diabetic retinopathy and CSMO has been documented, the balance of evidence does not show an increase in diabetic retinopathy or in the long-term incidence of CSMO following cataract extraction.

- Cataract extraction should not be delayed in patients with diabetes.
- Cataract extraction is advised when sight-threatening retinopathy cannot be excluded.

When cataract extraction is planned in the context of advanced eye disease that is not stabilized prior to surgery, the risk of disease progression and the need for close postoperative review should be discussed fully with the patient.

Pharmacological therapy

Fenofibrate reduces the risk of progression of retinopathy and the need for laser treatment in patients with type 2 diabetes. The outcomes were not explained by a change in the serum lipid profile and the effect was independent of its lipid-lowering properties.

Intravitreal triamcinolone may provide a short-term reduction in retinal thickness and a corresponding improvement in visual acuity. In the long term it does not appear to have any benefit over laser treatment. Triamcinolone may be useful in patients who do not respond to laser. There is a risk of raising intraocular pressure: in one study, 68% of patients were affected, with 44% requiring glaucoma medication and 54% of patients requiring cataract surgery.

A randomized clinical trial of patients with type 2 diabetes and raised serum lipid levels at baseline, found that atorvastatin reduced the severity of hard exudates following laser therapy ($P = 0.007$), although the clinical significance of this is not certain. A similar study showed a non-statistically significant improvement in visual acuity and reduction in clinically significant macular oedema in patients on simvastatin.

There is insufficient evidence to warrant routine usage of anti-VEGF therapies for the treatment of proliferative diabetic retinopathy or diabetic macular oedema, either as stand-alone therapy or as an adjuvant to laser therapy.

There is no good evidence for any additional benefit of angiotensin converting enzyme (ACE) inhibitors in diabetic eye disease.

An angiotensin receptor blocker (ARB) appeared to reduce significantly the incidence of new-onset retinopathy in patients with type 1 diabetes, by 35% when measured as a change of three steps in the ETDRS scale, rather than the two steps in the original study design. Treatment with the ARB enhanced regression of retinopathy by 34% in patients with type 2 diabetes with early retinopathy.

Rehabilitation

Patients should be registered by their ophthalmologist as partially sighted (best corrected acuity 6/60) or blind (3/60 or worse). They should be assisted to register as blind/partially sighted as soon as they fulfil the criteria. Recognized disability will allow direct referral to a local low-vision network and/or visual impairment team for assessment and ongoing support. Low-vision aids and adapted everyday appliances are available. Pen injectors and other devices may be useful for patients requiring insulin treatment. With instruction, self-monitoring of capillary glucose is possible; modified glucose meters are available, including devices providing an audible result.

Other potential support includes:

- Braille instruction
- large-print and audio books
- guide dog provision.

Depression is understandably common. Peer support organized through patient organizations can often be helpful.

CATARACT

A cataract is an opacity of the crystalline lens of the eye. It is usually asymptomatic in the early stages of development, but may progress to cause significant visual impairment or even blindness. The commonest variety of cataract is the so-called senile cataract. Cataracts are features of certain syndromes or therapies that may also be associated with diabetes, for example:

- myotonic dystrophy
- chronic corticosteroid therapy.

Epidemiological studies indicate that diabetes mellitus is a significant risk factor for cataract formation in patients aged up to 70 years. The incidence of cataract is increased several-fold compared with incidence in the non-diabetic population; the opacity also progresses more rapidly in diabetic patients. Good glycaemic control reduces the risk of cataract extraction.

Tip box

Cataracts are more common in diabetic patients and appear earlier than in non-diabetic people.

Rarely, diabetes is associated with the development of an acute form of rapidly developing lens opacity known as a 'snowflake cataract'. This usually occurs in young insulin-dependent patients and typically, though not invariably, follows a period of particularly poor glycaemic control. The cataract may appear and mature within weeks.

DIABETIC NEUROPATHY

The wide variability in symmetrical diabetic polyneuropathy prevalence data is due to lack of consistent criteria for diagnosis, variable methods of selecting patients for study, and differing assessment techniques. In addition, because many patients with diabetic polyneuropathy are initially asymptomatic, detection is extremely dependent on careful neurological examination by the primary care clinician.

In the UK, the prevalence of diabetic neuropathy among the hospital clinic population is thought to be around 30%. Using additional methods of detection, such as autonomic or quantitative sensory testing, the prevalence may be higher.

Race

No racial predilection has been demonstrated for diabetic neuropathy.

Sex

Male patients with type 2 diabetes appear to develop diabetic polyneuropathy earlier than female patients.

Age

Diabetic neuropathy can occur at any age, but is more common with increasing age and duration of diabetes.

Diabetic neuropathy can manifest with a wide variety of sensory, motor and autonomic symptoms:

- Sensory symptoms may be negative or positive, diffuse or focal.
- Motor problems may include distal, proximal, or more focal weakness.
- The autonomic nervous system is composed of nerves serving the heart, skin, eyes, gastrointestinal system and genitourinary system. Autonomic neuropathy can affect any of these organ systems.

CLASSIFICATION OF NEUROPATHY

A generally accepted classification of peripheral diabetic neuropathies divides them broadly into symmetrical and asymmetrical neuropathies. Development of symptoms depends on total hyperglycaemic exposure plus other risk factors such as raised lipid levels, BP, smoking, and high exposure to other potentially neurotoxic agents such as ethanol. Establishing the diagnosis requires careful evaluation, as patients with diabetes may present with a neuropathy from another cause.

Symmetrical polyneuropathies

Symmetrical polyneuropathies involve multiple nerves diffusely and symmetrically:

- Distal symmetrical polyneuropathy:
  - Most common manifestation of diabetic neuropathy.
  - Sensory, motor and autonomic functions affected in varying degrees, with sensory abnormalities predominating.
  - Chronic symmetrical symptoms affecting peripheral nerves in a length-dependent pattern (the longest nerves affected first).
  - Commonly presents as numbness and painful paraesthesias, which begin in the toes and ascend proximally in a stocking-like distribution over months and years.
  - When sensory symptoms reach the knees, the hands often develop similar symptoms, progressing proximally in a glove-like distribution.
  - Mild weakness of foot muscles and decreased ankle and knee reflexes occur commonly.
  - Loss of sensation predisposes to development of foot ulcers and gangrene.
  - With impaired proprioception and vibratory perception, gait may be affected, causing a sensory ataxia.
- Small-fibre neuropathy:
  - Distal symmetrical neuropathy involving predominantly small-diameter sensory fibres (Aδ and C fibres).
  - Manifests as painful paraesthesias that patients perceive as burning, stabbing, crushing, aching or cramp-like, with increased severity at night (particularly exacerbated by bedclothes).
  - Loss of pain and temperature sensation with relative sparing of distal reflexes and proprioception.
- Diabetic autonomic neuropathy:
  - Pure autonomic neuropathy is rare.
  - Diabetic autonomic neuropathy is relatively common if 'looked for'.
  - Some degree of autonomic involvement is present in most patients with diabetic polyneuropathy.
  - Signs and symptoms may include sudomotor symptoms (dry skin due to lack of sweating or excessive in certain areas),

orthostatic hypotension, resting tachycardia, loss of sinus arrhythmia, bowel or bladder dysfunction, and small pupils sluggishly reactive to light.

- Diabetic neuropathic cachexia:
  - Occurs more often in older men.
  - Precipitous and profound weight loss followed by severe and unremitting cutaneous pain, small-fibre neuropathy and autonomic dysfunction.
  - Symptoms usually improve with prolonged improved glycaemic control.
  - Symptoms are often refractory to other pharmacological treatment. Limited anecdotal improvement is reported with non-pharmacological treatments such as sympathectomy, spinal cord blockade and electrical spinal cord stimulation.
  - Recovery may be incomplete and prolonged over many months.

Asymmetrical neuropathies

Asymmetrical neuropathies include single or multiple cranial or somatic mononeuropathies. Syndromes include median neuropathy of the wrist (carpal tunnel syndrome), single or multiple somatic mononeuropathies, thoracic radiculoneuropathy, lumbosacral radiculoplexus neuropathy and cervical radiculoplexus neuropathy. These syndromes usually have a monophasic course, may appear acutely or subacutely, and have a weaker association with glycaemic control than symmetrical polyneuropathies.

- Cranial mononeuropathy:
  - Cranial nerves (CN) III, IV, VI, VII and II are most often involved.
  - CN III, IV and VI disease often manifests as acute or subacute periorbital pain or headache followed by diplopia. Muscle weakness is typically in the distribution of a single nerve, and pupillary light reflexes are usually spared. Complete spontaneous recovery usually occurs within 3 months.
  - Facial neuropathy manifests as acute or subacute facial weakness (taste is not normally involved) and can be recurrent or bilateral. Most recover spontaneously in 3–6 months.
  - Anterior ischaemic optic neuropathy manifests as acute visual loss or visual field defects (usually inferior altitudinal). The optic disc appears pale and swollen; flame-shaped haemorrhages may be present.

- Somatic mononeuropathies:
  - Focal neuropathies in the extremities caused by entrapment or compression at common pressure points or by ischaemia and subsequent infarction.
  - Entrapment and compression tend to occur in the same nerves and at the same sites as in individuals without diabetes.
  - Median nerve entrapment at the wrist (carpal tunnel syndrome) is more common in patients with diabetes and can be treated in the same manner as in patients without diabetes; the symptoms are often bilateral.
  - Neuropathy secondary to nerve infarction presents acutely with focal pain associated with weakness and variable sensory loss in the distribution of the affected nerve. Multiple nerves may be affected (mononeuritis multiplex).
- Diabetic thoracic radiculoneuropathy:
  - Patients older than 50 years are affected most often; it is more common in diabetes mellitus type 2 and is often associated with significant weight loss.
  - Coexisting diabetic distal symmetrical polyneuropathy is often present.
  - Burning, stabbing, boring, belt-like or deep aching pain usually begins unilaterally, then may become bilateral. Skin hypersensitivity and allodynia (pain with normally innocuous touch) may occur. Numbness in a dermatomal distribution, most prominent in distal distribution of intercostal nerves.
  - Single or multiple spinal roots are involved. Contiguous territorial extension of symptoms may occur in a cephalad, caudal or contralateral direction.
  - In the trunk, thoracoabdominal neuropathy or radiculopathy may cause chest and/or abdominal pain in the distribution of thoracic and/or upper lumbar roots.
  - Weakness presents in the distribution of the affected nerve root, for example bulging of the abdominal wall from abdominal muscle paresis (thoracic root).
- Diabetic radiculoplexus neuropathy:
  - Occurs in patients older than 50 years with poorly controlled diabetes and is more common in men than in women.
  - Significant weight loss occurs in 50% of patients.
  - The course is generally monophasic with improvement over many months; however, some residual deficits often remain.
  - The syndrome may occur in the cervical or lumbosacral distributions and is referred to in the literature by various designations including diabetic amyotrophy, Bruns–Garland syndrome and diabetic plexopathy, among others.

- The most frequent initial symptom is sudden, severe, unilateral pain in the hip/lower back or shoulder/neck. Weakness then develops days to weeks later. Atrophy of the limb musculature may occur. Allodynia, paraesthesias and sensory loss are common.
- Symptoms usually begin unilaterally and may later spread to the opposite side.
- Reflexes in the affected limb may be depressed or absent.

PHYSICAL SIGNS

The clinical signs and symptoms are usually in keeping with where the neuropathy fits into the classification described above.

Distal symmetrical sensorimotor polyneuropathy due to diabetes must occur in the presence of diabetes as outlined by the American Diabetes Association or World Health Organization. The severity of polyneuropathy should be commensurate with the duration and severity of the diabetes, and other causes of sensorimotor polyneuropathy should be excluded. Longer nerve fibres are affected to a greater degree than shorter ones, because nerve conduction velocity is slowed in proportion to a nerve's length.

The first clinical signs that usually develop is decrease or loss of vibratory and pinprick sensation over the toes. As disease progresses, the level of decreased sensation may move upward into the legs and then into the hands and arms, a pattern often referred to as 'stocking and glove' sensory loss. A glove–stocking distribution of numbness, sensory loss, dysaesthesia and night-time pain may develop. The pain can feel like burning, pricking sensation, achy or dull. Pins and needles sensation is common. Loss of proprioception, the sense of where a limb is in space, is affected early. These patients cannot feel when they are stepping on a foreign body, such as a splinter, or when they are developing a callous from an ill-fitting shoe. Consequently, they are at risk for developing ulcers and infections on the feet and legs.

Very severely affected patients may lose sensation in a shield distribution on the chest. Deep tendon reflexes are commonly hypoactive or absent, and weakness of small foot muscles may develop. More focal findings may be seen with injury to specific nerves as described above. Loss of motor function results in dorsiflexion, contractures of the toes and loss of the interosseous muscle function, and leads to contraction of the digits, so-called 'hammer toes'. These contractures occur not only in the foot but also in the hand, where the loss of the musculature makes the hand appear gaunt and skeletal.

TREATMENT

Despite advances in the understanding of the metabolic causes of neuropathy, treatments aimed at interrupting these pathological processes have been limited. Thus, with the exception of tight glucose control, treatments are for reducing pain and other symptoms.

Options for pain control include tricyclic antidepressants (TCAs), serotonin reuptake inhibitors (SSRIs) and antiepileptic drugs (AEDs). It is suggested that TCAs and traditional anticonvulsants are better for short-term pain relief than newer-generation anticonvulsants. A combination of medication may be superior to a single agent.

The only two drugs approved by the US Food and Drug Administration (FDA) for diabetic peripheral neuropathy are the antidepressant duloxetine and the anticonvulsant pregabalin (Fig. 5.1). Before trying a systemic medication, people with localized diabetic periperal neuropathy occasionally get relief from their symptoms with lidocaine patches.

In addition to pharmacological treatment there are several other modalities that help some patients. These have been shown to reduce

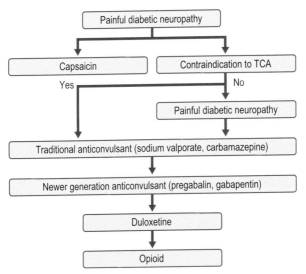

Figure 5.1 Treatment algorithm for management of painful diabetic peripheral neuropathy. TCA, tricyclic antidepressant. (Source: Wong et al (2007). Reproduced with permission.)

pain and improve quality of life, particularly for patients with chronic neuropathic pain: interferential stimulation, acupuncture, meditation, cognitive therapy, and prescribed exercise.

Tricyclic antidepressants

TCAs include imipramine, amitriptyline, desipramine and nortriptyline. These drugs are effective at decreasing painful symptoms but suffer from multiple side-effects that are dose-dependent. One notable side-effect is cardiac toxicity, which can lead to fatal arrhythmias. At low dosages used for neuropathy, toxicity is rare, but if symptoms warrant higher doses complications are more common. Among the TCAs, amitriptyline is most widely used for this condition, but desipramine and nortriptyline have fewer side-effects.

Serotonin reuptake inhibitors

SSRIs include fluoxetine, paroxetine, sertraline and citalopram. These agents have not been approved by the FDA to treat painful neuropathy because they have been found to be no more efficacious than placebo in several controlled trials. Side-effects are rarely serious, and do not cause any permanent disabilities. These drugs cause sedation and weight gain, which can worsen a diabetic's glycaemic control. They can be used at dosages that also relieve the symptoms of depression, a common concommitent of diabetic neuropathy.

The selective serotonin–noradrenaline reuptake inhibitor (SSNRI) duloxetine is approved for diabetic neuropathy. Typical dosages are 60 or 120 mg.

Antiepileptic drugs

AEDs, especially gabapentin and the related pregabalin, have emerged as first-line treatment for painful neuropathy. Gabapentin compares favourably with amitriptyline in terms of efficacy, and is clearly safer. Its main side-effect is sedation, which does not diminish over time and may in fact worsen. It needs to be taken three times a day, and sometimes causes weight gain, which can worsen glycaemic control. Carbamazepine is effective but is associated with side-effects at higher doses. Topiramate has not been studied in diabetic neuropathy, but has the beneficial side-effect of causing mild anorexia and weight loss, and is anecdotally beneficial (Table 5.5).

TABLE 5.5 Treatment options for painful diabetic neuropathy and their clinical efficacy

Approach	Compound/measure	Daily dose	Remarks	NNT
Optimal diabetes control	Lifestyle medication, OAD, insulin	Individual adaptation	Aim: HbA1c < 6.5% (48 mmol/L)	–
Pathogenetically oriented treatment	α-Lipoic acid (thioctic acid)*	600-mg IV infusion	Duration: 3 weeks	6.3‡
		1200–1800 mg orally	Favourable safety profile	2.8–4.2‡
Symptomatic treatment	First-line TCA			
	Amitriptyline	(10–)25–150 mg	NNMH: 15	2.1
	Desipramine	(10–)25–150 mg	NNMH: 24	2.2/3.2
	Imipramine	(10–)25–150 mg	CRR	1.3/2.4/3.0
	Clomipramine	(10–)25–150 mg	NNMH: 8.7	2.1
	Nortriptyline	(10–)25–150 mg	Plus fluphenazine	1.2§
	SNRI			
	Duloxetine†	60–120 mg	NNT with 120 mg, 60 mg	5.3, 4.9
	Anticonvulsants – calcium channel modulators (α₂δ ligands)			
	Gabapentin	900–3600 mg	High dose	3.8/4.0
	Pregabalin†	300–600 mg	NNT with 600 mg, 300 mg	5.9, 4.2
	Second-line weak opioids			
	Tramadol	50–400 mg	NNMH: 7.8	3.1/4.3
	Local treatment			
	Capsaicin (0.025%) cream	q.i.d. topically	Max. duration: 6–8 weeks	5.7

Continued

TABLE 5.5 Treatment options for painful diabetic neuropathy and their clinical efficacy—cont'd

Approach	Compound/measure	Daily dose	Remarks	NNT
Pain resistant to standard pharmacotherapy	Strong opioids Oxycodone ESCS		Add-on treatment Invasive, specialist required	2.6

CRR, concentration–response relationships; ESCS, electrical spinal cord stimulation; HbA1c, glycated haemoglobin; IV, intravenous; NNMH, number needed for major harm; NNT, number needed for treatments not significant; OAD, oral antidiabetic drugs; q.i.d., four times daily; TCA, tricyclic antidepressants; SNRI, selective serotonin–norepinephrine reuptake inhibitors.
* Available only in some countries
† licensed in USA and EU
‡ combined with fluphenazine
§ >50% symptom relief after 3 and 5 weeks.
Source: Holt et al (2010). © Wiley–Blackwell.

Other treatments

Transcutaneous electric nerve stimulation (TENS) may be effective in treating painful diabetic neuropathy.

Acupuncture may be of some benefit.

In more recent years, photo energy therapy devices have become more widely used to treat neuropathic symptoms. Photo energy therapy devices emit near infrared light (NIR therapy), typically at a wavelength of 880 nm. This wavelength is believed to stimulate the release of nitric oxide, an endothelium-derived relaxing factor, into the bloodstream, thus vasodilating the capillaries and venuoles in the microcirculatory system. This increase in circulation has been shown in various clinical studies to decrease pain in diabetic and non-diabetic patients. Photo energy therapy devices appear to address the underlying problem of neuropathy, poor microcirculation, which leads to pain and numbness in the extremities.

Sativex, a cannabis-based medication, has not been found to be effective for diabetic neuropathy.

Treatment based on pathogenetic mechanisms

α-Lipoic acid, an antioxidant that is a non-prescription dietary supplement, has shown benefit in a randomized controlled trial that compared once-daily oral doses of 600–1800 mg with placebo, although nausea occurred at the higher doses. The SYDNEY 2 trial suggested a possible benefit for α-lipioc acid in reducing pain, paraesthesia and numbness.

Benfotiamine is licensed for clinical treatment of diabetic peripheral neuropathy in several countries. However, the evidence is weak.

Of several aldose reductase inhibitors (ARIs), such as alrestatin, sorbinil and tolrestat only epalrestat is marketed (in India and Japan), with questionable benefits in diabetic peripheral neuropathy.

Tight glucose control

Treatment of early manifestations of sensorimotor polyneuropathy involves improving glycaemic control. Tight control of blood glucose can reverse the changes of diabetic neuropathy, but only if the neuropathy and diabetes are relatively recent in onset. Conversely, painful symptoms of neuropathy in poorly controlled diabetic patients tend to subside as the disease and numbness progress.

PROGNOSIS

The mechanisms of diabetic neuropathy remain poorly understood. However, the process is generally progressive.

At present, treatment alleviates pain and can control some associated symptoms. As a complication, there is an increased risk of injury to the feet because of loss of sensation. Minor infections can progress to ulceration, and this may lead to amputation.

DIABETIC AUTONOMIC NEUROPATHY

Autonomic dysfunction accounts for the most troublesome symptoms due to diabetic neuropathy. It can present with symptoms that affect cardiovascular, urogenital, gastrointestinal, pupillomotor regulatory and sudomotor functions. Simple non-invasive and sometimes bedside tests can help to diagnose autonomic dysfunction. In select cases highly specialized testing is required.

Cardiovascular system

It has been reported that there is an increased mortality rate in patients who have cardiac autonomic dysfunction due to diabetes. It is estimated that 5–10-year survival rates in such patients range from 25% to 60%. There is an increased risk of sudden cardiac death, possibly due to an increased risk of arrhythmias.

Loss of sinus arrhythmia with reduced 'R to R' variation is an early electrocardiographic feature. Increased resting heart rate may also occur and is thought to reflect unopposed sympathetic activity. Orthostatic hypotension is a common and disabling symptom of autonomic failure. The presenting symptoms depend on the degree of predominant denervation (either sympathetic or parasympathetic).

Gastrointestinal system

Disturbances can occur throughout the gastrointestinal system. Delay in gastric emptying time can occur in up to 50% of patients with type 1 diabetes. This results in gastroparesis diabeticorum and may present with nausea, postprandial vomiting, abdominal distension and discomfort, early satiety, and wide swings in glycaemic control due to mismatching of plasma glucose and insulin levels. On examination of the abdomen there may be a 'succussion splash'.

Diarrhoea and other lower gastrointestinal symptoms may occur. Diarrhoea may be due to altered motility, reduced fluid reabsorption, bacterial overgrowth, pancreatic exocrine deficiencies, coexistent coeliac disease and alterations in bile metabolism. Faecal incontinence is not uncommon and may be due to altered anal sphincter tone or anal sensation.

Urogenital system

Bladder dysfunction occurs in a significant proportion of patients with long-standing diabetes. This includes hesitancy, poor stream, inadequate emptying, retention and overflow incontinence, and is often associated with recurrent urinary tract infections.

Sexual dysfunction, including erectile dysfunction in men, is very common. The cause is multifactorial and includes alterations in endothelium-dependent relaxation of the corpus cavernosum. In addition, autonomic neuropathy may lead to retrograde ejaculation.

Sexual dysfunction occurs in women, is under-reported and poorly understood.

Sudomotor system

This generally manifests as anhidrosis or hyperhidrosis. Initially this may occur in a glove-and-stocking distribution, but may ultimately become global.

Gustatory sweating is the abnormal production of sweat that appears over the face, head, neck, shoulders and chest during or after eating. Symptoms are often worse when spicy food is consumed.

Treatment of autonomic dysfunction

Treatment of orthostatic hypotension

Diuretics, antihypertensives, antianginal drugs and antidepressants worsen symptoms and should be reduced or stopped if possible. Several agents have been tried with variable results. Fludrocortisone is the agent of choice and should be taken before bed. However, the presence of supine hypertension, hypokalaemia, fluid overload and ankle oedema needs to be monitored. Midodrine, a peripherally acting selective α-agonist, is also useful.

Treatment of gastroparesis diabeticorum

Small frequent meals and drug therapy may be useful. The dopamine agonist metoclopramide is usually used as a first-line agent. Domperidone is a useful alternative. Erythromycin, a motilin agonist, has also been tried. Strict glycaemic control has often helped to reverse gastroparesis. However, to achieve this insulin pump therapy is often the best option, wherein a delayed bolus is given with each meal. Recently implantations of gastric pacemakers have been tried, with variable success.

Treatment of erectile dysfunction

Several of the antihypertensive drugs worsen erectile dysfunction; such agents should be discontinued if possible. Phosphodiesterase-5 inhibitors, including sildenafil, tadalafil and vardenafil, are the most commonly used agents. However, some patients with diabetes do not respond to this intervention. It is to be noted that these drugs should not be used in individuals taking nitrates or in those with angina and congestive heart failure.

Other therapies include injecting papaverine, phentolamine and prostaglandin E1 into the corpus cavernosus. Penile prosthetic implants and vacuum devices are used very occasionally in patients who fail to respond to conventional therapies.

Treatment of hyperhidrosis

Sodium glycopyrrylate cream can be applied to the areas that are particularly severely affected. Anticholinergic agents such as trihexyphenidyl, propantheline and scopolamine have also been tried.

DIABETIC FOOT DISEASE

Diabetic patients have a 12–25% lifetime risk of developing a foot ulcer. The increasing prevalence of diabetes makes diabetic foot ulcers a major public health burden. Foot ulcers cause substantial morbidity, impair quality of life, engender high treatment costs and are the most important risk factor for lower-extremity amputations.

Diabetic foot infection is defined as an infection below the level of the malleoli in a diabetic patient. The spectrum of foot pathology include paronychia, foot ulcer with or without surrounding cellulitis, myositis, foot abscesses, necrotizing fasciitis, septic arthritis of the joints of the foot, tendon infections and osteomyelitis.

A number of factors contribute directly or indirectly towards the development of diabetic foot infections. Neuropathic ulcers, the most common type of diabetic foot ulcer, result from tissue-damaging mechanical loads applied to an insensate foot. Reduced sensation can substantially impair the patient's perception of touch, deep pressure, temperature and joint position. The foot injury that initiates ulcers often results from minor trauma, mechanical stress, repetitive or continuously applied unperceived pressure. Restricted joint mobility, poor foot care and foot deformity resulting in bony prominences, also contribute to the risk of ulceration. Thermal injury may also be a precipitating cause.

Motor neuropathy with the associated small muscle wasting can lead to clawing of toes and subluxation of the small joints that in turn cause pressure ulcers. Peripheral vascular disease in the form of macrovascular or microvascular disease is a component cause of one-third of foot ulcers, and is an important risk factor for recurrent ulcers. Patients with significant autonomic neuropathy may have bounding foot pulses yet severe microvascular disease in the distal limb (Table 5.6).

Moreover, initial colonization of these ulcers may subsequently lead to active infection because of impaired delivery of immune cells to the tissues. In addition, behavioural factors due to the chronic nature of the disease may lead to decreased compliance with therapy.

Microbial colonization of open ulcers is common and is a prerequisite for development of infection. Development of active infection depends upon several factors. These include:

- *Nature of the colonizing flora:* certain Gram-positive cocci such as *Staphylococcus aureus* and *Streptococcus pyogenes* secrete a number of toxins and adhesion factors that allow them to colonize, invade and damage the tissues. Other β-haemolytic streptococci, such as those belonging to Lancefield group C, F and G, can also cause pyogenic infections. On the other hand, coagulase-negative staphylococci are often harmless commensals. Gram-negative organisms such as *Pseudomonas aeruginosa* and *Proteus* spp can lead to active infection and impair wound healing.
- *Extent of tissue colonization:* microbes that commonly lead to superficial colonization can nonetheless cause infections at deeper sites. Thus, coagulase-negative staphylococci that commonly colonize skin and its appendages can cause serious bone and joint infections provided they get an entry into these deeper areas of the body.

TABLE 5.6 Signs of autonomic and motor neuropathy

Autonomic neuropathy	Motor neuropathy
Abnormal response to temperature	Intrinsic muscle weakness
Disorders of sweating	Claw toes
Brittle, dry skin	Retracted toes
Atrophy of fatty fibro-padding	Pes cavus
Oedema – arteriovenous shunting	Corn/callous

- *Host defence mechanisms:* if host defense mechanisms are compromised, a relatively non-virulent organism can occasionally cause quite severe infection.

Despite an overlapping range of pathology, certain types of infection are typically known to be caused by specific microbes. Thus, cellulitis is typically associated with isolation of *S. aureus* and *S. pyogenes*, whereas complicated ulcers often yield *P. aeruginosa*. Anaerobic organisms are often isolated from gangrenous lesions and from 'foetid foot'.

Foot infections are the most common cause of admission to hospital, and infection is the most important precipitating factor for lower limb amputation in diabetic patients.

EVALUATION/SCREENING OF PATIENTS OF THE DIABETIC FOOT

Patients with diabetic foot problems need to be assessed thoroughly in order to plan an appropriate management strategy. The medical history should include questions on previous ulcer/amputation, peripheral neuropathic symptoms, visual acuity, renal replacement therapy and smoking. General inspection should take place in a well-lit room and should include dermatological and musculoskeletal assessment. The patient's footwear should also be assessed, particularly for size and excessive wear. Sometimes just getting the patients to take their socks off can impress on them the importance of their feet in the context of diabetes.

Previous ulceration is particularly important, as recurrence is very common. Elderly, socially isolated patients who perhaps cannot inspect or even physically reach their feet are also at high risk. Oedema, from congestive cardiac failure, nephropathy, immobility or calcium antagonists, renders feet vulnerable.

The nature of the local pathology (both wound and the associated limb), assessment of the severity of infection, and presence of systemic illness each affect the ultimate outcome in an individual case. Earlier classification systems such as the Wagner dysvascular foot classification included all infections within a single category. More recently, the consensus classification developed by the International Working Group on the Diabetic Foot (Table 5.7) uses grades of severity as a tool in classifying the foot infections. Successful management of diabetic foot infections involves recognition that infection is by no means one entity. Rather, this patient-centred approach lays great emphasis on making distinctions based on response to infection, and not infection itself. For example,

TABLE 5.7 Clinical classification of diabetic foot infection

Clinical manifestation	Infection severity	PEDIS grade*
Wound lacking purulence or any manifestation of inflammation	Uninfected	1
Two or more manifestations of inflammation, but cellulitis or erythema extends ≤ 2 cm around the ulcer with infection limited to the skin or superficial subcutaneous tissues. No other local complications and no systemic illness	Mild	2
Infection as above in a patient who is systemically well and metabolically stable but with one or more of the following: cellulitis extending > 2 cm, lymphangitic streaking, spread beneath the superficial fascia, deep tissue abscess, gangrene, and involvement of muscle, tendons joint or bone	Moderate	3
Infection in a patient with systemic toxicity and metabolic instability (e.g. fever, chills, tachycardia, hypotension, confusion, vomiting, leukocytosis, acidosis, severe hyperglycaemia, azotaemia)	Severe	4

*PEDIS is an acronym for perfusion, extent, depth, infection, sensation.

systemic illness categorizes patients in grade 4 severity although the local wound may be only moderately inflamed. This classification also removes ambiguity with regards to terms such as 'complicated' wound.

Although very difficult to include in any classification, malodour can reflect poor hygiene and/or severe infection including anaerobic infection.

PREVENTIVE MANAGEMENT

Foot screening

Diabetic foot screening is very important in identifying the level of risk of developing foot ulceration. Risk stratification can identify those at increased risk of developing foot ulceration. Patients screened as being low risk have a greater than 99% chance of remaining free from ulceration and are more than 80 times less likely to ulcerate than the high-risk group. Patients who have intact protective sensation, adequate circulation, and no history of foot ulcers or amputation are at low risk. Patients with amputation or previous foot ulcer, decreased/loss of protective sensation and/or absent pedal pulses are at high risk. On examination, patients with high risk may have signs of ischaemia, including absent pulses, loss of protective sensation plus foot deformity or callus. Simple tests such as the use of the 10-g monofilament, palpation of pulses, presence of significant callus, presence of significant structural abnormality and previous ulceration are effective at predicting ulceration. A neurothesiometer can be used as part of a more formal assessment to detect peripheral neuropathy, as can Doppler ultrasonography to detect foot pulses. The ankle : brachial pressure index (ABPI) can be used to assess for peripheral arterial disease (PAD); however, the ABPI should be interpreted with caution in patients with diabetes as it is often falsely increased. Measurement of toe pressures is often of more value.

 All patients with diabetes should be screened to assess their risk of developing a foot ulcer.

Patient education

Patients should be given education about basic foot care including advice about footwear. This should include:

- buying well-fitting new shoes with low heels (no more than 1¼ inches)
- where possible the uppers should be made of natural materials (e.g. leather)
- trying on both shoes before purchase
- checking their shoes for sharp objects and for wear and tear, buying a well-fitting shoe, boot or trainer with laces or a strap fastening.

Patients should also be advised to:

- check their feet daily
- wash their feet daily
- moisturize their feet when necessary
- avoid walking barefoot
- change their socks, stockings or tights every day
- not undertake do it yourself (DIY) toenail cutting – amateur chiropody by the patient directed against lesions such as corns or deformed toenails should be discouraged (unless advised by the podiatrist)
- avoid extremes of temperature.

Podiatry education programmes should be structured. Easy access to a podiatrist improves self-care and reduces the number and size of foot calluses.

Patients should also be given ongoing advice on good glycaemic control, hyperlipidaemia, hypertension and smoking.

Tip box

Foot care education is recommended as part of a multidisciplinary approach in all patients with diabetes.

Preventive footwear and orthoses

Plantar pressure using ordinary shoes is similar to walking barefoot. Running-style, cushion-soled trainers can reduce plantar pressure more than ordinary shoes, but not as much as custom-built shoes.

The use of custom-made foot orthoses and prescription footwear reduces the plantar callus thickness and incidence of ulcer relapse. Patients who wear their prescription shoes and orthoses routinely are less likely to have ulcer relapse.

Tip box

Custom-built footwear or orthotic insoles should be used to reduce callus severity and ulcer recurrence.

MANAGEMENT OF ACTIVE FOOT DISEASE

Multidisciplinary foot clinic

Patients with active diabetic foot disease should be referred to a multidisciplinary diabetic foot care service.

A multidisciplinary foot team should include:

- podiatrist
- diabetes physician
- orthotist
- diabetes nurse specialist
- vascular surgeon
- orthopaedic surgeon
- radiologist.

Multidisciplinary foot care teams lead to quicker control of infection, intensive treatment and rapid access to vascular surgery that in turn will allow revascularization when needed. Wound healing and foot-saving amputations can then be achieved successfully, reducing the rate of major amputations. Adherence to locally established protocols may reduce length of hospital stay and major complication rates.

A multidisciplinary foot service should also address cardiovascular risk management. Aggressive cardiovascular intervention in the multidisciplinary diabetic foot care clinic reduces mortality rate at 5 years by 38% in patients with neuroischaemic ulcers and by 47% in patients with neuropathic ulcers.

Debridement

Local sharp debridement, surgical debridement, larvae therapy and hydrojet therapy used in different but appropriate settings are all useful in the management of patients with diabetic foot disease. Local sharp debridement should be considered first followed by others, depending on the clinical presentation or response of a wound.

Pressure relief

Total contact casting, prefabricated walkers and 'half-shoes' have all been shown in differing clinical situations to reduce the healing time of diabetic foot ulcers.

The walkers should be specifically designed for use with the diabetic foot and should always incorporate a total contact insole.

Antibiotic therapy

Only a small subgroup of patients with infected diabetic foot ulcers need to be treated with intravenous antibiotics; again, this is a decision made on clinical grounds. Some of the patients requiring intravenous antibiotic may not have responded to oral therapy, whereas for some others intravenous antibiotic therapy is required from presentation of the ulcer and again is usually followed by oral therapy.

No single broad-spectrum regimen, optimal duration or route of antibiotic therapy has been shown to be more effective than another in the treatment of patients with diabetic foot ulcers.

Treatment of a patient with an infected diabetic foot ulcer and/or osteomyelitis should be commenced immediately with an antibiotic in accordance with local/national protocols. Subsequent antibiotic regimens may be modified with reference to bacteriology and clinical response.

Negative-pressure wound therapy

Negative-pressure wound therapy (NPWT) has been used as an adjunct to standard wound care. Compared with advanced moist therapy, NPWT appears to increase the proportion of patients who achieve complete ulcer closure and lowers the rate of secondary amputation.

NPWT should be considered in patients with active diabetic foot ulcers or postoperative wounds. This therapy is less useful for plantar ulcers.

Arterial reconstruction/surgery

Patients with diabetes are more prone to peripheral artery disease (PAD) than patients without diabetes. This includes both proximal (aortoiliac and femoral) and distal (calf and foot) disease. Rates of limb salvage following bypass surgery and angioplasty are high. Salvage rates of around 80% are reported in the presence of tissue loss (gangrene and ulceration).

All patients with critical limb ischaemia, including rest pain, ulceration and tissue loss, should be considered for arterial reconstruction.

Removal of digits may suffice; however, an inadequate peripheral blood supply may result in a slow-healing or non-healing amputation site. A ray amputation of the second, third or fourth toes, taking the associated metatarsal head, may result in a very satisfactory outcome, although healing will often take many weeks. If possible forefoot and mid-foot amputations are generally avoided. Below- rather than through- or above-knee amputation is the best option if major amputation is required.

CHARCOT NEUROARTHROPATHY OF THE FOOT

Charcot neuroarthropathy of the foot is a neuroarthropathic process with osteoporosis, fracture, acute inflammation and disorganization of foot architecture.

During the acute phase, Charcot neuroarthropathy of the foot can be difficult to distinguish from infection. The clinical diagnosis of acute Charcot neuroarthropathy is based on the appearance of a red, swollen, oedematous and possibly painful foot in the absence of infection. The foot skin temperature is often 2–8 °C higher than that of the contralateral foot.

Acute Charcot neuroarthropathy is associated with increased bone blood flow, osteopenia, and fracture or dislocation. The disease process can progress with increased bone formation, osteosclerosis, spontaneous arthrodesis and ankylosis.

Diagnosis of Charcot neuroarthropathy of the foot should be made by clinical examination. Magnetic resonance imaging (MRI) cannot reliably distinguish early changes of Charcot neuroarthropathy from osteomyelitis. However, it may provide information that cannot be identified by X-ray (especially the presence of marrow oedema).

Suspected Charcot neuroarthropathy of the foot is an emergency and the patient should be referred immediately to the multidisciplinary foot team. Treatment of patients with contact casting is associated with a reduction in skin temperature, in bone activity and fewer diabetic foot deformities. Intravenous bisphosphonate therapy may reduce skin temperature and bone turnover in active Charcot neuroarthropathy.

PREVENTION OF RECURRENCE

Education of the patient and the relevant carers, provision of special footwear, home help and careful follow-up in the foot clinic helps to prevent recurrence. For patients with severe deformities, assessment by an orthotist is essential. Ready-to-wear boots may be helpful in the short term but are unaesthetic. Shoes made to order may be required to accommodate insoles. Devices are available that identify high-pressure sites, thereby aiding insole design.

REHABILITATION

Major amputation is usually a devastating event. The prospects for successful rehabilitation are often remote. Using a below-knee prosthesis, walking energy expenditure is increased by 50%, an impossible target in elderly or debilitated patients. The risk of ulceration in the contralateral foot may be increased owing to altered weight-bearing, and confinement to a wheelchair may be the unfortunate consequence.

DIABETIC NEPHROPATHY

DEFINITIONS

Diabetic kidney disease is usually classified on the basis of the extent of urine protein excretion – microalbuminuria or nephropathy.

Microalbuminuria is defined by a rise in urinary albumin loss to between 30 and 300/mg day. Timed urine collections may be inaccurate and therefore a urinary albumin/creatinine ratio (ACR) > 2.5 mg/mmol in men and > 3.5 mg/mmol in women is often used to define microalbuminuria. This is the earliest sign of diabetic kidney disease and predicts end-stage renal failure, cardiovascular morbidity and mortality, and increased total mortality.

Diabetic nephropathy is defined by a raised urinary albumin excretion of > 300 mg/day (indicating clinical proteinuria) in a patient with or without a raised serum creatinine level. Providing other causes have been excluded, an ACR > 30 mg/mmol in a spot urine sample is consistent with a diagnosis of diabetic nephropathy. This represents a more severe and established form of renal disease and is more predictive of total mortality, cardiovascular mortality and morbidity, and end-stage renal failure than microalbuminuria.

The presence of retinopathy has often been taken as a prerequisite for making a diagnosis of diabetic nephropathy, but diabetic nephropathy can occur in the absence of retinopathy. Very occasionally, patients can have persistent albuminuria and no retinopathy with glomerulonephritis or normal glomerular structure.

Glomerular filtration rate (GFR) is defined as the volume of plasma that is filtered by the glomeruli per unit of time, and is usually measured by estimating the rate of clearance of a substance from the plasma. GFR varies with body size and conventionally is corrected to a body surface area (BSA) of 1.73 m^2, the average BSA of a population of young men and women studied in the mid-1920s.

In most individuals the diagnosis of diabetic kidney disease is made clinically, as biopsy may not alter management. Classical diabetic kidney disease is characterized by specific glomerular pathology. It is important to note that there are other reasons why an individual with diabetes may develop proteinuria and/or a declining GFR, notably hypertensive nephropathy and renovascular disease. In many individuals, kidney disease will be due to a combination of one or more of these factors.

With the advent of reporting of estimated GFR (eGFR), increasing numbers of people are being identified with a sustained low GFR. Chronic kidney disease (CKD) in the absence of proteinuria would not previously be classified as having diabetic kidney disease (Table 5.8).

PREVALENCE AND PROGRESSION OF KIDNEY DISEASE IN DIABETES

Estimates of prevalence from individual studies must be interpreted in the context of their patient population, such as levels of deprivation and the proportion of individuals from ethnic minorities.

TABLE 5.8 Stratification of chronic kidney disease

Stage	Description	GFR (ml per min per 1.73 m²)
1	Kidney damage* with normal or raised GFR	≥90
2	Kidney damage* with mild decrease in GFR	60–89
3A	Moderately lowered GFR	45–59
3B		30–44
4	Severely lowered GFR	15–29
5	Kidney failure (endstage renal disease)	<15

*Kidney damage defined as abnormalities on pathologic, urine, blood, or imaging tests.
If proteinuria (24-h urine > 1 g per day or urine protein/creatinine ratio (PCR) > 100 mg/mmol) is present, the suffix P may be added. Patients on dialysis are classified as stage 5D. The suffix T indicates patients with a functioning renal transplant (can be stages 1–5).
GFR, glomerular filtration rate.

The racial differences in CKD are not accounted for simply by the increased risk and prevalence of diabetes in minority ethnic populations. The higher incidence of stage 4 and 5 CKD in minority ethnic populations may, in part, reflect reduced access to health care and genetic differences between populations.

The number of patients with diabetes requiring renal replacement therapy (RRT) is increasing.

MICROALBUMINURIA AND PROTEINURIA

In people with type 1 diabetes, the cumulative incidence of microalbuminuria at 30 years' disease duration is approximately 40%. For microalbuminuric patients, the relative risk of developing proteinuria is 9.3 compared with that in normoalbuminuric patients. Some 25% of individuals who were in the conventional arm of the Diabetes Control and Complications Trial (DCCT) had proteinuria, raised serum creatinine levels (> 177 µmol/L) and/or were on RRT after 30 years of diabetes. Data from type 2 patients is available from the UKPDS and is presented in Table 5.9.

Remission of microalbuminuria may occur, and so the presence of microalbuminuria does not necessarily imply an inexorable progression to nephropathy. There are data to suggest that there has been a decrease in the incidence of diabetic nephropathy in people with type 1 diabetes diagnosed more recently, with earlier aggressive BP and glycaemic control.

TABLE 5.9 Proteinuria and microalbuminuria in people with newly diagnosed type 2 diabetes measured over a 15-year follow-up

Follow-up (years)	No. of patients	Microalbuminuria (%)	Proteinuria (%)
Baseline	994	12.8	2.1
3	1048	14.5	2.5
6	938	18.3	3.5
9	721	25.4	6.5
12	348	34.2	10.3
15	95	39.0	12.6

Source: UK Prospective Diabetes Study.

In the general population, particularly in people with diabetes, an eGFR <60 mL per min per 1.73 m^2 is associated with an increased risk of the major adverse outcomes of CKD (impaired kidney function, progression to kidney failure and premature death from cardiovascular disease).

Microalbuminuria is associated with an approximately 2-fold increase in cardiovascular morbidity and mortality. The 4-year mortality rate for patients with type 2 microalbuminuria is 32%, and 50% for those with type 2 proteinuria. When proteinuria and hypertension are present, the standardized mortality ratio is increased 5-fold in men and 8-fold in women with type 2 diabetes, and 11-fold in men and 18-fold in women with type 1 diabetes.

SCREENING FOR KIDNEY DISEASE IN DIABETES

Prediction equations

Prediction equations improve the inverse correlation between serum creatinine and GFR by taking into account confounding variables such as age, sex, ethnic origin and body weight. The formula developed by Cockcroft and Gault to estimate creatinine clearance, and the four-variable formula derived from the Modification of Diet in Renal Disease (MDRD) study to estimate GFR, are the most widely used of these prediction equations. The Cockcroft–Gault formula incorporates age, sex and weight in addition to creatinine, whereas the four-variable MDRD formula incorporates age, sex and ethnicity, but not weight.

eGFR should be assessed on an annual basis in people with diabetes. More frequent assessment may be necessary in adults with established CKD.

Microalbuminuria

Microalbuminuria is the earliest, clinically detectable manifestation of classical diabetic kidney disease. Conventional urine dipstick testing cannot reliably be used to diagnose the presence or absence of microalbuminuria. There is a daily variability in urinary albumin loss and so the ACR is best measured on an early morning specimen of urine. ACR may be measured on a spot sample if a first-pass sample is not provided (but should be repeated on a first-pass specimen if abnormal).

Urine albumin excretion may be increased temporarily by other factors, such as intercurrent illness and diabetic ketoacidosis. Therefore, it is usual to require multiple positive tests, usually two or three over a period of months, before microalbuminuria is confirmed.

The literature is confusing in relation to the timing of commencing screening in young people with diabetes. Early microvascular abnormalities may occur before puberty, which then appears to accelerate these abnormalities. For clarity and simplicity it is suggested that screening for kidney disease should commence at 12 years of age in both boys and girls.

Proteinuria

Proteinuria is associated with cardiovascular and renal disease and is a predictor of end-organ damage in patients with hypertension. Detection of an increase in protein excretion is known to have both diagnostic and prognostic value in the initial detection and confirmation of renal disease.

In evaluating the diagnostic accuracy of tests of proteinuria, measurement of protein (or albumin) excretion in a timed urine collection over 24 h has been used as a reference standard.

Protein/creatinine ratio (PCR) measured in early morning or random urine samples correlates closely with 24-h proteinuria and is at least as good as 24-h urine protein estimation at predicting the rate of loss of GFR in patients with CKD.

MANAGEMENT OF DIABETIC NEPHROPATHY

Prevention of nephropathy

Prevention in type 1 diabetes

Good glycaemic control, as in the DCCT trial, reduced the risk of development of microalbuminuria by 39% and of proteinuria by 54%. BP control, especially by effects on the renin–angiotensin system, has significantly lowered the risk of microalbuminuria in patients with type 1 diabetes.

Prevention in type 2 diabetes
Tight glycaemic control has been demonstrated to lead to lower incidence of nephropathy. Studies in support of this include the UKPDS, ADVANCE and Kumamoto studies. Angiotensin receptor blockers (ARBs) have been shown to be effective, but most clinicians assume that ACE inhibitors are equally effective at delaying diabetic nephropathy.

MANAGEMENT OF ESTABLISHED DIABETIC KIDNEY DISEASE

Physicians need to exclude non-diabetic causes of renal disease before assuming that the cause of renal dysfunction in a diabetic individual is indeed due to diabetes. Absence of retinopathy, rapid decline in renal function, presence of systemic disorders known to cause renal dysfunction, presence of asymmetrical kidneys, presence of active sediments and short duration of type 1 diabetes all point to possible renal disorder other than that due to diabetes, and must be investigated and managed appropriately.

Good glycaemic control

Long-term follow-up studies have conclusively shown the benefit of good glycaemic control in patients with type 1 and type 2 diabetes. In a highly selected group of patients undergoing pancreatic transplant it has been demonstrated that renal structural changes can be reversed.

Inhibition of renin–angiotensin system and blood pressure control
ACE inhibitors, ARBs and recently the direct renin inhibitor, aliskiren, have been demonstrated to reduced microalbuminuria, macroproteinuria and even established overt nephropathy.

Low protein diet

A Cochrane meta-analysis concluded that reducing dietary protein intake may reduce progression to end-stage renal disease. However, dietary protein should not be restricted to less than 0.7 g per kg body weight per day.

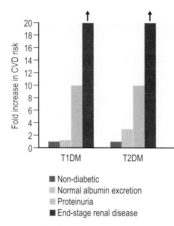

Figure 5.2 Increasing risk of cardiovascular disease (CVD) with the development of nephropathy in type 1 diabetes mellitus (T1DM) and type 2 diabetes mellitus (T2DM). (Source: Holt et al (2010). © Wiley-Blackwell.)

Cardiovascular risk modification

Aggressive cardiovascular risk modification is warranted in patients with renal dysfunction (Fig. 5.2). This includes smoking cessation, BP control, lipid modification, antiplatelet use, weight reduction and regular exercise schedule.

DIABETIC CARDIOVASCULAR DISEASE

EPIDEMIOLOGY

Morbidity and mortality from cardiovascular disease (CVD) are 2–5 times higher in patients with diabetes than in non-diabetic subjects. Women with diabetes have been shown to have a higher relative risk of death from CVD than men, although the absolute risk is lower. This excess in mortality occurs even in areas with high background death rates from CVD, and is evident in all age groups, most pronounced in young people with type 1 diabetes, and exacerbated by socioeconomic deprivation. The life expectancy of both men and women diagnosed as having type 2 diabetes at age 40 years is reduced by 8 years relative to people without diabetes. There is an increased prevalence of CVD in South Asian individuals with diabetes.

CARDIOVASCULAR RISK FACTORS

Dyslipidaemia

Dyslipidaemia is commonly present in patients with type 2 diabetes. The most common type of dyslipidaemia in type 2 diabetes is the combination of raised triglycerides, low HDL and small dense LDL.

An increased concentration of LDL cholesterol or total cholesterol is an independent risk factor for cardiovascular morbidity and mortality. A 1-mmol/L reduction of LDL cholesterol represents a 21% reduction in risk of CVD.

Triglycerides are an independent marker of increased risk of CVD in type 2 diabetes.

Hypertension

Hypertension is positively related to risk of CVD death, with a progressive increase in risk with rising systolic pressures. Each 10-mmHg reduction in systolic pressure is associated with a 15% reduction in the risk of CVD death over 10 years.

Hyperglycaemia

Increasing glycaemia (measured as HbA1c) was associated with an increased risk of CVD morbidity and mortality in observational data from UKPDS. Each 1% (11 mmol/mol) reduction in HbA1c was associated with a 21% lower risk of diabetes-related death and specifically a 14% lower risk of myocardial infarction (MI) over 10 years. No lower threshold was demonstrated. Intensive glycaemic control reduced the risk of CVD by approximately 10% compared with standard care (with borderline statistical significance), but did not have a significant effect on all-cause or CVD mortality.

In addition to its role in identifying patients at risk of diabetic nephropathy, microalbuminuria is an independent marker associated with a doubling in cardiovascular risk. There is insufficient evidence to determine whether reducing albumin excretion rate specifically reduces cardiovascular morbidity or mortality.

LIFESTYLE MODIFICATION

Lifestyle modification is recommended to reduce cardiovascular risk factors. However, no studies identifying obesity as an independent risk factor in established diabetes are available.

PHARMACOLOGICAL THERAPY

Antihypertensive therapy

BP lowering in people with diabetes reduces the risk of macrovascular and microvascular disease. Hypertension should be treated aggressively with lifestyle modification and drug therapy.

The lowering of BP to 80 mmHg diastolic is of benefit in people with diabetes. In the Hypertension Optimal Treatment (HOT) study, the lowest incidence of major cardiovascular events in all patients occurred at a mean achieved diastolic BP of 82.6 mmHg, and further reduction below this BP was safe in patients with diabetes. There was a 51% reduction in major cardiovascular events in the BP target group ≤ 80 mmHg compared with the target group ≤ 90 mmHg ($P = 0.005$).

Tip box

Target diastolic blood pressure in people with diabetes is < 80 mmHg.

In the HOT study, although diastolic BP was measured accurately, systolic BP was consistently underestimated. The reported achieved systolic BP of 139.7 mmHg in patients with a diastolic target of ≤ 80 mmHg is likely to have been closer to 146 mmHg. In the UKPDS, the achieved systolic BP of 144 mmHg in patients located to 'tight control' was observed when aiming for a systolic BP of < 150 mmHg. The long-term follow-up of these patients emphasized the need for maintenance of good BP control. In an epidemiological analysis, lowest risk was observed in those with a systolic BP < 120 mmHg.

Tip box

Target systolic blood pressure in people with diabetes is < 130 mmHg.

When starting antihypertensive treatment, calcium channel blockers, diuretics and ACE inhibitors are equally effective. There was no significant difference in outcome among the three treatment groups in the Antihypertensive and Lipid-Lowering Treatment to Prevent Heart Attack Trial (ALLHAT). A subgroup analysis of ALLHAT found an increase in heart failure in patients treated with an alpha-blocker as first line versus a diuretic, although this may simply reflect an increase in the prevalence of ankle swelling (relative risk of heart failure in patients with diabetes, 1.85).

The Anglo-Scandinavian Cardiac Outcomes Trial (ASCOT) found that amlodipine (a calcium channel blocker) based treatment (with an ACE inhibitor as add-on treatment) reduced the incidence of total cardiovascular events and procedures compared with an atenolol (beta-blocker) regimen (with a thiazide diuretic as add-on treatment). This study demonstrated increased cardiovascular mortality in patients treated with beta-blockers in comparison with those treated with renin–angiotensin blocking agents.

There is also evidence from two studies for the use of combination of ACE inhibitor and diuretic. In one study, ACE inhibitor and diuretic reduced BP (5.6/2.2 mmHg) and the relative risk for deaths, cardiovascular deaths and major vascular events by 14%, 18% and 9%, respectively, independent of the initial BP level. A second study found that ACE inhibitor and diuretic reduced BP by 9.4/4.6 mmHg. The reduction in risk of further stroke for those patients with diabetes was 38% – equivalent to one stroke avoided for every 16 patients treated for 5 years.

Angiotensin-II receptor blockers (ARBs) are equally effective alternative antihypertensive agents in patients with ACE inhibitor-induced cough or rash. They also have similar renal benefits in patients with microalbuminuria.

The British Hypertension Society A/CD algorithm (Fig. 5.3) has been accepted as the best method of defining combination drug therapy. It specifies the use of ACE inhibitors (or ARBs if intolerant), calcium channel blockers and thiazide-type diuretics.

Patients with diabetes requiring antihypertensive treatment should be commenced on:

- an ACE inhibitor (ARB if ACE inhibitor intolerant), or
- a calcium channel blocker, or
- a thiazide diuretic.

Beta-blockers and alpha-blockers should not normally be used in the initial management of BP in patients with diabetes.

An algorithm such as the A/CD should be followed, unless there is a specific indication that a particular specific class be used first (e.g. ACE inhibitor or ARB in those aged under 55 years or with nephropathy; beta-blockers in ischaemic heart disease). The expectation should be that most patients end up on more than one agent.

Antiplatelet therapy

The role of aspirin in primary prevention of vascular disease in patients with diabetes remains uncertain.

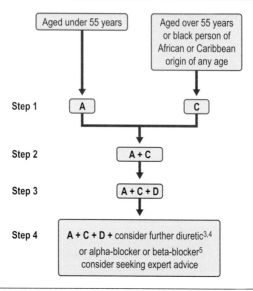

Key

A – ACE inhibitor or angiotensin II receptor blocker (ARB)[1]

C – Calcium-channel blocker (CCB)[2]

D – Thiazide-like diuretic

[1] Choose a low-cost ARB

[2] A CCB I preferred but consider a thiazide-like diuretic if a CCB is not tolerated or the person has oedema, evidence of heart failure or a high risk of heart failure.

[3] Consider a low dose of spironolactone4 or higher doses of a thiazide-like diuretic.

[4] At the time of publication of this algorithm by BHS/NICE (August 2011) spirolactone did not have UK marketing authorization for this indication. Informed consent should be obtained and documented.

[5] Consider an alpha-blocker or beta-blocker if further diuretic therapy is not tolerated, or is contraindicated or ineffective.

Figure 5.3 The British Hypertension Society (BHS) A/CD algorithm. ACE, angiotensin converting enzyme; NICE, National Institute for Health and Clinical Excellence. (Source: National Prescribing Centre, 2011. Reproduced with permission.)

Lipid lowering

Three large randomized clinical trials – the Collaborative Atorvastatin Diabetes Study (CARDS), ASCOT and the Heart Prevention Study (HPS) – examined the effects of statins versus placebo in people with diabetes and no existing cardiovascular risk. Statin therapy significantly reduced cardiovascular events comprising stroke, acute coronary events and coronary revascularizations: percutaneous coronary intervention (PCI) and coronary artery bypass grafting (CABG).

The reduction of events in patients with type 1 diabetes did not differ from that in patients with type 2 diabetes. Reduction in cardiovascular events was seen regardless of baseline cholesterol concentrations. People with diabetes experienced no more side-effects from statins than people without diabetes.

Lipid-lowering drug therapy with simvastatin 40 mg or atorvastatin 10 mg is recommended for primary prevention in patients with type 2 diabetes aged above 40 years regardless of baseline cholesterol level.

Lipid-lowering drug therapy with simvastatin 40 mg should be considered for primary prevention in patients aged over 40 years with type 1 diabetes.

Patients aged under 40 years with type 1 or type 2 diabetes and other important risk factors, such as microalbuminuria, should be considered for primary prevention lipid-lowering drug therapy with simvastatin 40 mg.

ACUTE CORONARY SYNDROMES

Acute coronary syndromes are a common cause of death in people with diabetes. However, the case fatality rate from MI is double that in the non-diabetic population.

Glycaemic control

Raised blood glucose concentration at hospital admission is a strong independent risk marker for patients with MI.

In the Diabetes mellitus Insulin–Glucose infusion in Acute Myocardial Infarction (DIGAMI) trial (620 patients), intensive metabolic control using insulin and glucose infusion in patients with diabetes mellitus or a blood glucose level > 11.0 mmol/L conferred a marked mortality benefit at 1 year (18.6% versus 26.1%).

The subsequent DIGAMI 2 trial (1253 patients) investigated whether long-term insulin therapy should be considered in patients with type 2 diabetes mellitus and acute MI. The trial demonstrated that long-term insulin was of no additional benefit, although there was extensive use of insulin at discharge in all treatment groups, making interpretation difficult. For patients with type 2 diabetes, most clinicians would not recommend that insulin is not routinely required beyond the first 24 h.

Primary coronary angioplasty

Primary angioplasty is equally successful in patients with and without diabetes, and may be more effective than thrombolytic therapy in patients with diabetes, either with or without acute MI.

Primary PCI is superior to thrombolysis for the treatment of patients with ST elevation acute coronary syndrome. In comparison with thrombolysis, primary PCI reduced short- and long-term mortality, stroke, reinfarction, recurrent ischaemia and the need for CABG surgery, as well as the combined endpoint of death or non-fatal reinfarction. This benefit was consistent across all patient subgroups and was independent of the thrombolytic agent used. The greatest benefit was seen in patients treated within 12 h of symptom onset.

Patients with ST elevation acute coronary syndrome should be treated immediately with primary PCI.

Thrombolysis

Thrombolytic therapy has been shown to reduce mortality after acute MI in patients with diabetes by up to 42%, and the indications and contraindications for thrombolysis in patients with diabetes are the same as for non-diabetic patients. Thrombolytic therapy should not be withheld because of concern about retinal haemorrhage in patients with retinopathy.

Compared with primary PCI, the benefit of thrombolysis on the 6-month mortality rate is more time-dependent, and is associated with a lesser degree of myocardial salvage at all time points.

When primary PCI cannot be performed within 90 min of diagnosis, thrombolytic therapy should be administered. This is based upon the assumptions that there is a 30-min delay to the administration of thrombolysis and that the superiority of primary PCI is most clear when the time difference between administration of thrombolysis and balloon inflation is ≤ 60 min.

When primary PCI cannot be provided within 90 min of diagnosis, patients with ST elevation acute coronary syndrome should receive immediate thrombolytic therapy.

Antiplatelet therapy

Platelet inhibitor therapy results in a 31% reduction in non-fatal reinfarction, a 42% reduction in non-fatal stroke and a 13% reduction in cardiovascular mortality.

Aspirin should be given routinely and continued long-term in patients with diabetes and coronary heart disease (CHD).

In the Clopidogrel in Unstable Angina to prevent Recurrent Events (CURE) trial, clopidogrel (75 mg daily) was administered for between 3 and 12 (median 9) months after non-ST elevation acute coronary syndrome. The clinical benefits were seen predominantly in the first 3 months of therapy. Clopidogrel therapy reduced the primary composite endpoint of cardiovascular death, MI or stroke, but this was principally driven by a reduction in recurrent non-fatal MI. There was no demonstrable effect on mortality. However, the bleeding risks with clopidogrel were consistently higher.

In addition to long-term aspirin, clopidogrel therapy should be continued for 3 months in patients with non-ST elevation acute coronary syndromes.

In addition to long-term aspirin, clopidogrel therapy should be continued for up to 4 weeks in patients with ST elevation acute coronary syndrome. Patients prescribed clopidogrel have a reduced relative risk of death, reinfarction or stroke.

Glycoprotein IIb/IIIa antagonist

These antagonists have become an important therapeutic modality in the treatment of unstable angina and non-Q MI. They have been shown to be of equal, if not greater, benefit in patients with diabetes compared with those without diabetes. The PRISM-PLUS study, EPILOG study and EPISTENT study all provide evidence for their use.

Beta-blockers

Diabetes is not a contraindication to the use of beta-blockers, which reduce mortality, sudden cardiac death and reinfarction when given after acute MI.

Long-term beta-blocker therapy after MI resulted in a 23% relative risk reduction in total mortality and a 32% relative risk reduction in sudden death. The Carvedilol Post-Infarct Survival Control in Left ventricular Dysfunction (CAPRICORN) trial in 1959 patients with low ejection fraction (< 0.40) following MI showed that delayed (3–14 days) and cautious uptitration (over 4–6 weeks postinfarction) of carvedilol resulted in an absolute risk reduction of 3% (relative risk reduction 23%) in all-cause mortality compared with placebo. Although immediate beta-blocker therapy should be avoided in patients with acute pulmonary oedema and acute left ventricular failure, subsequent cautious introduction of beta-blockade is associated with major benefits.

> **Tip box**
>
> Patients with clinical myocardial infarction should be maintained on long-term beta-blocker therapy.

Blockers of the renin–angiotensin system

The major morbidity and mortality benefits of ACE inhibitor therapy have been widely established in patients with heart failure or left ventricular dysfunction following MI.

Patients with clinical MI should be commenced on long-term ACE inhibitor therapy within the first 36 h. It has been confirmed that ACE inhibitors reduce mortality and that most of the benefits occur during the first few days, when the mortality rate is highest. Patients at higher risk appear to obtain a greater absolute benefit.

Lipid lowering

Statin therapy in people with diabetes appears to be associated with a statistically significant reduction in the relative risk of various clinical endpoints, including all-cause mortality and fatal and non-fatal MI.

In people with diabetes, the use of atorvastatin 80 mg was associated with a significant reduction in major cardiovascular events (25% relative risk reduction in CHD death, MI, cardiac arrest or stroke). A marked reduction in cardiovascular events was particularly evident in diabetic patients with CKD.

> **Tip box**
>
> Intensive lipid-lowering therapy with atorvastatin 80 mg should be considered for patients with diabetes and acute coronary syndromes where there is objective evidence of coronary heart disease on angiography, or following coronary revascularization procedures.

In the Veterans Affairs High-Density Lipoprotein Intervention Trial (VA-HIT), 2531 patients with diabetes (not on baseline standard statin therapy) were randomized to gemfibrozil or placebo. Gemfibrozil reduced the primary endpoint of non-fatal MI or cardiovascular death (relative risk reduction 22%). Stroke and transient ischaemic attacks were reduced by 31% and 59%, respectively. The Fenofibrate Intervention and Event Lowering in Diabetes (FIELD) study randomized 9795 patients with diabetes not on baseline standard statin therapy to fenofibrate or placebo. The primary endpoint of coronary events was not reduced.

There is presently insufficient evidence to recommend fibrates, ezetimibe or nicotinic acid for the primary or secondary prevention of cardiovascular outcomes in patients with type 1 or 2 diabetes treated with statins.

Fibrate treatment can be considered in patients who are intolerant of statins. However, addition of fibrate to statin is probably of little/no benefit, as demonstrated in the Action to Control Cardiovascular Risk in Diabetes (ACCORD) study. The combination may be of benefit only in a select subgroup of patients with increased triglycerides along with associated low HDL.

CONGESTIVE HEART FAILURE

Blockers of the renin–angiotensin system

ACE inhibitors were first shown to be effective in heart failure in the 1980s. Many randomized clinical trials have confirmed their benefit on mortality and morbidity in patients with chronic heart failure, left ventricular diastolic dysfunction (LVSD), or both, after MI, and in patients with asymptomatic LVSD.

In patients with chronic heart failure, treatment with an ACE inhibitor reduced relative risk of mortality by 23% and admission for heart failure was reduced by 35%. In a further meta-analysis in patients with LVSD, heart failure, or both, after MI, relative risk of death was reduced by 26% and hospital admission by 27%.

ACE inhibitors should be considered in patients with all New York Heart Association (NYHA) functional classes of heart failure due to left ventricular systolic dysfunction.

Beta-blockers

There was an approximately one-third reduction in total mortality with bisoprolol, extended release metoprolol succinate and carvedilol in heart failure. Treatment with nebivolol resulted in a significantly reduced composite outcome of death or cardiovascular hospitalizations in elderly patients with heart failure.

There is consistent evidence for positive benefits from beta-blockers in patients with heart failure, with risk of death from cardiovascular causes reduced by 29%, mortality owing to pump failure reduced by 36% and all-cause mortality reduced by 23%.

Benefits were seen with beta-blockers with different pharmacological properties, whether β1-selective (bisoprolol, metoprolol, mebivolol) or non-selective (carvedilol).

Beta-blockers produce benefit in the medium to long term. In the short term they can produce decompensation with worsening of heart failure and hypotension. They should be initiated at low dose and only gradually increased with monitoring up to the target dose. Beta-blockers are contraindicated in patients with asthma, second- or third-degree atrioventricular heart block or symptomatic hypotension, and should be used with caution in those with low initial BP (systolic BP <90 mmHg). There is some evidence that cardioselective beta-blockers can be used safely in patients with chronic obstructive pulmonary disease (COPD) and heart failure.

Tip box

Beta-blockers reduce mortality in diabetic patients with heart failure.

Other measures

A 1% reduction in HbA1c has been found to decrease the risk of congestive heart failure by 16%. Thiazolidinediones can provoke or worsen heart failure and should be avoided. Metformin in the past was not used in patients with heart failure owing to the fear of lactic acidosis. However, recent observational studies demonstrated that metformin use was associated with a reduction in readmission rates for heart failure and diabetes.

MANAGEMENT OF PATIENTS WITH DIABETES AND STABLE ANGINA

Antiplatelet therapy

In the context of stable angina it has been shown that antiplatelet therapy, mainly with aspirin, given in a dose ranging from 75 to 150 mg daily, leads to a significant reduction in serious vascular events, non-fatal MI, non-fatal stroke and vascular mortality.

Enteric-coated products do not prevent the major gastrointestinal complications of aspirin therapy and are significantly more expensive than the standard dispersible formulation.

Lipid lowering with statins

Statin therapy is associated with a significant reduction in all-cause and coronary mortality, MI, need for coronary revascularization plus fatal or non-fatal stroke.

> **Tip box**
>
> All patients with stable angina due to atherosclerotic disease should receive long-term standard aspirin and statin therapy.

Blockers of the renin–angiotensin system

In patients with coronary artery disease and preserved left ventricular systolic function, ACE inhibitors significantly reduce all-cause mortality, non-fatal MI and stroke.

Patients with LVSD or heart failure are at higher risk and gain relatively more benefit from ACE inhibitor therapy (risk reduction ranges from 3.8% to 6%). All patients with stable vascular disease are likely to derive some benefit from ACE inhibitors, to a degree approximately proportional to the level of baseline risk.

> **Tip box**
>
> All patients with stable angina should be considered for treatment with ACE inhibitors.

Other than a significant reduction in stroke events with losartan in patients with left ventricular hypertrophy, studies of angiotensin-II receptor blockers have failed to show cardiovascular benefit on their own, or in combination with an ACE inhibitor.

CORONARY REVASCULARIZATION

Patients with diabetes are at increased risk of complications during revascularization procedures, increased risk of death following both coronary bypass surgery and angioplasty; there is also a substantially increased risk of restenosis following angioplasty in diabetic patients, partly ameliorated by the use of coronary stents. Much of this increased risk is due to confounding associations, including female sex, diffuse coronary disease, impaired left ventricular function and renal impairment, rather than the diabetic state itself. Indications for coronary angiography in patients with diabetes with symptomatic coronary disease are similar to those in non-diabetic subjects.

> **Tip box**
>
> For patients with diabetes and multivessel disease, coronary artery bypass grafting with use of the internal mammary arteries is preferred over percutaneous transluminal coronary angioplasty.

Stenting improves the outcome after angioplasty. Platelet glycoprotein-IIb/IIIa receptor antagonists (e.g. abciximab) also reduce mortality after angioplasty with or without stenting in patients with diabetes.

Drug-eluting stents (DES) reduce in-stent restenosis and target lesion revascularization when compared with bare metal stents (BMS) for revascularization in patients with diabetes.

In patients with diabetes, DES are recommended rather than BMS in patients with stable CHD or non-ST elevation MI to reduce in-stent restenosis and target lesion revascularization.

DIABETIC CARDIOMYOPATHY

The entity remains controversial. Patients with diabetes have greater left ventricular mass, higher resting heart rates and greater propensity for heart failure. Several metabolic abnormalities have been postulated to contribute to the development of these abnormalities. Patients with diabetes have a higher risk of:

● diastolic dysfunction
● prolonged isovolumetric relaxation time
● decreased diastolic filling
● abnormal transmitral flow.

ACUTE STROKE

The relative risk of stroke in patients with diabetes is twice as high as in the non-diabetic population, and the mortality rate following stroke is increased compared with that in non-diabetic patients. Stroke is considered conventionally a macrovascular complication of diabetes. However, small-vessel strokes (i.e. lacunar infarcts) are the commonest subtype of stroke occurring in patients with diabetes. These tend to occur almost a decade earlier than in non-diabetic individuals. It is thought that large-vessel disease tends to unmask the small-vessel disease earlier in patients with diabetes.

Management of stroke is similar to that in non-diabetic patients. Routine glucose control should be maintained. Rehydration and intravenous insulin may also be required.

Patients with diabetes who have no cerebrovascular disease but have one or more risk factors should be advised how this may affect the likelihood of their developing cerebrovascular disease.

Patients should be given information to help them recognize the following risk factors:

- smoking
- dyslipidaemia
- hypertension
- hyperglycaemia
- carotid artery disease
- atrial fibrillation
- central obesity.

Primary prevention of stroke

Glycaemic control
Evidence from the DCCT and UKPDS (the follow-up studies) showed that there was a reduction in combined endpoints of MI, stroke, cardiac death or revascularization procedures but not in the individual endpoints.

RAS blockers
The ACE inhibitor ramipril (in the Heart Outcomes Prevention Evaluation (HOPE) study) and losartan (in the Losartan Intervention For Endpoint reduction in Hypertension (LIFE) study) were shown to be of benefit in lowering the relative risk of stroke in patients with diabetes.

Treatment of acute stroke

Thrombolytic therapy
Thrombolysis for acute ischaemic stroke has been shown to be effective if given within a few hours after symptom onset. Thrombolysis in patients with diabetes is not as successful as in the general population.

Glycaemic control
Hyperglycaemia results in a greater chance of re-occlusion after thrombolysis, a greater risk of haemorrhagic transformation in infarction and a worse neurological functional outcome. Intensive treatment of hyperglycaemia (similar to that demonstrated in acute MI) may be associated with better outcome. Further studies are needed.

Blood pressure control
This is an area of debate. Hypertension should probably be treated if the systolic pressure rises above 220 mmHg or diastolic pressure is greater than 120 mmHg.

Medical management

Prevention of aspiration, pressure sores, nutrition, prevention of deep vein thrombosis, management of infections and hyperthermia are important issues in management of stroke.

Secondary treatment

- Patients with diabetes and new or established CVD should be offered treatment similar to the secondary prevention of coronary artery disease.
- Patients should be encouraged to take advantage of all cardiac rehabilitation programmes offered.
- The Clopidogrel Versus Aspirin in Patients at Risk of Ischemic Events (CAPRIE) study showed that the combination of clopidogrel with aspirin was superior to aspirin alone.
- Aggressive lipid lowering with LDL targets < 100 mg/dL (4 mmol/L) and preferably < 70 mg/dL (2 mmol/L) have been advocated.
- Patients with carotid artery disease benefit from carotid end-arterectomy or stenting if the degree of stenosis is > 70%.
- Patients with diabetes with atrial fibrillation should be anticoagulated.

PERIPHERAL VASCULAR DISEASE

Peripheral vascular disease (PVD) is common in diabetes and affects up to 30% of all diabetics. Amputation is 5–8 times commoner in diabetics than in those without diabetes. The atherosclerotic lesions in diabetes are usually located more peripherally (below the knee) and therefore more difficult to treat surgically.

The World Health Organization (WHO) defines PVD using an ABPI of < 0.9. The patient may be completely asymptomatic or may complain of claudication, rest pain or non-healing ulcers.

Diagnosis is made from history and objective findings on examination. Hand-held Doppler ultrasonography helps in measuring ABPI. However, the ABPI can be falsely high in patients with diabetes owing to calcification of arteries in diabetics. Alternatively, toe pressure measurement is useful. Angiography is useful when intervention is contemplated.

Treatment of peripheral vascular disease

Treatment of symptoms

Graded exercise therapy has been shown to improve symptoms; it especially increases pain-free walking distance. Medical treatment includes use of drugs such as cilostazol, naftidrofuryl and statins.

Interventional treatment

Interventional treatment is indicated when other treatment options have failed and the patient has claudication that is incapacitating, rest pain or critical limb ischaemia. It is also warranted for non-healing ulcers. Surgical intervention including bypass or angioplasty is often less successful in diabetic patients, particularly due to the peripheral location of lesions.

DERMATOLOGICAL FEATURES OF DIABETES MELLITUS

Various skin conditions occur frequently in diabetes, although common lesions may be associated by chance. Skin disorders affect about 30% of diabetic patients and therefore the association may be due to chance alone and not necessarily causally related. For example, generalized pruritus was previously widely regarded as a marker of diabetes. A recent study found that, although localized vulval pruritus (associated with candidiasis) was three times more common in diabetic than in non-diabetic women, the prevalence of generalized pruritus was the same (3%) in the diabetic as in the general population.

Necrobiosis lipoidica diabeticorum consists of non-scaling plaques with atrophic epidermis, thick degenerating collagen in the dermis, surface telangiectasia with a violaceous or sometimes raised erythematous border, and usually in the pretibial region. It has an incidence of 3 per 1000 diabetic patients per year; three-quarters of cases are in women, with an average age of onset of 34 years. The lesions vary in size, small papules often coalescing to form large irregular plaques, sometimes several centimetres in diameter. One-third of the lesions ulcerate. Multiple or bilateral lesions occur in most cases, and sites other than the pretibial are affected in 15% of patients.

'Necrobiosis' refers to degeneration and thickening of collagen bundles in the dermis. Acellular necrobiotic foci are associated with granular debris scattered throughout the dermis and surrounded by a mixed cellular infiltrate. Overall, the association between necrobiosis lipoidica diabeticorum and diabetes seems weaker than previously assumed, and necrobiosis lipoidica diabeticorum may not be a specific marker for diabetes. There is a 20% spontaneous remission rate.

Granuloma annulare is an annular or arciform lesion with a raised flesh-coloured papular border and hyperpigmented flat centre, usually found on the dorsum of the hands and arms. The feet, legs and trunk are involved much less frequently. Granuloma annulare differs histologically from necrobiosis lipoidica diabeticorum in that the epidermis is normal and the necrobiotic collagen is localized to the mid-dermis and associated with abundant mucin. Clinically, it can be difficult to distinguish granuloma annulare from necrobiosis lipoidica diabeticorum. Both diabetes and granuloma annulare are relatively common, and chance associations are therefore likely.

'Diabetic thick skin' includes both the rare scleroderma (affecting the neck, upper back and arms) and the common diabetic hand syndrome (Dupuytren's contracture, sclerosing tenosynovitis, knuckle pads and carpal tunnel syndrome).

'Scleroderma' describes a rare condition with marked non-pitting induration and thickening of the skin. Two types have been described. The first, scleroderma of Bushke, is not significantly associated with diabetes and may follow acute viral or streptococcal infection. The second type, scleroderma diabeticorum, which tends to be more persistent, is associated with type 1 diabetes mellitus. Both forms can involve the back of the neck and the upper part of the back, but that associated with diabetes frequently extends to involve the upper limbs and hands, and can result in joint contractures. The more common 'diabetic thick skin' syndromes appear to share a similar pathophysiological mechanism with scleroderma. The diabetic thick skin syndrome includes fibroproliferative complications of the diabetic hand, namely Dupuytren's contractures, sclerosing tenosynovitis of the palmar flexor tendons, Garrod's knuckle pads and carpal tunnel syndrome.

Acanthosis nigricans is characterized by brown, velvety, hyperkeratotic plaques that most often affect the axillae, back of the neck and other flexural areas. The lesions range in severity from minimal discoloration that spares the skin creases to thicker, more extensive, hyperkeratotic areas.

Histologically, the epidermis is extensively folded, slightly thickened and has increased cell density. The dark colour is caused by an increased number of melanocytes.

Acanthosis nigricans is associated with a large heterogeneous group of disorders with the common feature of insulin resistance, ranging from asymptomatic hyperinsulinaemia to overt diabetes. High circulating insulin concentrations associated with insulin resistance appear to promote epidermal growth.

- Type A – genetic defects in the insulin receptor or postreceptor mechanisms
- Type B – acquired insulin resistance, due to autoantibodies directed against the insulin receptor.

Acanthosis and insulin resistance can also be associated in obesity, where receptor and postreceptor defects have been shown to play a role in the insulin-resistant state, and in various endocrinopathies.

'Diabetes dermopathy' is also known as 'shin spots' or 'pigmented pretibial patches'. There is no strong evidence for an association with the chronic complications of diabetes and the condition is not pathognomonic of the diabetes, having been reported in approximately 2% of healthy students. Initially, lesions are round or oval, red or brownish papules that slowly evolve into discrete, sharply circumscribed, atrophic, hyperpigmented or scaly lesions. Lesions are bilateral but often not symmetrical. Dermopathy occurs in about 60% of diabetic men older than 50 years and in around 30% of similarly aged female patients.

Bullosis diabeticorum is a very rare condition that affects men more than women and has a predilection for patients with long-standing diabetes complicated by neuropathy. One or more tense blisters on a non-inflammatory base appear suddenly, often overnight, with no preceding trauma, and heal over some weeks with or without scarring. The condition is usually confined to the feet and lower legs but may involve the hands. It can be diagnosed only in diabetic patients in whom other bullous disorders have been excluded by the absence of immunoglobulin deposition.

Complications of sulphonylureas include various cutaneous reactions and may occur with the first dose. Further complications of diabetic treatment include insulin allergy and injection-site lipodystrophy.

The rare glucagonoma syndrome (associated with an A-cell glucagon-secreting islet-cell pancreatic tumour) presents with a migratory erythematous eruption, peripheral scaling and vesiculation leading to erosions and ulceration. Patients develop a polymorphous, erythematous eruption with peripheral scaling that waxes and wanes in cycles of 7–14 days and may remit and relapse spontaneously. Superficial vesiculation can lead to erosions and necrosis. The eruption is usually worst around the mouth, groin, perineum and genitals. It is often associated with painful glossitis, weight loss, relatively 'mild diabetes', intermittent diarrhoea, mood changes and venous thrombosis.

Cutaneous reactions to insulin previously occurred in half of the patients treated, but have become much less frequent since purified pork and human insulins were introduced.

Insulin allergy

This may be local or systemic and develops within 1–4 weeks of starting treatment. Local allergy was extremely common in the 1960s with the use of 'impure' insulins, but the reported prevalence in patients receiving monocomponent porcine insulin was zero in one study and 5% in another.

Lipodystrophy

Lipodystrophy and insulin hypertrophy are complications of insulin injections. Lipodystrophy presents as circumscribed depressed areas of skin at the injection site and occasionally at distant sites as well.

Insulin hypertrophy (lipodystrophy) presents as a soft dermal nodule with normal surface epidermis at the injection site, which has often been used for many years.

Idiosyncratic reactions

Pigmentation can occur at the injection site and, rarely, keloids may form.

MUSCULOSKELETAL AND CONNECTIVE TISSUE DISEASE

A variety of musculoskeletal disorders are found in individuals with diabetes. They may cause pain and disability, and are considered to be microvascular complications of diabetes.

FIBROPROLIFERATIVE DISORDERS OF SOFT TISSUE

Limited joint mobility (cheiroarthropathy)

Diabetes of long duration may result in thickening of the subcutaneous tissues producing limited mobility and stiffness around the joints. The 'prayer' sign may be elicited when the patient is unable closely to oppose some or all fingers when palms are placed together. In addition, the skin of affected patients may have a waxy appearance similar to scleroderma (scleroderma diabeticorum).

Adhesive capsulitis

This commonly occurs in the shoulder (frozen shoulder) or rarely in hips and is associated with diabetes. Treatment includes physiotherapy, analgesics and intra-articular corticosteroids.

Dupuytren's contracture

This is a fibroproliferative disorder of palmar fascia leading to the formation of palmar nodules, and to flexion contractures especially of the ring and little finger. Rarely, similar lesions lead to plantar fibromatosis. Surgical treatment is the mainstay of therapy.

Stenosing tenosynovitis

This condition is commoner in individuals with diabetes.
Corticosteroid injection is useful.

Carpal tunnel syndrome

This syndrome is commoner in diabetics. Surgery is mainstay of
treatment.

DISORDERS OF JOINTS

Charcot joint

See in section on foot ulceration.

Gout

An increase in serum uric acid concentration is a marker for CHD
and is associated with metabolic syndrome and hyperglycaemia.
In non-diabetic individuals, plasma uric acid levels are inversely
related to rates of insulin-mediated glucose disposal as determined
using the glucose clamp technique.

Osteoarthritis and rheumatoid arthritis

Both of these conditions are commoner in diabetes. Increased weight
(body mass index) is probably the reason for greater risk of
osteoarthritis in diabetics, whereas rheumatoid arthritis and type 1
diabetes share several genetic associations.

SKELETAL DISEASE IN DIABETES

Diffuse idiopathic skeletal hyperostosis (DISH)

This is characterized by increased bone formation and increased risk
of enthesitis. Ossification of ligaments may occur.

Localized osteopenia

This is of importance in the pathogenesis of Charcot
neuroarthropathy. Increased local blood flow is thought to be an
important contributory factor.

Osteopenia/osteoporosis and fracture risk

Meta-analyses of observational studies show that bone mineral
density (BMD) is decreased in type 1 diabetes, possibly due to lower
body weight, lower levels of insulin-like growth factor-1 and local

osteopenia due to neuropathy. In type 2 diabetes, bone density may be lowered due to concomitant use of glitazones. Bone quality is also altered due to advanced glycation endproduct formation.

Patients with diabetes are at increased risk of falls due to diabetes-related complications, hypoglycaemia and drug-related hypotension. It has been demonstrated that, once fracture occurs, the fracture-healing rate in diabetics is abnormal.

MUSCLE INVOLVEMENT IN DIABETES

Spontaneous myonecrosis

This is a rare condition that presents with acute severe pain and swelling in thigh or calf muscle. MRI demonstrates intramuscular oedema and inflammation. Treatment of uncomplicated cases is symptomatic with bed rest and analgesia. An acute compartmental syndrome may complicate the condition when urgent surgical decompression is warranted.

Rhabdomyolysis

This very rare complication can be associated with statin therapy.

INFECTION AND DIABETES

PREVALENCE OF INFECTION AND DIABETES

Although fungal and bacterial infections may be encountered more frequently in diabetic patients, particularly when metabolic control is poor, it remains uncertain whether the overall incidence of infection is increased. Diabetes has long been considered a risk factor for pulmonary tuberculosis. Recurrent cutaneous or urogenital infections, such as vulvovaginal candidiasis or balanitis, may be the presenting feature of diabetes and their occurrence should prompt appropriate investigations.

Tip box

Recurrent cutaneous or urogenital infections may be the presenting feature of diabetes.

PREDISPOSING FACTORS

● *Physical factors*. Severe invasive infections may develop because of particular predisposing factors that arise from the diabetic state. For example, chronic complications such as foot ulcers provide a portal of entry of microorganisms to soft tissues and bone. Polymicrobial infections are usual in this situation. Autonomic neuropathy (see p. 187) predisposes to urinary stasis and ascending infections. Pyelonephritis is occasionally complicated by necrosis and sloughing of renal papillae demonstrable on retrograde pyelography. Necrotizing otitis externa may be encountered, particularly in elderly diabetic patients.

● *Metabolic factors*. The ability of neutrophil leukocytes to migrate, ingest and kill organisms may be compromised by hyperglycaemia; overactivity of the polyol pathway is implicated. Through stimulation of counter-regulatory hormone secretion and cytokine release (tumour necrosis factor-α and interleukins induce insulin resistance), infections may lead to a deterioration in metabolic control; infections are the commonest identifiable precipitating cause of diabetic ketoacidosis (DKA) (see p. 143).

> **Tip box**
> Acute infections may lead to deterioration in metabolic control.

Attainment of good metabolic control is therefore important in the management of infections in diabetic patients; this may necessitate temporary insulin therapy in diet- or tablet-treated patients with type 2 diabetes. The association between the rare and serious complication of invasive infection with the saprophytic *Mucor* species (rhinocerebral mucormycosis) with DKA (see p. 143) is noteworthy; this condition is encountered in some other states associated with severe metabolic acidosis.

VIRAL INFECTIONS

As discussed in Section 1, some viruses (rubella, mumps, Coxsackie B4) have been implicated in the aetiology of type 1 diabetes. Intrauterine rubella infection leads to autoimmune type 1 diabetes in 20–40% of children. Recent concerns that immunization against common childhood infections might lead to an increased risk of type 1 diabetes have not been substantiated.

PERIODONTAL DISEASE AND DIABETES

Periodontal disease has been recognized as a common complication of diabetes mellitus. In fact, signs and symptoms of periodontal disease may be the first manifestation of diabetes. There are two main types of periodontal disease: gingivitis, in which the gingiva surrounding the teeth is reddened and inflamed and bleeds easily, and periodontitis, in which the infection and inflammation surrounding the teeth destroys the ligamentous attachment of the teeth as well as the alveolar bone surrounding the teeth.

Periodontal disease is commoner in diabetics, and the relationship between diabetes and periodontal disease is a two-way relationship. Diabetic patients with periodontal disease have worse glycaemic control and it has also been reported that treatment of periodontal disease leads to better glycaemic control. Recently it has been reported that periodontal disease is an independent risk factor for heart disease and stroke.

SPECIAL TOPICS

CHILDHOOD AND ADOLESCENCE

Diabetes is one of the most common chronic diseases of childhood; 1 in 300 in Europe and North America develop diabetes by the age of 20 years. Over the past few decades the incidence has been increasing by 3–5% per year.

Type 1a (autoimmune) diabetes mellitus (T1aDM) accounts for the vast majority of children with diabetes. Newborn babies and infants rarely develop the disease (1 in 250 000 in those younger than 6 months) and the aetiology is usually monogenic, not autoimmune. T1aDM is believed to be caused by the interplay of genetic and environmental factors. The initial step is the development of islet autoimmunity, which is marked by the presence of islet autoantibodies. This is thought to be driven by one or more environmental triggers. After this initiation of islet autoimmunity, most patients have a long preclinical period that does offer the opportunity for secondary prevention of the progression to clinical diabetes. The presence of more than one of the autoantibodies combined with susceptibility human leukocyte antigen (HLA)-DR and HLA-DQ genotypes identifies those at high risk of developing diabetes.

Type 1b diabetes has the same clinical presentation as T1aDM, but islet autoantibodies are absent.

The diagnosis of diabetes in children is based on polyuria, polydipsia, weight loss, fatigue and random blood glucose level above 11.1 mmol/L (200 mg/dL). With the increased community recognition of diabetes, most children present with mild hyperglycaemia of short duration. However, 75% of children have the symptoms for more than 2 weeks, suggesting that the diagnosis could be made earlier in many cases. The diagnosis of diabetes should be considered in all sick children; urine or blood testing for glucose and ketones leads to an early diagnosis. Young children may have a non-specific presentation, possibly presenting with enuresis, vomiting or rapid breathing during the course of an infection. Nearly all patients admitted with severe diabetic ketoacidosis (DKA) have been seen hours or days earlier by health-care providers who missed the diagnosis. Most children do not require intravenous (IV) fluids or insulin infusion at the diagnosis of diabetes.

The availability of outpatient care centres has helped to decrease hospitalization at diagnosis. Admission with DKA is more often found among younger children and in children with lower socioeconomic status who encounter possible barriers in accessing medical care.

A family history of an autosomal dominant inheritance of diabetes appearing under the age of 25 years is highly suggestive of maturity-onset diabetes of the young (MODY). It is not uncommon for young people with MODY to be diagnosed when they present with an intercurrent illness.

The principal aims of treatment of diabetes in childhood are:

- achievement of good metabolic control
- attainment of normal growth and development
- avoidance of serious hypoglycaemia
- prevention of long-term complications of diabetes.

The difficulties posed by insulin treatment in children and adolescents mean that these ideals can be difficult to achieve. Emphasis should, however, be placed on the favourable prospects for the child with diabetes; diabetes should be a bar to few recreational activities or occupations.

MANAGEMENT OF DIABETES IN CHILDHOOD

Diabetic ketoacidosis

The principles of therapy are similar to those for adults. Soluble insulin is infused IV at a rate of 0.1 units per kg per h. Particular care should be exercised with IV fluid replacement in view of the risk to children of the uncommon but potentially fatal complication of cerebral oedema during treatment. Hydration status should be assessed, and fluid deficit and osmolality calculated to help guide fluid and electrolyte replacement. Serum electrolytes, glucose, blood urea nitrogen (BUN), creatinine, calcium, magnesium, phosphorus and blood gas testing should be repeated every 2–4 hours, or more frequently in severe cases.

Cerebral oedema

Subclinical cerebral oedema occurs in most children with DKA. Severe clinical oedema affects 0.5–1% and is fatal in over 20%. Neurological status should be monitored at frequent and regular intervals. Typically, cerebral oedema occurs at 4–12 hours and potential risk factors for symptomatic cerebral oedema in children include:

- more profound dehydration, hyperventilation and acidosis at presentation
- bicarbonate therapy
- excessive and rapid fluid administration, especially if initial serum osmolality is greater than 320 mOsm/L

- failure of serum sodium level to rise as hyperglycaemia resolves
- initial IV insulin bolus or too early initiation of insulin infusion.

Signs and symptoms of cerebral oedema include headache, change in mental status or behaviour, incontinence, focal neurological findings, sudden normalization of heart rate in a previously tachycardic dehydrated patient, or a worsening clinical course in a patient with improved laboratory values. Bradycardia, hypertension and irregular respiration (Cushing triad) are signs of greatly increased intracranial pressure. Early intervention is essential and treatment includes:

- administration of mannitol (1 g/kg over 30 min)
- decreasing fluid rate to 75% or less of maintenance rate
- elevation of head of bed.

Mannitol therapy may need to be repeated. IV hypertonic saline has also been used as an alternative to mannitol. Radiographic imaging (such as computed tomography of the head) should be obtained after, rather than during, treatment of cerebral oedema.

Insulin therapy

Injection regimens should be individualized and include:

- Basal bolus regimen: 40–60% of the total daily dose as a basal insulin analogue (glargine, detemir) in 1–2 doses a day plus a rapid-acting insulin analogue with each meal (in some patients after the meal); soluble human insulin requires administration at least 20–30 min before each meal
- Intermediate-acting human (or neutral protamine Hagedorm; NPH) insulin twice daily and soluble human insulin 20–30 min before each meal
- Two injections daily of a (pre-mixed) mixture of short or rapid and intermediate-acting insulin before breakfast and before the evening meal
- Three injections using some variation of the following: a mixture of short- or rapid-acting and intermediate-acting insulin before breakfast, rapid-acting or soluble human insulin before the afternoon snack or evening meal, and intermediate or basal/long-acting insulin before bed.

Intermediate-acting insulins such as NPH are often mixed with soluble human (regular) or rapid-acting analogues (aspart, lispro or glulisine). Patients and families should be taught how to mix the insulin properly, in order to avoid contamination. It is generally taught to draw up clear (regular or short-acting) insulin before drawing up cloudy insulin (NPH).

Pre-mixed insulins contain a mixture of regular (or rapid-acting) insulin and NPH insulin in various fixed ratios. These preparations may be useful for children who do not want to draw insulin from separate vials before injecting. They may also be useful in reducing the number of injections when compliance is an issue, especially among teenagers. Pre-mixed insulins are also available for use in pen injector devices. The main disadvantage to using pre-mixed insulin preparations is the lack of flexibility in adjusting the separate insulin doses, which is often necessary with varied food intake or during illness or exercise.

Glargine or detemir insulins should not be mixed with any other insulin.

Insulin pump therapy

Insulin pump therapy is the best way to restore the body's physiological insulin profile. Rapid-acting insulin analogues perform better in pumps than regular insulin, in terms of both mimicking the first-phase insulin release after meals and avoidance of postprandial hypoglycaemia. The user initiates bolus doses before meals and to correct hyperglycaemia. Even with the analogues, however, insulin has to be administered at least 10–15 min before a meal in order to reach effective levels in time. The pump delivers a variable programmed basal rate that corresponds to the diurnal variation in insulin needs.

Currently, the most frequent complications of insulin treatment include failures of insulin delivery because of a displaced or obstructed infusion set, local skin infections and DKA. Patients and their families must be instructed on troubleshooting and treatment of hyperglycaemia, particularly if ketones are present, as this may be an indication of pump malfunction. Syringes should always be available so that insulin may be administered via injection in the event of a pump failure.

Most clinical trials have demonstrated that, compared with multiple daily injections (MDI), pump therapy delivers better glycated haemoglobin (HbA1c), less severe hypoglycaemia, and can improve the quality of life in children.

Insulin pump treatment is significantly more expensive than regimens based on injections. For some patients, pumps may be too difficult to operate or comply with the multiple testing and carbohydrate counting requirements, or may be unacceptable because of body image issues or extreme physical activity (e.g. swimming, contact sports).

Paediatric diabetes outpatient care

Diabetes is managed primarily in the outpatient setting by a team including:

- a paediatrician specializing in diabetes
- a diabetes specialist nurse
- a diabetes dietitian
- a paediatric psychologist with knowledge of childhood diabetes and chronic illness
- possibly a paediatric social worker trained in childhood diabetes.

Health-care providers and the diabetes care team should be aware of and sensitive to the cultural needs and barriers to care that may arise with children from minority ethnic groups.

Tip box

Anxieties and feelings of guilt are common in parents and require considerate and informed handling.

Education

Initial education should provide a basic understanding of the pathophysiology of diabetes and its treatment to ensure that families feel confident in providing diabetes care at home. In most centres where appropriate outpatient resources are available, diabetes education and initiation of insulin therapy can occur as an outpatient, which has been shown to be cost-effective.

In the first few months following diagnosis, close contact in the form of frequent outpatient visits, home visits, telephone communication and other methods of communication is essential to address the frequently changing requirements.

Diabetes education is a continuous process and must be repeated to be effective. It must be adapted and appropriate to the age of the child. Infants and toddlers often have unpredictable eating and activity patterns.

Needle phobia can present a significant issue with the perception of pain inflicted by the caregiver.

Hypoglycaemia is more common in this age group and the prevention, recognition and management of hypoglycaemia is a priority.

Education should also focus on age-appropriate stepwise handover of diabetes responsibilities. This becomes particularly important in adolescence, during which there is a critical balance between promoting independent responsible management of diabetes while maintaining parental involvement.

Once established, it is common practice for children to be seen in the diabetes clinic at least every 3 months; visits should be more often if the patient does not meet the treatment goals or treatment requires intensified, for example if insulin pump treatment is initiated. During these visits:

- overall health and well-being is assessed
- growth and vital signs are monitored
- routine screening for diabetes-associated complications and comorbidities is performed
- blood glucose records (including HbA1c) are assessed
- medications and school plans need to be reviewed.

The advent of new technology, including downloadable glucometers, insulin pumps and continuous glucose sensors, has made it increasingly possible for the diabetes care team to gain insight into the home management of diabetes.

The dietitian should review dietary habits and provide ongoing nutrition education as needed.

Diabetes management in school

Children with diabetes spend a significant portion of their day in school; therefore, diabetes management in school is a critical portion of their diabetes management plan. A school health plan should be in place and should include:

- contact information for the child's family as well as their diabetes care providers
- information regarding routine management of diabetes (blood sugar monitoring, insulin administration and dosing, snack times)
- an emergency plan for management of hypoglycaemia and hyperglycaemia.

Extracurricular activities are an important component of a child's school experience, and children with diabetes should be allowed to participate and their needs accommodated accordingly.

Nutrition

Nutritional management in children with diabetes remains a key component of diabetes care and education. The management does not require a restrictive diet, just a healthy dietary regimen that the children and their families can benefit from. A thorough dietary history should be obtained including the family's dietary habits and traditions, the child's typical meal times and patterns of food intake. Current guidelines target optimal glycaemic control, reduction of cardiovascular risk, psychosocial well-being and family dynamics. Insulin pump and MDI therapy utilize carbohydrate counting in which the grams of carbohydrate to be eaten are counted and a matching dose of insulin is administered. This plan allows for the greatest freedom and flexibility in food choices, but it requires expert education and commitment, and may not be suitable for many families or situations (e.g. school lunches, teenagers).

Principles of dietary planning in children with diabetes can be found in Appendix 6.1.

Exercise

Children with diabetes derive the same benefits from exercise as children without diabetes and therefore should be allowed to participate with equal opportunities and safety. When children without diabetes exercise, there is a decrease in pancreatic insulin secretion and an increase in counter-regulatory hormones resulting in an increase in liver glucose production. This matches skeletal muscle uptake of glucose during exercise, maintaining stable blood glucose concentrations. In children with T1DM, there is no pancreatic regulation of insulin in response to exercise and there may be impaired counter-regulation. These factors combine to increase the risk of hypoglycaemia. It can be helpful to keep a record of the insulin doses, timing and type of exercise, blood glucose levels before and after exercise, snacks eaten and the time of any episode of hypoglycaemia.

Hypoglycaemia

Hypoglycaemia is the most common acute complication in the treatment of T1DM and is responsible for a significant proportion of deaths in people with diabetes aged under 40 years.

Ideally, blood glucose levels should be checked before, during and after the exercise. Children should consume carbohydrates prior to exercise, with the amount depending on the blood sugar level before the exercise and the duration and intensity of exercise. The site of insulin injection should also be taken into account. Exercise increases blood flow in the part of the body being used, increasing insulin absorption if that area is where the insulin injection was administered. For example, before running, insulin should not be administered in the legs. Hypoglycaemia can occur several hours after exercise secondary to increased glucose transport into the skeletal muscle, the late effect of increased insulin sensitivity, and the delay in replenishing liver and muscle glycogen stores. Blood glucose levels must be monitored for several hours after exercise, at bedtime, and sometimes during the night on days with strenuous exercise.

For anticipated exercise, the dose of insulin can be reduced depending on the intensity of the exercise. The details are beyond the scope of this book. Reduction of insulin administered should mean less carbohydrate intake and may aid weight loss.

Monitoring and goals of diabetes management

Self-monitoring of blood glucose (SMBG) provides an immediate measure of hyperglycaemia and hypoglycaemia, helps to determine immediate and daily insulin requirements, detects hypoglycaemia and assists in its management.

Increased HbA1c levels predict an increased risk of long-term microvascular and macrovascular complications. HbA1c levels, in terms of the optimal glycaemic control, should be considered along with quality of life and documented hypoglycaemia.

The safest recommendation for glycaemic control in children is to achieve the lowest HbA1c that can be sustained without severe hypoglycaemia or frequent moderate hypoglycaemia. Each child should have targets individually determined.

Sick-day management

Children with diabetes with good metabolic control should not experience more illness than non-diabetic children. Health-care providers should equip patients and their carers with the tools necessary to avoid dehydration, uncontrolled hyperglycaemia/ketoacidosis, and hypoglycaemia in the face of intercurrent illnesses.

- Face to face education
- Written instructions are important
- Most parents require telephone advice when first facing sickness in their child and some may need repeated support.

Over time, most parents should be able to manage sick days independently as well as identify when it is appropriate to seek help from their diabetes provider or emergency services.

Insulin therapy must *never* be stopped during a sick day, although the dose may need to be decreased if the child is vomiting or eating less than usual.

However, infections and other illnesses may be associated with an increase in insulin requirements.

Psychological care

The diagnosis of T1DM changes the lives of affected families and can pose significant problems. It is impossible to take a 'holiday' from diabetes. Persisting problems with adjusting to T1DM may trigger underlying dysfunction or psychopathology of the child or the family/caregiver. Young people with T1DM are diagnosed with and treated for psychiatric disorders, eating disorders, neurocognitive problems, learning problems, family dysfunction and poor coping skills more frequently than the general population.

Coeliac disease

Many children with diabetes are asymptomatic but are positive for specific serological markers of coeliac disease, such as autoantibodies to tissue transglutaminase. The prevalence of biopsy-confirmed coeliac disease in patients with T1DM is around 5%, compared with less than 1% in the general population.

Thyroid disease

Hypothyroidism is present in approximately 15% of children with T1DM. Long-term follow-up suggests that as many as 30% of people with T1DM develop autoimmune thyroiditis. The presence of hypothyroidism is associated with thyroid autoantibodies, female sex, increasing age and diabetes duration.

Addison's disease

Addison's disease affects approximately 1 in 10 000 of the general population, but 1% of subjects with T1DM. The autoimmune process resulting in Addison's disease can be identified by the detection of autoantibodies reacting to 21-hydroxylase (21-OH).

TRANSITION TO THE ADULT DIABETES CLINIC

The terms 'transition' and 'transfer' have been used interchangeably in the literature when referring to adolescents moving between diabetes services. Transition may be interpreted as simply a process of physical transfer of a patient to a different service with a failure to acknowledge the psychosocial needs of the adolescent and family members/carers.

Adolescence is a period characterized by transition and change regardless of health status. Diabetes in adolescence is a life-changing condition requiring very careful and consistent management by a multidisciplinary team of clinicians, in addition to the support provided by the family unit/carers. Many young people with diabetes establish a long-term relationship with their paediatric health-care team and the transition to an adult diabetes service provider is an enormous event. The seamless transfer of adolescents with diabetes from paediatric to adult services is a challenge for diabetes teams.

Adolescence is a transitional stage of human development that:

- occurs between childhood and adulthood
- is characterized by significant and complex biological, social and psychological changes.

During this time the adolescent is developing a sense of self and identity, establishing autonomy and understanding sexuality. It is usually accompanied by an increase in independence and generally less overall supervision. This is true too of adolescents transferring to an adult care service. The intention is to provide the adolescent with the practical and cognitive skills required for diabetes self-care and the capability to interact with others such as health-care providers. Age itself may not be a reliable indicator, as adolescents may have different needs and mature at different rates. The parents of the adolescent must also be prepared to relinquish some of the responsibility for diabetes care that they may have undertaken for many years. For some parents, this shift in responsibility can be a time of high anxiety. Fundamental to a successful transition programme is to work with parents to help them find a balance between shifting the responsibility to the adolescent and continuing to maintain an appropriate level of interest.

Transition should be planned, coordinated, and viewed holistically as opposed to focusing solely on the referral from one medical doctor to another. Transition should promote better management for adolescents with T1DM by developing their capacity to self-care through healthy choices.

A powerful predictor of good self-care is self-efficacy. Adolescents should be encouraged to have confidence in their capability to make decisions and take actions that demonstrate good diabetes self-care (see Appendix 6.1: Principles of dietary planning in children with diabetes).

DIABETES IN THE ELDERLY

Diabetes, mainly type 2 diabetes, is particularly common in the elderly; more than 50% of patients in the UK are over 60 years of age (the majority having type 2 diabetes). In many countries diabetes affects 10–25% of elderly people (>65 years), with particularly high rates in populations such as Pima Indians, Mexican Americans and

---

TABLE 6.1 Factors contributing to glucose intolerance in old age

Impaired glucose disposal and utilization
- Insulin-mediated uptake into skeletal muscle
- Insulin-mediated vasodilatation in muscle
- Non-insulin-mediated glucose uptake (NIMGU)

NIMGU accounts for 70% of glucose uptake under fasting conditions (primarily into the CNS) and for 50% of post-prandial glucose uptake (especially into skeletal muscle)

Impaired glucose-induced insulin secretion
- Obesity
- Physical inactivity
- Reduced dietary carbohydrate
- Diabetogenic drugs (thiazides, glucocorticoids)

South Asians. Glucose tolerance worsens with age, the main factor being impairment of insulin-stimulated glucose uptake and glycogen synthesis in skeletal muscle; progressive insulin resistance also contributes (Table 6.1). Symptoms of diabetes may be non-specific, vague or absent.

AIMS OF TREATMENT

The management of T2DM and its common comorbidity of cardiovascular disease is complicated because of the added effects of ageing on metabolism and renal function, the use of potentially diabetogenic drugs, and low levels of physical activity. Cardiovascular risk is particularly high because many risk factors of the metabolic syndrome can be present for up to a decade before T2DM is diagnosed. Management strategies for many elderly people with diabetes are the same as those for the younger population, with similar lipid-lowering and antihypertensive treatment schedules, and aspirin or clopidogrel for patients with increased cardiovascular risk. Effective delivery of diabetes care depends on close cooperation between hospital and community, the involvement of diabetes teams and practice nurses, and attention to all causes of disability and ill-health (Table 6.2).

COMORBIDITY

Coexisting cardiovascular and cerebrovascular disease are especially common; polypharmacy is often necessary and carries risks of adverse effects and drug interactions. Degrees of renal impairment, arising for a multiplicity of reasons (e.g. diuretic therapy, prostatic

TABLE 6.2 Special characteristics of older subjects with diabetes
• High level of associated medical comorbidities
• Increased risk of cognitive dysfunction
• Mood disorder
• Varying evidence for impaired activities of daily living and lower limb function
• Increased vulnerability to hypoglycaemia
• Increased risk of inpatient mortality
• Increased need to involve spouses/family and carers in management

obstruction), are relatively common in the elderly population; care must be exercised with renally excreted drugs. In addition, impaired hepatic function (e.g. hepatic congestion secondary to cardiac failure) may render certain antidiabetic medications inappropriate.

The prevalence of hypertension rises with age together with the risk of cardiovascular events. Attention should be directed towards modifiable cardiovascular risk factors, notably hypertension and dyslipidaemia. Cardiovascular events may present with atypical symptoms in the elderly (e.g. acute confusion).

ORAL ANTIDIABETIC AGENTS

Care should be exercised with sulphonylureas because severe hypoglycaemia, although uncommon, carries a relatively high mortality rate. Agents with a short duration of action are preferred.

INSULIN TREATMENT

Although the majority of elderly patients have type 2 diabetes, insulin therapy becomes necessary in a significant proportion as oral agents lose their capacity to provide adequate glycaemic control. Other patients will require insulin because of contraindications to oral agents arising from comorbidity (see above). Avoidance of insulin-induced hypoglycaemia is often paramount for the very elderly and those living alone. Insulin may be appropriately commenced during an intercurrent illness and continued thereafter when oral agents may suffice.

INSTITUTIONAL CARE OF THE ELDERLY DIABETIC

Elderly people with diabetes in care homes are particularly vulnerable and require greater diabetes specialist input. High levels of disability are common in older people with diabetes and lead to heavy usage of health-care resources and premature death. The burden of hospital care is increased 2–3-fold in those with diabetes compared with the general aged population, with more frequent clinic visits and a 5-fold higher admission rate.

About 16% of elderly people with diabetes in the UK are registered blind or partially sighted (8-fold high than in the non-diabetic population); this justifies regular screening for undetected eye disease.

Risk factors for foot ulceration affect 25% of elderly people with type 2 diabetes.

Older people with diabetes use primary care services two to three times more often than their counterparts without diabetes.

Hospital admissions last twice as long for older patients with diabetes compared with age-matched control groups without diabetes.

MANAGEMENT OF DIABETES IN WOMEN OF CHILDBEARING AGE

An optimal outcome may be obtained from pregnancy in women with diabetes if excellent glycaemic control is achieved before and during pregnancy. However, type 1 and 2 diabetes are high-risk states for both the woman and her fetus. There is an increased risk of complications of diabetes, including severe hypoglycaemia and progression of microvascular complications.

 Ketoacidosis must be avoided.

There are also increased risks of obstetric complications, such as miscarriage, maternal infection, pre-eclampsia, premature labour, polyhydramnios and failure to progress in first or second stage. Fetal and neonatal complications include congenital malformation, later intrauterine death, fetal distress, hypoglycaemia, respiratory distress syndrome and jaundice. Rates of fetal and neonatal loss and congenital malformation are increased by at least 2–3-fold. The prevalence of type 2 diabetes is increasing in women of reproductive age, and outcomes may be equivalent or worse than in those with type 1 diabetes. Management before and during pregnancy should follow the same intensive programme of metabolic, obstetric and neonatal supervision.

An experienced multidisciplinary team, led by a named obstetrician and physician with an interest in diabetes, and including a diabetes specialist nurse, diabetes specialist midwife and dietitian, should provide comprehensive care from pre-pregnancy to postnatal review.

PRE-PREGNANCY AND PREGNANCY CARE

Contraception

Contraception should be discussed on an individual basis with all women of childbearing age with diabetes. There is little evidence on choice of contraceptive method specifically for a woman with diabetes. The contraceptive advice should follow that in the general population. The combined oral contraceptive (COC) may be contraindicated in women with diabetes according to the presence and severity of diabetic complications and/or other risk factors for vascular disease. Progestogen-only preparations, oral or intramuscular, are suitable in these women. World Health Organization (WHO) evidence-based guidance for medical eligibility criteria for contraceptive use makes recommendations for women with diabetes.

Long-acting methods such as implants, intrauterine systems (IUS) and copper intrauterine devices (IUD) are safe methods of contraception that may be particularly suitable for use in women with diabetes as they are as effective as sterilization and produce low circulating hormone levels.

Pregnancy should be planned; good contraceptive advice and pre-pregnancy counselling are essential.

Health-care professionals should refer to the WHO medical eligibility criteria for contraceptive use prior to offering contraceptive advice to women with diabetes.

Pre-pregnancy clinic

Attendance at a pre-pregnancy clinic is associated with a reduction in the rate of miscarriage and complications of pregnancy; babies have fewer problems and are kept in special care units for shorter periods than infants of non-attending mothers.

Tip box

Pre-pregnancy care for women with diabetes should be provided by a multidisciplinary team.

The essential components of a pre-pregnancy care programme include review and consideration of the medical (including pharmacological treatment) obstetric and gynaecological history; advice on glycaemic control to optimize HbA1c levels; screening for complications of diabetes; and counselling for maternal and fetal complications.

Tip box

Women contemplating pregnancy should have access to structured education in line with the recommendations for adults for diabetes.

All health-care professionals in contact with women of childbearing age with diabetes should be aware of the importance of pre-pregnancy care and local arrangements for its delivery, and should share this information with the woman.

Pre-pregnancy targets for blood sugar

Observational evidence has found an association between maternal glycaemia (before and during pregnancy) and the increased risk of congenital malformation and miscarriage. The risk of congenital anomaly in the offspring of women with pre-pregnancy diabetes is increased with an increasing level of HbA1c. No HbA1c threshold for such effects has been identified (Table 6.3).

Pre-pregnancy glycaemic control should be maintained as close to the non-diabetic range as possible, taking into account risk of maternal hypoglycaemia.

TABLE 6.3 Derived absolute risk of major or minor congenital anomaly in association with the number of standard deviations (SD) of glycosylated haemoglobin above normal, and the approximate corresponding HbA1c concentration, measured periconceptually

SD of GHb	Corresponding HbA1c		Absolute risk of congenital anomaly (%)
	%	mmol/mol	
0	5.0	31	2.2 (0.0 to 4.4)
2	6.0	42	3.2 (0.4 to 6.1)
4	7.0	53	4.8 (1.0 to 8.6)
6	8.0	64	7.0 (1.7 to 12.3)
8	9.0	75	10.1 (2.3 to 17.8)
10	10.0	86	14.4 (2.8 to 25.9)
≥12	≥11	≥97	20.1 (3.0 to 37.1)

Values in parentheses are 95% confidence intervals. GHb, glycosylated haemoglobin. © ADA 2007. Reprinted with permission.

The target for pre-pregnancy glycaemic control for most women should, as a minimum, be an HbA1c of less than 7% (53 mmol/mol), although lower targets of HbA1c may be appropriate if maternal hypoglycaemia can be minimized.

Oral medication before and during pregnancy

Folic acid

Neural tube defects in high-risk pregnancies are associated with lower levels of folate. All women with diabetes should be prescribed high-dose pre-pregnancy folate supplementation, continuing up to 12 weeks' gestation.

Folic acid 5-mg tablets are readily available, suitable, and should be provided wherever pre-pregnancy care is delivered.

Metformin and sulphonylureas

Metformin and sulphonylureas are not shown to be associated with an increase in congenital malformation or early pregnancy loss. Sulphonylureas other than glibenclamide are unsafe due to placental passage. Recent evidence suggests that metformin may be used in pregnancy (after discussion with patient)-NICE & IDF guidelines.

Statins

The *British National Formulary* recommends that statins (atorvastatin, fluvastatin, pravastatin and simvastatin) should be avoided during pregnancy and lactation. Congenital malformations have been reported and decreased synthesis of cholesterol may further affect fetal development. The malformations include major defects of the central nervous system.

Angiotensin converting enzyme inhibitors

Angiotensin converting enzyme (ACE) inhibitors have been associated with an increased risk of congenital malformation. and both ACE inhibitors and angiotensin receptor blocking medications should be avoided throughout pregnancy.

Tip box

The use of statins, ACE inhibitors and angiotensin receptor blocking medications should be reviewed in women pre-pregnancy, and avoided during pregnancy.

Nutritional management

It is good clinical practice to provide dietary advice to women before, during and after pregnancy.

Advice on diet and exercise should be offered in line with recommendations for adults with diabetes.

Tip box

Dietetic advice should be available in all diabetic antenatal clinics.

Optimization of glycaemic control

Glucose monitoring

Optimal glucose control before pregnancy reduces congenital malformations and miscarriage, while during pregnancy it reduces macrosomia, stillbirth, neonatal hypoglycaemia and respiratory distress syndrome.

All women with pre-gestational diabetes should be encouraged to achieve excellent glycaemic control.

During pregnancy, preprandial testing and where appropriate postprandial testing may be advised. A reduced incidence of pre-eclampsia is associated with postprandial monitoring and targeting.

In women with gestational diabetes, measurement and targeting of postprandial glucose is associated with improved outcomes (including birth weight, reduced perinatal morbidity and macrosomia).

Postprandial glucose monitoring should be carried out in pregnant women with gestational diabetes and may be considered in pregnant women with type 1 or type 2 diabetes.

Tip box

Postprandial glucose monitoring should be carried out in pregnant women with gestational diabetes and should be considered in pregnant women with either type 1 or type 2 diabetes.

In women with type 1 or type 2 diabetes, as long as hypoglycaemia can be minimized, aim to achieve blood glucose:

- between 4 and 6 mmol/L preprandially
- <8 mmol/L 1 hour postprandially, or
- <7 mmol/L 2 hours postprandially
- <6 mmol/L before bed.

There is limited evidence that continuous glucose monitoring may be of benefit to women during pregnancy.

Diabetes specialist nurses and midwives have an important role in educating women on the need for home blood glucose monitoring and intensive insulin regimens. Intensive basal bolus regimens are commonly used and insulin analogues are increasingly used, although research on their role and safety in pregnancy is limited.

Insulin therapy

Intensive insulin therapy is beneficial in terms of maternal and neonatal outcomes. Use of insulin analogues is associated with limited evidence in terms of reduction in hypoglycaemia. The choice of insulin therapy should be discussed as part of pre-pregnancy counselling.

Lispro and aspart are associated with an improved glycaemic profile with a trend towards reduced major hypoglycaemia and nocturnal hypoglycaemia. There is a lack of high-quality evidence regarding outcomes of pregnancy using basal insulin analogue therapy or continuous subcutaneous insulin infusion (CSII) in women who are pregnant. Current evidence also suggests neither benefit nor harm with CSII.

NPH insulin should remain the basal insulin of choice in pregnancy unless the clinical benefit of a basal insulin analogue has been demonstrated on an individual basis. Rapid-acting insulin analogues (lispro and aspart) appear safe in pregnancy and may be considered in individual patients where hypoglycaemia is problematic.

Women should be advised that, although most commonly used regular human insulins are licensed for use during pregnancy, other insulins and oral glucose-lowering agents (e.g. metformin, glibenclamide, other sulphonylureas, detemir) are not.

Complications during pregnancy

Obstetric complications

There is no specific evidence on management of obstetric complications, including pregnancy-induced hypertension and increased risk of thromboembolism, in women with diabetes. These risks should be managed as for other pregnant women.

Metabolic complications

During pregnancy, hypoglycaemic unawareness and severe hypoglycaemia are common. Diabetic ketoacidosis can develop more rapidly, at lower levels of blood glucose and in response to therapeutic glucocorticoids. Women and their partners need education on the management of hypoglycaemia, including the use of glucagon; avoiding hypoglycaemia while driving; and on the recognition and prevention of ketoacidosis. Ketoacidosis may result in fetal death. Local emergency contact arrangements must also be explicit.

Microvascular complications

Diabetic retinal and renal disease can deteriorate during pregnancy. The presence of retinopathy alone is not associated with a poorer pregnancy outcome for the fetus, unless concurrent nephropathy is evident.

Retinopathy

Poor glycaemic control in the first trimester and pregnancy-induced or chronic hypertension are independently associated with the progression of retinopathy.

Nearly 40% of women with baseline retinopathy will progress during pregnancy, although sight-threatening retinopathy is rare (around 2% of pregnancies).

Examination of the retina prior to conception and during each trimester is advised in women with type 1 or type 2 diabetes. More frequent assessment may be required in those with poor glycaemic control, hypertension or pre-existing retinopathy.

Multidisciplinary teams should have locally agreed protocols for the grade of retinopathy required for referral. Owing to the potential for rapid development of neovascularization, early referral of pregnant women with referable retinopathy to an ophthalmologist is recommended.

Parous women with type 1 diabetes have significantly lower levels of retinopathy compared with nulliparous women. Women should be reassured that tight glycaemic control during and immediately after pregnancy can effectively reduce the long-term risk of retinopathy.

Nephropathy

There is an association between pre-existing nephropathy (microalbuminuria or albuminuria) and a poorer pregnancy outcome, although this is not due to any increase in congenital malformations. Proteinuria increases transiently during pregnancy, returning to a pre-pregnancy level within 3 months of delivery. The incidence of worsening chronic hypertension or pregnancy-induced hypertension/pre-eclampsia is high in women with both incipient and overt nephropathy, occurring in over 50% of women where overt nephropathy is present. Nephropathy and superimposed pre-eclampsia are the most common causes of pre-term delivery in women with diabetes.

Women with diabetic nephropathy require careful monitoring and management of blood pressure.

ACE inhibitors and angiotensin receptor blocking medications should be avoided as they may adversely affect the fetus.

Appropriate antihypertensive agents that may be used during pregnancy include methyldopa, labetalol and nifedipine.

Fetal assessment

An early pregnancy scan is considered good practice to confirm viability in women with pre-existing diabetes, particularly when changes in medication are required or diabetic control is suboptimal.

There is evidence of an increased incidence of congenital malformations in women with pre-existing diabetes (type 1 and type 2). In general, the sensitivity of ultrasound scanning for detecting structural abnormalities increase with gestational age. It is not possible to determine when during the second trimester scanning should take place to maximize detection rates. A detailed anomaly scan, including evaluation of the four-chamber heart and outflow tracts, undertaken at around 20 weeks (18–22 weeks) enables detection of many major structural abnormalities.

All women should be offered scanning to include:

- an early viability scan
- a gestational age scan between 11 and 13 weeks (+6 days) in association with biochemical screening and nuchal translucency measurement to risk assess for trisomies
- a detailed anomaly scan including four-chamber cardiac view and outflow tracts between 20 and 22 weeks.

In pregnancies complicated by maternal diabetes, the fetus is at risk of both macrosomia and intrauterine growth restriction (IUGR). The risk of macrosomia is greater when there has been poor glycaemic control. The risk of IUGR is greater in women with vascular complications of diabetes (retinopathy, nephropathy) or when pre-eclampsia develops.

Fetal monitoring includes cardiotocography (CTG), Doppler ultrasonography and ultrasound measurement of fetal growth and liquor volume. Although regular fetal monitoring is common practice, no evidence has been identified on the effectiveness of any single or multiple techniques, and therefore the clinical judgement of an obstetrician experienced in diabetic pregnancy is essential.

When IUGR is suspected, additional monitoring with serial ultrasonography and umbilical arterial Doppler velocimetry is associated with improved outcomes (fewer inductions of labour and hospital admissions, with a trend to improved perinatal mortality rates).

The evidence for the accuracy of ultrasonography in predicting macrosomia (birth weight above 4000 g) is mixed. The accuracy of fetal weight estimation in women with diabetes is at least comparable to that in women who are not diabetic. The negative predictive value of ultrasonography is high (80–96%), and therefore it is feasible that the true value of ultrasonography in the management of these women is its ability to rule out the diagnosis of macrosomia.

There is evidence to suggest that the incorrect diagnosis of a large-for-gestational-age fetus increases the induction and caesarean section rate without improving clinical outcome. Numerous studies have concluded that the reliability of ultrasound estimation of fetal weight is suboptimal. The ability to predict shoulder dystocia in the non-diabetic population is poor and evidence in the diabetic population limited. However, the determination of polyhydramnios is clinically useful as it may be associated with an adverse clinical outcome.

Trials report either equivalent outcomes or improved outcomes (birth weight, macrosomia, large-for-gestational-age infants) in women with gestational diabetes. Improved outcomes were associated with abdominal circumference (AC) being ascertained early (rather than late) in the third trimester and intensively managed thereafter. Where outcomes were equivalent this was achieved with fewer women requiring insulin or a change of treatment assignment. Although the rates of large-for-gestational-age infants were reduced with insulin therapy, there were no immediate clinical benefits observed from this reduction and there was an increase in the caesarean section rate.

Where IUGR is suspected, regular monitoring including growth scans and umbilical artery Doppler monitoring should be carried out.

Gestational diabetes

Gestational diabetes can be defined as carbohydrate intolerance of variable severity with onset or first recognition during pregnancy. This definition will include women with abnormal glucose tolerance that reverts to normal after delivery, those with undiagnosed type 1 or type 2 diabetes, and rarely women with monogenic diabetes. If type 1 or type 2 diabetes is presumed, for example due to early presentation or grossly raised blood glucose levels, urgent action is required to normalize metabolism.

Randomized controlled trials (RCTs) have shown that intervention in women with gestational diabetes with dietary advice, monitoring and management of blood glucose is effective in reducing birth weight, macrosomia, neonatal hypoglycaemia and the rate of large-for-gestational-age infants, as well as perinatal morbidity. More recent RCTs of the detection and management of GDM have found no change in the rate of caesarean section.

Tip box

A suitable programme to detect and treat gestational diabetes should be offered to all women in pregnancy.

The most appropriate strategies for screening and diagnosing GDM remain controversial. There is a continuous relationship between maternal glucose level (fasting, 1 h and 2 h after a 75-g oral glucose tolerance test; OGTT) at 24–28 weeks and pregnancy outcomes (macrosomia, fetal insulin, clinical neonatal hypoglycaemia and caesarean section). Studies showing a benefit of screening-detected GDM have used a variety of strategies.

Screening for GDM

Early pregnancy

An important aim of screening, particularly in early pregnancy, is to identify women with undiagnosed type 2 diabetes. Clinical suspicion that type 1 or type 2 diabetes is present or developing in pregnancy may be raised by persistent heavy glycosuria in pregnancy (2+ on more than two occasions), random glucose > 5.5 mmol/L 2 hours or more after food or ≥7 mmol/L within 2 hours after food.

The International Association of Diabetes and Pregnancy Study Group consensus document suggests that all or high-risk women should be offered screening with HbA1c, fasting or random glucose at the first gestational visit. Although the characteristics of HbA1c in early pregnancy should be close to those outwith pregnancy, it should be noted that normal HbA1c falls in later pregnancy, potentially resulting in false-negative results. Levels of glucose tolerance diagnostic of diabetes (HbA1c ≥6.5% (48 mmol/mol), fasting ≥7.0 mmol/L or 2-h glucose ≥11.1 mmol/L) can be interpreted in early pregnancy, but the clinical interpretation of intermediate levels of glucose tolerance (HbA1c 6.0–6.4% (42–46 mmol/mol), fasting glucose 5.1–6.9 mmol/L, 2-h glucose 7.8–11.0 mmol/L) encompassing current definitions of gestational diabetes, impaired fasting glucose and impaired glucose tolerance remain to be defined.

Later pregnancy

Controversy remains over the best screening strategy for detection of GDM, and the most clinically and cost-effective strategy is likely to vary depending on the population. A number of risk factors can be identified and health economic analysis supports screening of women with risk factors using a 75-g OGTT at 24–28 weeks of gestation. Measurement of fasting glucose provides a good predictor of adverse outcomes.

Strategies to detect previously existing but undetected diabetes in early pregnancy, and strategies to screen for gestational diabetes at 24–28 weeks, will be refined as information on the characteristics of this testing becomes apparent for the local population. Strategies are likely to be simplified for women believed to be at low risk based on risk factors (Table 6.4).

Screening at first antenatal visit

At booking, all women should be assessed for the presence of risk factors for gestational diabetes. All women with risk factors should have HbA1c or fasting glucose levels measured.

Women in early pregnancy with levels of HbA1c $\geq 6.5\%$ (48 mmol/mol), fasting glucose ≥ 7.0 mmol/L or 2-h glucose ≥ 11.1 mmol/L, diagnostic of diabetes, should be treated as having pre-existing diabetes.

Women with intermediate levels of glucose (HbA1c 6.0–6.4% or 42–46 mmol/mol), fasting glucose 5.1–6.9 mmol/L or 2-h glucose 8.6–11.0 mmol/L should be assessed to determine the need for immediate home glucose monitoring and, if the diagnosis remains unclear, assessed for gestational diabetes by a 75-g OGTT at 24–28 weeks.

Screening later in pregnancy

All women with risk factors should have a 75-g OGTT at 24–28 weeks.

Fasting plasma glucose at 24–28 weeks is recommended in low-risk women.

Diagnosis of GDM

There is a continuous relationship between maternal glucose level (fasting, 1 h, 2 h after a 75-g OGTT) and fetal growth.

Appropriate RCTs are not available to guide decision-making regarding the level of glucose at which different health benefits

---

TABLE 6.4 Risk factors for gestational diabetes

BMI > 30 kg/m^2
Previous macrosomic baby weighing 4.5 kg or more
Previous gestational diabetes
Family history of diabetes (first-degree relative with diabetes)
Family origin with a high prevalence of diabetes:
- South Asian (specifically women whose country of family origin is India, Pakistan or Bangladesh)
- Black Caribbean
- Middle Eastern (specifically women whose country of family origin is Saudi Arabia, United Arab Emirates, Iraq, Jordan, Syria, Oman, Qatar, Kuwait, Lebanon or Egypt)

TABLE 6.5 Screening for and diagnosis of GDM

- Perform a 75-g OGTT, with plasma glucose measurement fasting and at 1 and 2 h, at 24–28 weeks of gestation in women not previously diagnosed with overt diabetes.
- The OGTT should be performed in the morning after an overnight fast of at least 8 h.
- The diagnosis of GDM is made when any of the following plasma glucose values are exceeded:
  - Fasting >92 mg/dL (5.1 mmol/L)
  - 1 h >180 mg/dL (10.0 mmol/L)
  - 2 h >153 mg/dL (8.5 mmol/L)

OGTT, oral glucose tolerance test; GDM, gestational diabetes mellitus.

---

accrue. It is suggested that criteria are set at a level where there is an impact not only on birth weight but also on other outcomes, including shoulder dystocia and caesarean section.

A recent international consensus suggested criteria that result in a diagnosis of gestational diabetes in 16–18% of the pregnant population, where all women are tested with a 75-g OGTT. Women diagnosed using these criteria have a 1.75-fold increased risk of macrosomia. It is suggested that these international consensus criteria be adopted.

Depending on individual clinical circumstance, it is accepted that dietary intervention in women with lower glucose levels (2-h glucose 7.8–8.5 mmol/L) may help to reduce birth weight, and dietary advice and intervention on an individual basis might be considered (for example, in previous macrosomia or previous complicated delivery).

The adoption of internationally agreed criteria for gestational diabetes using the 75-g OGTT is recommended (Table 6.5):

- when fasting venous plasma glucose ≥ 5.1 mmol/L
- when 1-hour glucose is ≥ 10 mmol/L, or
- 2 hours after OGTT ≥ 8.5 mmol/L.

Women with frank diabetes by non-pregnant criteria (fasting venous glucose ≥ 7 mmol/L, 2-h glucose ≥ 11.1 mmol/L) should be managed within a multidisciplinary clinic as they may have type 1 or type 2 diabetes and be at risk of pregnancy outcomes similar to those of women with pre-gestational diabetes.

Management of GDM

Management with dietary change to lower blood glucose levels and, if necessary, treatment with insulin improves outcomes in gestational diabetes. Glycaemic management should be tailored to control preprandial and postprandial blood sugar levels. The majority of women with gestational diabetes can be managed with dietary therapy alone. If, after nutritional advice, preprandial and postprandial glucose levels are normal and there is no evidence of excessive fetal growth, the pregnancy can be managed as for a normal pregnancy.

Controlled trials suggested that management strategies using metformin or glibenclamide can achieve similar outcomes to initial management with insulin, although 20–40% of women will still eventually require insulin therapy. Metformin crosses the placenta and glibenclamide appears not to.

If blood glucose levels are in the range for established diabetes, intensive specialist management and initial therapy with insulin is required.

Pregnant women with GDM should be offered dietary advice and blood glucose monitoring, and treated with glucose-lowering therapy depending on fasting and postprandial targets.

Glucose-lowering therapy should be considered in addition to diet where fasting or 2-hour glucose levels are above target, for example where two or more values per fortnight are:

- ≥ 5.5 mmol/L preprandially or ≥ 7 mmol/L 2 h postprandially on monitoring at ≤ 35 weeks
- ≥ 5.5 mmol/L preprandially or ≥ 8 mmol/L 2 h postprandially on monitoring at > 35 weeks, or
- any postprandial value > 9 mmol/L.

After discussion with the patient, metformin should be considered as the initial pharmacological glucose-lowering treatment in women with gestational diabetes.

DELIVERY

The timing of delivery should be determined on an individual basis. Delivery in women with diabetes is generally expedited within 40 weeks of gestation. However, no clear evidence has been identified to inform the optimal timing for delivery.

Women who are at risk of pre-term delivery should receive antenatal corticosteroids. If corticosteroids are indicated clinically for pre-term labour, supervision by an experienced team is essential to regulate diabetic control.

Women with diabetes have a higher rate of caesarean section even after controlling for confounding factors.

Women with diabetes requiring insulin or oral glucose-lowering medication who have a pregnancy that is otherwise progressing normally should be assessed at 38 weeks' gestation with delivery shortly afterwards, and certainly by 40 weeks.

Women with diabetes should be delivered in consultant-led maternity units under the combined care of a physician with an interest in diabetes, obstetrician and neonatologist.

Women with diabetes should have a mutually agreed written plan for insulin management at the time of delivery and immediately afterwards.

The progress of labour should be monitored as for other high-risk women, including continuous electronic fetal monitoring.

IV insulin and dextrose should be administered as necessary to maintain blood glucose levels between 4 and 7 mmol/L.

INFANTS OF MOTHERS WITH DIABETES

Labour and delivery should be undertaken only in a maternity unit supported by neonatal intensive care facilities. There is no need for routine admission of the infant to the neonatal unit. There is insufficient evidence on the preferred method of cotside blood glucose measurement in neonates; however, whichever method is used, the glucose values should be confirmed by laboratory measurement. Neonatal hypoglycaemia is defined as a blood glucose level < 2.6 mmol/L, and is associated with adverse short- and long-term neurodevelopmental outcomes.

Neonatal hypoglycaemia has been associated with adverse neurodevelopmental outcomes and impaired cognitive development.

In pre-term infants, significant hypoglycaemia (< 2.6 mmol/L) is associated with reductions in Bayley motor and developmental scores of 13 and 14 points, respectively, at 18 months' corrected age. An association between recurrent exposure to hypoglycaemia and a 3.5-fold increase in the incidence of cerebral palsy and developmental delay in infants was also found. Recurrent episodes of blood glucose < 2.6 mmol/L in small-for-gestational-age (SGA) pre-term infants were associated with measurable neurodevelopmental deficits affecting fine motor ability and perceptual performance that were still apparent at 5 years of age. Repeated episodes of hypoglycaemia have also been shown to produce a reduction in occipitofrontal circumference, a surrogate marker of brain growth, at 12, 18 and 60 months of age.

Tip box

Early feeding is advised to avoid neonatal hypoglycaemia and to stimulate lactation.

Glycaemic control at 6 weeks in women with type 1 diabetes who exclusively breastfeed their babies has been found to be significantly better that those who bottlefeed. There are further well-documented health benefits for infants who are breastfed. Although breastfeeding is recommended for infants of mothers with diabetes, mothers should be supported in the feeding method of their choice.

Most medicines are not licensed for use in lactation. Specialist reference sources provide information on suitability of medicines in breastfeeding. Insulin, metformin and glibenclamide are considered compatible with breastfeeding, although the infant should be observed for signs of hypoglycaemia. The antihypertensives commonly used in pregnancy (labetalol, nifedipine and methyldopa) are found in breast milk in low concentration and these agents are considered appropriate for use in breastfeeding mothers, although with labetalol the infant should be monitored for bradycardia and hypotension. Of the ACE inhibitors, enalapril and captopril are considered safer. There is no information available on angiotensin-II receptor antagonists. Statins are not recommended when breastfeeding. Information on use of aspirin is conflicting, with some sources advising that low-dose aspirin is safe in breastfeeding, whereas others advise cautious use owing to potential for toxicity (possible Reye syndrome).

Specialist advice should be sought if the baby is premature or unwell.

POSTNATAL CARE

Women with type 1 or type 2 diabetes may require adjustment of their treatment regimen postnatally. Women with gestational diabetes should be investigated postnatally to clarify the diagnosis and exclude type 1 or type 2 diabetes. The opportunity should also be taken to provide lifestyle advice to reduce the risk of subsequent type 2 diabetes.

Postnatal follow-up should be seen as an opportunity to initiate pre-pregnancy care for any subsequent pregnancy. Appropriate contraception should be provided and the importance of good glycaemic control emphasized.

Breastfeeding should be encouraged to benefit mother and baby, but it may necessitate insulin dose adjustment and a dietetic review.

FOLLOW-UP OF WOMEN WITH GESTATIONAL DIABETES

A diagnosis of GDM identifies women at increased risk of developing type 2 diabetes in future. Rates of progression to type 2 diabetes in women with previous GDM vary widely (between 15%

and 50% cumulative incidence at 5 years) and will be influenced by other risk factors such as ethnicity, obesity and exercise.

A Cochrane review concluded that diet combined with exercise or diet alone enhances weight loss postpartum. Both intensive lifestyle and pharmacological interventions reduce the onset of type 2 diabetes in people with impaired glucose tolerance, including women with previous gestational diabetes.

> **Tip box**
> Women who have developed GDM should be given diet, weight control and exercise advice.

There is no robust evidence to determine when follow-up testing should be carried out. Women who have developed GDM should also be reminded of the need for pre-conception counselling and appropriate testing to detect progression to type 2 diabetes.

Where diabetes is not apparent immediately after delivery, glucose tolerance should be reassessed at least 6 weeks postpartum with a minimum of fasting glucose and with a 75-g OGTT if clinically indicated.

An annual assessment of glycaemia using fasting glucose or HbA1c should be carried out thereafter.

A checklist for provision of information to women with GDM can be found in Appendix 6.2.

SURGERY AND DIABETES

Careful attention needs to be paid to the metabolic status of people with diabetes undergoing surgical procedures. Elective surgery in people with uncontrolled diabetes should preferably be scheduled after acceptable glycaemic control has been achieved. Admission to hospital 1–2 days before scheduled surgery is advisable for such patients. Whenever feasible, emergency surgery should be delayed to allow stabilization of diabetic patients. In addition, to avoid protracted fasting, the operation should be scheduled for early in the day.

Patients with diabetes have an increased requirement for surgical procedures and increased postoperative morbidity and mortality rates.

The stress response to surgery and the resultant hyperglycaemia, osmotic diuresis and hypoinsulinaemia can lead to perioperative ketoacidosis or hyperosmolar non-ketotic (HONK) syndrome (hyperglycaemic hyperosmolar state (HHS)).

The management goal is to optimize metabolic control through close monitoring, adequate fluid and the judicious use of insulin.

Major surgical operations require a period of fasting during which oral antidiabetic medications cannot be used.

The stress of surgery itself results in metabolic perturbations that alter glucose homeostasis; persistent hyperglycaemia is a risk factor for endothelial dysfunction, postoperative sepsis, impaired wound healing and cerebral ischaemia.

The stress response itself may precipitate diabetic crises (DKA, HONK syndrome) during surgery or postoperatively, with negative prognostic consequences. HHS is a well-known postoperative complication following certain procedures, including cardiac bypass surgery, where it is associated with a greater than 40% mortality rate.

The actual treatment recommendations for a given patient should be individualized. However, the recommendations should be based on:

- diabetes classification
- usual diabetes regimen
- state of glycaemic control
- nature and extent of the surgical procedure.

In addition, gastrointestinal instability provoked by anaesthesia, medications and stress-related vagal overlay can lead to nausea, vomiting and dehydration. This compounds the volume contraction that may already be present from the osmotic diuresis induced by hyperglycaemia, thereby increasing the risk of ischaemic events and acute renal failure. Subtle to gross deficits in key electrolytes (principally potassium, but also magnesium) may pose an arrhythmogenic risk, which often is superimposed on a milieu of endemic coronary artery disease in middle-aged or older people with diabetes.

Anaesthesia and surgery cause a stereotypical metabolic stress response, which could overwhelm homeostatic mechanisms in patients with pre-existing abnormalities of glucose metabolism. The features of the metabolic stress response include release of the catabolic hormones:

- adrenaline (epinephrine)
- noradrenaline (norepinephrine)
- cortisol
- glucagon
- growth hormone
- plus the inhibition of insulin secretion and action.

ANTI-INSULIN EFFECTS OF SURGICAL STRESS

In addition to insulin resistance induced by circulating stress hormones, surgical stress has a deleterious effect on pancreatic β-cell functions. Plasma insulin levels fall and insulin secretory responses to glucose become impaired during surgery.

These anti-insulin effects of the metabolic stress response essentially reverse the physiological anabolic and anti-catabolic actions of insulin. The important anabolic actions of insulin that may be reversed or attenuated during the stress of surgery include:

- stimulation of glucose uptake and glycogen storage
- stimulation of amino acid uptake and protein synthesis by skeletal muscle
- stimulation of fatty acid synthesis in the liver and storage in adipocytes
- renal sodium reabsorption and intravascular volume preservation.

The anti-catabolic effects of insulin include:

- inhibition of hepatic glycogen breakdown
- inhibition of gluconeogenesis
- inhibition of lipolysis
- inhibition of fatty acid oxidation and ketone body formation
- inhibition of proteolysis and amino acid oxidation.

DIRECT CATABOLIC EFFECTS OF STRESS HORMONES

The neuroendocrine response to the stress of general anaesthesia and surgery leads to activation of potent counter-regulatory hormones. The catecholamine noradrenaline (norepinephrine) is augmented mostly during surgery, whereas after surgery adrenaline (epinephrine) stimulates gluconeogenesis and glycogenolysis. Catecholamines also inhibit glucose utilization by peripheral tissues and inhibit insulin secretion.

These effects predispose to severe hyperglycaemia, which is further exacerbated by the stimulatory effect of adrenaline and noradrenaline on glucagon secretion. Other catabolic effects of catecholamines include stimulation of lipolysis and ketogenesis. The activated hormone-sensitive lipase promotes lipolysis and release of free fatty acids into the circulation.

Glucagon, the level of which is augmented by catecholamines, exerts catabolic effects similar to those of the catecholamines: stimulation of hepatic glucose production and ketogenesis, and inhibition of insulin action in peripheral tissues. Growth hormone and glucocorticoids potentiate the catabolic effects of catecholamines and glucagon. Glucocorticoids increase hepatic glucose production and induce lipolysis and negative nitrogen balance by stimulating proteolysis. The products of lipolysis and proteolysis provide substrates for increased gluconeogenesis by the liver.

APPROACHES TO MANAGEMENT

Operationally, all patients with type 1 diabetes undergoing minor or major surgery and patients with type 2 diabetes undergoing major surgery are considered appropriate candidates for intensive perioperative diabetes management. The management approach in these categories of patients always includes insulin therapy in combination with dextrose and potassium infusion.

The aims of perioperative management are:

- to avoid hypoglycaemia particularly during anaesthesia
- to avoid excess metabolic decompensation
- to achieve a locally agreed care pathway with which health professionals are familiar.

Tip box

Major surgery is defined as one requiring general anaesthesia of ≥ 1 h.

Patients managed by diet alone

People whose diabetes is well controlled by a regimen of dietary modification and physical activity may require no special preoperative intervention for diabetes. The fasting blood glucose level should be measured on the morning of surgery and intraoperative blood glucose monitoring is desirable if the surgical procedure is lengthy (> 1 h). If surgery is minor, no specific therapy is required. If surgery is major or if diabetes is poorly controlled (blood glucose ≥ 11 mmol/L), an IV infusion of insulin and dextrose should be considered (see below) and hourly intraoperative glucose monitoring is recommended.

Patients treated with oral antidiabetic agents

Second-generation sulphonylureas (gliclazide, glipizide and glibenclamide) should be discontinued 1 day before surgery. Other oral agents can be continued until the day of surgery. Although metformin has a short half-life of about 6 h, it is sensible to withhold therapy for 1–2 days before surgery, especially in sick patients and those undergoing procedures that increase the risk of renal hypoperfusion, tissue hypoxia and possible lactate accumulation.

At a minimum, blood glucose should be monitored before and immediately after surgery in all patients. Those undergoing extensive procedures should have hourly glucose monitoring during and immediately after surgery. Bedside capillary blood glucose meters are adequate for these monitoring requirements. However, extremely high or low values should be repeated immediately before instituting remedial action, and a simultaneous blood specimen should be sent for laboratory corroboration.

Patients treated with oral antidiabetic agents

Second-generation sulphonylureas (gliclazide, glipizide, glibenclamide) should be discontinued 1 day before surgery. Other oral agents can be continued until the day of surgery. Although metformin has a short half-life of about 6 h, it is prudent temporarily to withhold therapy 1–2 days before surgery, especially in sick patients and those undergoing procedures that increase the risk of renal hypoperfusion, tissue hypoxia and lactate accumulation.

At a minimum, blood glucose should be monitored before and immediately after surgery. Those undergoing extensive procedures should have hourly glucose monitoring during and immediately after surgery. Bedside capillary blood glucose meters are adequate for these monitoring requirements. However, extremely high or low values should be repeated immediately and a simultaneous blood specimen should be sent for laboratory corroboration before instituting remedial action.

For minor surgery, perioperative hyperglycaemia (>11 mmol/L) can be managed with small subcutaneous doses (4–10 units) of short-acting insulin. Care must be taken to avoid hypoglycaemia. After minor procedures, most usual antidiabetic medications can be restarted once the patient starts eating. In patients treated with metformin, the drug should be withheld for about 72 h after surgery or iodinated radiocontrast procedures. Metformin therapy can be restarted after documentation of normal renal function and absence of contrast-induced nephropathy. The recommended treatment for patients undergoing major surgery and for those with poorly controlled type 2 diabetes is IV insulin infusion, with glucose, using one of two standard regimens.

Insulin-treated patients

Minor surgery

Patients treated with long-acting insulin (e.g. glargine, detemir) should be switched to intermediate-acting forms before elective surgery. Close perioperative blood glucose monitoring is crucial to avoid extremes of glycaemia. IV insulin–glucose–potassium should be commenced before surgery. Blood glucose levels should be monitored hourly during and immediately after surgery. The infusion should be stopped and usual insulin treatment resumed once oral intake is established. There should be a 1-h overlap between stopping IV insulin and reinstituting subcutaneous insulin.

Major surgery

Insulin-treated patients undergoing major elective surgery should preferably be admitted 2–3 days before surgery, if glycaemic control is suboptimal (HbA1c > 8%). If admission is not feasible, a diabetes specialist nurse should work with the patient to optimize self-monitoring of blood glucose (SMBG) values in the days. SMBG should be performed at least before each meal and also at bedtime, with target preprandial values of 80–120 mg/dL and bedtime values of 100–140 mg/dL.

The preoperative evaluation should include a thorough physical examination (with particular focus on autonomic neuropathy and cardiac status), measurement of serum electrolytes and creatinine and urine ketones. The presence of autonomic neuropathy mandates increased surveillance for hypotension, respiratory arrest and haemodynamic instability during surgery. Gross metabolic and electrolyte abnormalities (e.g. hyponatraemia, dyskalaemia, acidosis) should also be corrected before surgery.

Insulin

Several reports have emphasized the advantages of the insulin infusion regimen over subcutaneous delivery.

Two main methods of insulin delivery have been used:

● combining insulin with glucose and potassium in the same bag (the GKI regimen)
● delivering insulin separately with an infusion pump.

The combined GKI infusion is efficient, safe and effective in many patients but does not permit selective adjustment of insulin delivery without changing the bag. The glucose component can be either 5% or 10% dextrose. The latter provides more calories.

Regardless of whether separate or combined infusions are given, close monitoring is required to avoid catastrophe during these infusion regimens. A sample regimen for separate insulin infusion is indicated below.

Blood glucose level (mmol/L)	Infusion rate (units/h)
<4	0
4.1–7.0	1
7.1–11.0	2
11.1–17.0	3
17.1–22.0	4
>22	5
Check capillary blood glucose level hourly initially and then 2 hourly.	

These recommendations must be interpreted flexibly, given the individual variability in insulin requirements and metabolic profiles. In the absence of strict evidence-based guidelines, the consensus approach is to avoid extremes of glycaemia (aiming for 120–180 mg/dL) and to tailor therapies to individual patients based on feedback from glucose monitoring.

The initial infusion rate can be estimated as between one-half and three-quarters of the patient's total daily insulin dose, expressed as units per hour. Regular insulin, 0.5–1 units/h, is an appropriate starting dose for most type 1 diabetic patients. Patients treated with oral antidiabetic agents who require perioperative insulin infusion, as well as insulin-treated type 2 diabetic patients, can be given an initial infusion rate of 1–2 units/h.

An infusion rate of 1 unit/h is obtained by mixing 25 units of regular insulin in 250 mL saline (0.1 unit/mL) and infusing at a rate of 10 mL/h. Alternatively, 50 units of regular insulin is made up to 50 mL with saline and given by syringe pump at 1–2 mL/h. Adjustments to the insulin infusion rate are made to maintain blood glucose between 120 and 180 mg/dL.

The duration of insulin (and dextrose) infusions depends on the clinical status of the patient. The infusions should be continued postoperatively until oral intake is established, after which the usual diabetes treatment can be resumed. It is prudent to give the first subcutaneous dose of insulin 30–60 min before disconnecting the IV line.

Glucose

Adequate fluids must be administered to maintain intravascular volume. Fluid deficits from osmotic diuresis in poorly controlled diabetes can be considerable. The preferred fluids are normal saline and dextrose in water. Fluids containing lactate (i.e. Ringer's lactate, Hartmann's solution) cause exacerbation of hyperglycaemia.

Adequate glucose should be provided to prevent:

- catabolism
- starvation
- ketosis
- insulin-induced hypoglycaemia.

The physiological amount of glucose required to prevent catabolism in an average non-diabetic adult is approximately 120 g/day (or 5 g/h). With preoperative fasting, surgical stress and ongoing insulin therapy the caloric requirement in most diabetic patients averages 5–10 g/h glucose. This can be given as 5% or 10% dextrose. An infusion rate of 100 mL/h with 5% dextrose delivers 5 g/h glucose.

The usual range of perioperative blood glucose that clinicians are comfortable with is about 6.5–10 mmol/L. The insulin and glucose infusion rates should be adjusted accordingly. Insulin requirements are higher in:

- patients with sepsis
- obese patients
- unstable patients
- patients treated with steroids
- patients undergoing cardiopulmonary bypass surgery.

Potassium
The infusion of insulin and glucose induces an intracellular translocation of potassium, resulting in a risk of hypokalaemia. If renal function is normal and the patient has initially normal serum potassium, potassium chloride (10 mmol/L) should be added routinely to each 500 mL dextrose to maintain normokalaemia. Hyperkalaemia (confirmed with repeat measurement and electrocardiogram) plus renal insufficiency are contraindications to potassium infusion.

Emergency surgery

Unfortunately, many patients who require emergency surgery will have suboptimal glycaemic control. However, this is not necessarily a contraindication to undertaking potentially life-saving surgery. IV access should be secured and immediate blood specimens sent for glucose, electrolyte and acid–base assessment. Gross derangements of volume and electrolytes (e.g. hypokalaemia, hypernatraemia) should be corrected.

Surgery should be delayed, whenever feasible, in patients with DKA, so that the underlying acid–base disorder can be corrected or, at least, ameliorated. Patients with HHS are markedly dehydrated and should be restored quickly to good volume and improved metabolic status before surgery. Blood glucose should be monitored hourly at the bedside, and insulin, glucose and potassium infusion should be administered, as appropriate, to maintain blood glucose in the 6.5–10 mmol/L range. Serum potassium should be checked frequently (every 2–4 h) and potassium supplementation should be adjusted to ensure that the patient remains eukalaemic throughout surgery and postoperatively.

The initial evaluation of a diabetic patient with a suspected surgical emergency must include a thorough medical history and physical examination. Particular care must be taken to exclude DKA and other conditions that are likely to be mistaken for surgical emergencies. For example, patients with DKA and prominent abdominal symptoms have undergone needless surgical exploration for a non-existent acute abdominal emergency. Functional syndromes due to diabetic autonomic neuropathy of the gastrointestinal tract (gastroparesis, gastroenteropathy, intractable or cyclical vomiting) may mimic anatomical surgical emergencies. Similarly, the rare diabetic pseudotabes syndrome, characterized by sharp neuropathic pain along thoracolumbar dermatomes, can be confused with visceral disorders. Patients with pseudotabes typically have pupillary and gait abnormalities from associated cranial and peripheral neuropathy.

The glucose–potassium–insulin (GKI) regimen in adults (≥ 16 years of age)

The GKI regimen should be considered in the following situations:

- patients with insulin-requiring diabetes who need surgery
- patients with type 2 diabetes who need major surgery
- patients with poorly controlled type 2 diabetes who require surgery
- patients with insulin-requiring diabetes who need to fast for procedures (e.g. endoscopy or radiology procedures)
- patients with diabetes who are unable to eat or are nil by mouth (e.g. vomiting due to autonomic neuropathy)
- patients in the later stages of treatment for DKA.

The following regimen will work only if the initial blood glucose level is approximately in the target range of 6–11 mmol/L. If the initial blood glucose is greatly in excess of this range then IV insulin by infusion pump should be given at a rate of 6 units/h, with half-hourly monitoring of glucometer readings, until blood glucose level is less than 15 mmol/L.

Instructions

1. No subcutaneous insulin to be given on morning of operation or procedure.
2. Prior to setting up the GKI infusion, *send blood to the laboratory* for urgent glucose and urea and electrolytes and glucose estimation (use an emergency form).
3. Set up the GKI infusion at 8 a.m.:

500 mL 10% glucose with 10 mmol KCl (10% glucose and 0.15% potassium chloride IV infusion BP) *plus* 15 units Actrapid insulin added to bag and mixed well	**To be administered over 5 hours (100 ml/h)**

The giving set should be run through with 20–30 mL of the GKI mixture before being connected to the patient.

4. The glucose and insulin infusion must be continued, regardless of whether other IV fluids are required.
5. Subsequent adjustment of the insulin regimen should be as follows:

Blood glucose result	Action
6–11 mmol/L	**Continue** infusion as above
>11 mmol/L	**Increase** insulin concentration by discarding original bag and making up a new bag with 20 units Actrapid added
<6 mmol/L	**Decrease** the insulin concentration by discarding original bag and making up a new bag with 10 units Actrapid added

See Section 2, page 87 on adjustment of insulin dose if further dosage change becomes necessary.

Frequency of glucose monitoring:

- In theatre and recovery area: as decided by the anaesthetist
- Thereafter:
  - immediately on return to ward
  - 2 h and 4 h after return to ward
  - then every 2–4 h
  - once blood glucose level is stable, every 4 h.
- *At least* two blood glucose measurements during 24 h must be sent to the laboratory.

Urea and electrolytes should be measured on return from theatre and thereafter once daily. If the patient is on a GKI regimen for more than 24 h, ensure that 0.9% sodium chloride is also given to avoid hyponatraemia. If the potassium replacement requires adjustment on the basis of urea and electrolytes testing, do this by altering the potassium content of other IV fluids, such as sodium chloride 0.9%. *Do not* adjust the potassium content of the GKI.

Infusion should continue whilst light diet is started. Once the patient is eating reliably, subcutaneous insulin can be restarted. The glucose–insulin infusion should not be stopped until *1 hour after* the first subcutaneous injection.

Adjustment of insulin dose in GKI regimen

In clinical trials, 80% of truly insulin-dependent diabetics undergoing surgery were controlled within the target limits of blood glucose using a regimen starting with 15 units insulin per 500-mL bag of 10% glucose with 10 mmol KCl and adjusted if necessary within the following limits:

- Measure blood glucose every 2 h initially – frequency of monitoring is variable and depends on the clinical situation; levels can usually be measured less frequently as time progresses.
- Adjust infusion as follows: continue to adjust in 5 units insulin per 500 mL glucose 10% with 10 mmol KCl (1 unit insulin per h) increments/decrements as necessary. However, if moving outwith the range of 10–20 units insulin/500 mL (2–4 units/h) *consider the factors listed below before making change.*

Blood glucose result	Action
6–11 mmol/L	**Continue** usual GKI regimen: 15 units per 500 mL 10% glucose (3 units/h)
>11 mmol/L	**Increase** to 20 units per 500 mL 10% glucose (4 units/h)
<6 mmol/L	**Decrease** to 10 units per 500 mL 10% glucose (2 units/h)

Where target blood glucose levels are not achieved using the above algorithm, consider:

1. The GKI regimen assumes that metabolism is in a steady state. It will work only if the *initial* blood glucose level was in the target range. It should not be used for patients who are severely hyperglycaemic at the onset (when a separate insulin infusion is better suited), or when they have started to eat again. If the initial

blood glucose level is outwith the target range, appropriate measures must be taken to bring it within the range before using the GKI regimen.

2. Check that the IV cannula (Venflon) is patent and functioning, and consider that the GKI solution may have been constituted incorrectly.

3. *The constant infusion of glucose at the rate specified is an essential part of the regimen.* The insulin regimen cannot be applied when an infusion fluid other than 10% or 5% glucose administered over 5 h is being used (although additional 0.9% sodium chloride can be infused at the same time as 10% glucose when required).

4. In the following situations, altered insulin requirement is likely to occur:

Condition	Insulin requirement
Patients with subcutaneous insulin requirement <30 units per day; thin elderly type 2 diabetics	May require reduced insulin – start at 10 units per 500-mL bag 10% glucose and 0.15% KCl IV infusion (2 units/h)
Obesity	May require increased insulin – start at 15 units per 500-mL bag 10% glucose and 0.15% KCl IV infusion (3 units/h), but be aware of possibility of increased requirement
Severe infection	May require increased insulin – may need as much as 25–40 units per 500-mL bag 10% glucose and 0.15% KCl IV infusion (5–8 units/h), or more
Any severe illness, infusion of catecholamines or inotropes	Often marked increase in insulin requirement – consider using infusion pump for insulin rather than adding to bag of glucose. Insulin infusion requirement of $\geq$6–12 units/h possible. More frequent monitoring and adjustment required
Steroid therapy	May require increased insulin

5. Insulin-dependent diabetics never require no insulin (other than very transiently). The half-life of IV insulin is approximately 4 min, and that of its biological effect approximately 20 min. The presence of an apparently zero insulin requirement therefore implies a tissue depot of insulin, such as a recent subcutaneous administration of insulin, or persistence of a depot of long-acting insulin (e.g. Lantus®).

6. Check daily for dilutional hyponatraemia.

'Sliding scales' with wide doses ranging from zero to high infusion rates (as published in some clinical handbooks):

- risk 'roller-coastering' – wild fluctuations in blood glucose levels with over-frequent adjustments in dosage
- frequently 'work' satisfactorily by good fortune when they are employed in the middle of their dose range.

It is therefore better to use the GKI dosage algorithm and, where dosages lie outside the algorithm limits, bracket the patient's requirements as in the notes above.

Sliding-scale intravenous regimen

Add 50 units soluble insulin (Actrapid or Humulin S) to 50 mL 0.9% saline in a 50-mL syringe. Infuse IV using a pump and adjust according to the sliding scale. Sliding-scale regimens need to be re-evaluated frequently as insulin dosages need to be adjusted to achieve target glycaemic control.

 If blood glucose IS regularly outwith the range of 6–12 mmol/L, insulin doses should be reassessed and the diabetes/medical team contacted.

INTERCURRENT ILLNESSES

TYPE 1 DIABETES: SICK-DAY RULES

As people with type 1 diabetes are at risk of developing DKA, it is important to take action at the earliest possible sign of any form of illness such as a cold, infection or virus. Regular monitoring of blood glucose levels is advised and insulin doses may need to be increased if necessary. Those with type 1 diabetes are also advised to check for the presence of ketones.

How can I test for ketones?

It is possible to check for ketones in the urine or blood. The ketones build up in the bloodstream and spill over into the urine causing 'ketonuria', which can be detected by dipping a test strip in the urine and reading the colour. The test strips are available on prescription.

Many people with type 1 diabetes can benefit from measuring blood ketones using a special meter that can detect levels of ketones in the blood. It is advisable to contact a diabetes nurse or doctor for further advice on this method of testing for ketones. Again, the strips are available on prescription.

People with type 1 diabetes should test their urine or blood for ketones if their blood glucose levels are high (usually over 14 mmol/L) or if they are developing symptoms of ketoacidosis. DKA or ketoacidosis can develop and progress quickly. Treatment for advanced DKA may require admission to hospital. However, it is possible to prevent ketoacidosis by recognizing the warning signs, checking the urine and blood regularly for ketones and glucose, and treating with extra insulin.

What action should be taken if blood glucose levels are high?

Guidelines

Guidelines for extra insulin to treat hyperglycaemia or raised ketones depend upon the total daily dose of insulin taken by the individual. This can be calculated by adding together all the long- and short-acting insulin taken over 24 hours. The table below provides guidance for people with type 1 diabetes who are having four or more injections a day (known as the basal-bolus or basal-prandial regimen).

What action should be taken for a positive ketone test?
- Take extra rapid-acting insulin as soon as possible (see table above).
- Drink plenty of water and unsweetened fluids.
- Test blood glucose every 1–2 h and repeat the extra insulin (see table above) until blood/urine is negative to ketones.
- Try to identify cause of high blood glucose level and seek treatment if necessary.
- Contact diabetes team if high glucose and ketone levels persist.
- Contact GP/accident and emergency department if you are vomiting, as dehydration may occur.
- Continue with the usual amount of background insulin.

REMEMBER – drink at least a cupful of unsweetened fluid every 15 min (about 500 mL per hour) while blood glucose levels are high.
ALWAYS – take insulin during times of illness.

BARIATRIC SURGERY

EFFICACY OF WEIGHT LOSS HEALTH OUTCOMES

Bariatric surgery is an effective weight loss intervention. Patients with a body mass index (BMI) ≥ 35 kg/m^2 receiving bariatric surgery (laparoscopic banding, biliopancreatic diversion $\pm$ Roux-en-Y gastric bypass) will lose between 50% and 80% excess weight at 10 years postsurgery. Laparoscopic adjustable banding in diabetic patients with a BMI >35 kg/m^2 results in greater excess weight loss at 2 years compared with intensive diet, lifestyle and medical therapy (87.2% versus 21.8%, respectively; $P < 0.001$).

The overall mortality rate is 29–40% lower 7–10 years after bariatric surgery (adjustable or non-adjustable gastric banding, vertical banded gastroplasty or gastric bypass) compared with that in BMI-matched subjects not having surgery. More than 70% of recently diagnosed type 2 diabetic patients (less than 2 years since diagnosis) undergoing bariatric surgery with adjustable gastric banding are likely to go into remission with reduction of other cardiovascular risk factors, compared with 10% of the control group (where the focus is on weight loss by lifestyle change). Surgical and control/lifestyle groups lose approximately 20% and 2% of their weight, respectively, at 2 years, with no serious complications in either group. Remission of diabetes appears to be related to the degree of weight loss and lower baseline HbA1c levels. There is also a significantly higher level of withdrawal of diabetic medications following surgery.

Rates of many adverse maternal (e.g. gestational diabetes and pre-eclampsia) and neonatal (e.g. macrosomia and low birth weight) outcomes are lower in women who become pregnant after having had bariatric surgery, compared with rates in pregnant women who are obese.

There are greater improvements at 10 years in current health perceptions, social interactions, obesity-related problems and depression in patients who had bariatric surgery compared with those having the best available medical weight management. However, individuals who chose to have bariatric surgery had worse health-related quality-of-life scores at baseline.

There is a significantly higher mortality rate from non-disease causes (accidents, poisoning, and suicide) at 10 years postsurgery in patients receiving bariatric surgery compared with severely obese individuals from the general population. The reasons are not clear, although the individuals who seek bariatric surgery have differing baseline psychological status (e.g. increased anxiety levels) than those with similar obesity levels who do not seek surgery.

FACTORS INFLUENCING THE EFFICACY OF SURGERY

Predictors of efficacy of bariatric surgery, particularly laparoscopic adjustable gastric banding, include lower age of patient, lower BMI and male sex. Surgical experience is also a predictor of successful outcome. Predictors of mortality from gastric bypass include BMI $> 50 \text{ kg/m}^2$, male sex, hypertension, high risk of pulmonary thromboembolism and age above 45 years.

Presence of depression does not influence efficacy of surgery. Increased psychological dysfunction, dysfunctional eating behaviour, binge-eating disorder and a past history of intervention for substance misuse are not associated with poorer weight loss outcomes. Data are available for up to 6 years postoperatively.

HARMS AND THE BALANCE OF RISK

Postoperative mortality in the bariatric surgery group is approximately 0.25% at 90 days. This included bleeding (0.5%), thromboembolic events (0.8%), wound complications (1.8%), deep infection, abscess or leak (2.1%), and pulmonary complications (6.2%); reoperation was necessary in approximately 2% of patients.

Men who undergo bariatric surgery (adjustable or non-adjustable gastric banding, vertical banding gastroplasty or gastric bypass) have a 4.2-fold increased incidence of cholelithiasis, 4.5-fold increased incidence of cholecystitis and a 5.4-fold increased incidence of cholecystectomy. There is no difference in the frequency of biliary disease in women following bariatric surgery.

NUTRITION/SUPPLEMENTATION

Plasma vitamin D concentrations are low in obese patients before bariatric surgery and are associated with increased parathyroid hormone levels (secondary hyperparathyroidism). Postsurgery vitamin D concentrations are either unchanged or occasionally increased.

 Obese adults with type 2 diabetes should be offered individualized interventions to encourage weight loss (including lifestyle, pharmacological or surgical interventions), in order to improve metabolic control.

MALE AND FEMALE SEXUAL DYSFUNCTION

ERECTILE DYSFUNCTION (TABLES 6.6–6.9)

The prevalence of erectile dysfunction (ED) in men with diabetes increases with age and is about 35–50% overall. Tumescence is a vascular process under the control of the autonomic nervous

TABLE 6.6 Key features in the clinical history of erectile dysfunction in diabetes

- Onset usually gradual and progressive
- Earliest feature often inability to sustain erection long enough for satisfactory intercourse
- Erectile failure may be intermittent initially
- Sudden onset often thought to indicate a psychogenic cause
- Preservation of spontaneous and early morning erections does not necessarily indicate a psychogenic cause
- Loss of libido is consistent with hypogonadism
- Impotent men often understate their sex drive for a variety of reasons

TABLE 6.7 Medications associated with erectile dysfunction

Antihypertensives
- Thiazide diuretics
- Beta-blockers
- Calcium-channel blockers
- Angiotensin converting enzyme (ACE) inhibitors
- Central sympatholytics (methyldopa, clonidine)

Antidepressants
- Tricyclics
- Monoamine oxidase inhibitors
(NB: selective serotonin reuptake inhibitors can cause ejaculatory problems)

Major tranquillizers
- Phenothiazines
- Haloperidol

Hormones
- Luteinizing hormone-releasing hormone (goserelin, buserelin)
- Oestrogens (diethylstilbestrol/stilbestrol)
- Anti-androgens (cyproterone)

Miscellaneous
- 5α-reductase inhibitors (finasteride)
- Statins (simvastatin, atorvastatin, pravastatin)
- Cimetidine
- Digoxin
- Metoclopramide
- Allopurinol
- Ketoconazole
- Non-steroidal anti-inflammatory agents
- Fibrates

Drugs of 'abuse'/'social' drugs
- Alcohol, tobacco, marijuana
- Amphetamines
- Anabolic steroids
- Barbiturates
- Opiates

TABLE 6.8 Conditions associated with erectile dysfunction

Psychological disorders
- Anxiety about sexual performance
- Psychological trauma or abuse
- Misconceptions
- Sexual problems in the partner
- Depression
- Psychoses

Vascular disorders
- Peripheral vascular disease
- Hypertension
- Venous leak
- Pelvic trauma

Neurological disorders
- Stroke
- Multiple sclerosis
- Spinal and pelvic trauma
- Peripheral neuropathies

Endocrine and metabolic disorders
- Diabetes
- Hypogonadism/hyperprolactinaemia/hypopituitarism
- Thyroid dysfunction
- Hyperlipidaemia
- Renal disease/liver disease

Miscellaneous
- Surgery and trauma
- Smoking
- Drug and alcohol abuse
- Structural abnormalities of the penis

TABLE 6.9 Investigation of erectile dysfunction in diabetes

Serum testosterone if libido reduced or hypogonadism suspected (ideally taken at 9 a.m.)
Serum prolactin and luteinizing hormone if serum testosterone subnormal
Assessment of cardiovascular status if clinically indicated:
- Electrocardiography (ECG)
- Serum lipids
Glycosylated haemoglobin, serum electrolytes if clinically indicated

system. The erectile tissue of the corpus cavernosum behaves as a sponge and erection occurs when it becomes engorged with blood. This leads to compression of the outflow venules against the rigid tunica albuginea. Smooth muscle relaxation is the key phenomenon in this process. The process is under the control of parasympathetic fibres; the neurotransmitter involved is now known to be nitric oxide (NO). NO is produced in the parasympathetic nerve terminals and is generated by NO synthase in the vascular endothelium. Within the smooth muscle cell of the corpus cavernosum, NO stimulates guanylate cyclase, leading to increased production of the second messenger, cyclic guanosine monophosphate (cGMP), which induces smooth muscle relaxation, probably by opening up calcium channels. There is also evidence that neuronally derived NO is important in initiation, whereas NO from the endothelium is responsible for maintenance of the erection.

In men with diabetes there is evidence that ED is caused by failure of NO-induced smooth muscle relaxation caused by both autonomic neuropathy and endothelial dysfunction.

More recently, other potential abnormalities have been described that may contribute to the development of ED in diabetes:

- Endothelium-derived hyperpolarizing factor (EDHF) has a role in endothelium-dependent relaxation of human penile arteries, and this is significantly impaired in penile resistance arteries in men with diabetes.
- The formation of products of non-enzymatic glycosylation to produce advanced glycosylation end-products generates reactive oxygen species that impair NO bioactivity.
- Non-enzymatic glycation of proteins has been reported to impair endothelium-dependent relaxation of aorta in rats.

Erectile dysfunction as a risk factor for cardiovascular disease

There is an association between ED and cardiovascular disease, presumably because they share common risk factors:

- increased waist measurement
- reduced physical activity
- hyperlipidaemia.

There is also evidence that ED is an early marker of endothelial dysfunction.

Cigarette smoking almost doubles the risk of developing ED after about 7 years.

Tip box

Erectile dysfunction significantly worsens quality of life.

Oral agents

Phosphodiesterase-5 inhibitors

Phosphodiesterase type 5 (PDE-5) is an enzyme found in smooth muscle, platelets and the corpus cavernosum. The mechanism of action of PDE-5 inhibitors is as follows: during tumescence, there is an increase in the intracellular concentrations of NO, which produces smooth muscle relaxation via the second messenger, cGMP, which is degraded by PDE-5.

Adverse effects include headache, dyspepsia and flushing. Dyspepsia is usually mild. Abnormal vision is experienced by about 6% of men taking sildenafil, possibly because the drug has some activity against PDE-6, a retinal enzyme. Significant autonomic neuropathy or endothelial dysfunction reduces the efficacy of PDE-5 inhibitors.

PDE-5 inhibitors are not associated with increased cardiovascular risk.

Restoring sexual function, however, is not completely without risk. Sexual activity, like any form of physical activity, can precipitate cardiovascular events in those at risk. Nitrate therapy should not be given within 24 h of taking sildenafil or vardenafil, and within at least 48 h of taking tadalafil.

PDE-5 inhibitors should be used with caution in patients who take alpha-blockers, because the combination may lead to symptomatic hypotension.

Other therapies

Apomorphine

Apomorphine has been in use for many years. It is a centrally acting D1/D2 dopamine agonist that acts on the paraventricular nucleus of the thalamus early in the cascade that leads to erection.

Intracavernosal injection therapy

The technique of intracavernosal self-injection was first described in 1982 using phentolamine. Papaverine is more effective than phentolamine, but is an unlicensed treatment. It has been superseded by alprostadil (prostaglandin E), which was licensed for the treatment of ED in 1996.

Many men find injection therapy unacceptable because it requires injecting the penis. Transurethral administration of the vasoactive agent appears largely to overcome this problem.

Vacuum therapy

Vacuum devices became widely available in the 1970s. They consist of a translucent tube, which is placed over the penis, and an attached vacuum pump. The air is pumped out of the tube and the negative pressure draws blood into the erectile tissue, producing tumescence. A constriction band (which has previously been placed over the base of the tube) is then slipped off to remain firmly around the base of the penis so as to maintain the erection, and the tube is then removed.

Surgery

In spite of recent advances in the management of ED, some men will not be able to use the available treatment options. There will therefore always be a limited role for surgery.

The surgical options available are:

- the insertion of penile prostheses
- corrective surgeries for associated Peyronie's disease or postinjection corporal fibrosis
- venous and arterial surgery.

Patients must be warned regarding postoperative pain or discomfort and the potential for reoperation. The risk of infection is probably no higher in diabetes after insertion of a penile prosthesis, but, should infection occur, it is more serious.

FEMALE SEXUAL DYSFUNCTION

There has been considerably more interest in, and research into, the sexual dysfunction of men compared with women. It appears that women with diabetes admit to specific sexual dysfunctions when they are asked, but it is the universal experience of diabetologists that women with diabetes rarely complain of sexual problems.

The female equivalent of male ED is reduced vasocongestion of the vulva and vagina, leading to impaired arousal and reduced vaginal lubrication. If vaginal lubrication is the female equivalent of tumescence, then vaginal dryness and impaired arousal is probably related to failure of NO-mediated smooth muscle relaxation secondary to endothelial dysfunction and autonomic neuropathy.

Most studies report that the prevalence of impaired sexual arousal and inadequate lubrication is between 14% and 45% in women with diabetes. In contrast, there is little evidence of an increased risk of dyspareunia or problems with orgasm in women with diabetes.

The mechanism of action of PDE-5 inhibitors would suggest that they might improve arousal and vaginal lubrication; however, trials of sildenafil for this purpose in non-diabetic women have shown conflicting results.

Topical oestrogen or simple lubricant gels are usually effective.

Managing loss of libido in women with diabetes is more complex.

PSYCHOSOCIAL AND LEGAL ASPECTS

EMPLOYMENT

With a few provisos, diabetes is not a bar to most occupations, and people with diabetes are protected in many countries by legislation against discrimination on the grounds of disability. However, there remains some prejudice against people with diabetes, and access to employment may be limited through discriminatory employment practices and restrictions posed by employers (rather than by legislation). There may be perceived problems associated with diabetes or job-sensitive issues related to the potential risks of hypoglycaemia or visual impairment. Diabetes can also affect employment through increased sick leave and absenteeism, and by adversely influencing productivity. Employment is generally restricted where hypoglycaemia could be hazardous to the worker with diabetes, their colleagues or the general public (Table 6.10). In fact, severe hypoglycaemia in the

---

TABLE 6.10 Forms of employment from which insulin-treated people with diabetes are generally excluded in the UK

Vocational driving
- Large goods vehicles (LGV)
- Passenger-carrying vehicles (PCV)
- Locomotives and underground trains
- Professional drivers (chauffeurs)
- Taxi drivers (variable, depends on local authority)

Civil aviation
- Commercial pilots and flight engineers
- Aircrew
- Air traffic controllers

National and emergency services
- Armed forces (army, navy, airforce)
- Police force
- Fire brigade or rescue services
- Merchant navy
- Prison and security services

Dangerous areas for work
- Offshore: oil rigs, gas platforms
- Moving machinery
- Incinerators and hot-metal areas
- Work on railway tracks
- Coal mining
- Heights: overhead lines, cranes, scaffolding

workplace is uncommon and shift work seldom compromises glycaemic control.

Employment-related issues are not confined to people with T1DM. The rising prevalence of T2DM in the population of working age, along with the increasing use of insulin, has become an issue for occupational health assessment. Diabetes in general has a negative long-term influence on the economic productivity of the individual; studies in the UK found that relatively more people with diabetes were not earning because of inability to work, health-related disabilities, intercurrent illness, or early retirement on medical grounds.

> **Tip box**
>
> Depressive illness and poor glycaemic control are associated with higher unemployment and sickness absence in people with diabetes.

DRIVING

Driving demands complex psychomotor skills, visuospatial coordination, vigilance and satisfactory judgement. Motor accidents are common, although medical disabilities are seldom responsible. In most countries, the duration of the licence of a driver with diabetes is period-restricted by law, and its renewal is subject to review of medical fitness to drive. The main problems for the driver with diabetes are:

- hypoglycaemia
- visual impairment resulting from cataract or retinopathy
- rarely, peripheral neuropathy
- peripheral vascular disease
- lower limb amputation can present mechanical difficulties with driving – these problems may be overcome by adapting the vehicle and using automatic transmission systems.

Despite these challenges, drivers with diabetes do not appear to be involved in more accidents than their non-diabetic counterparts. Accident rates are probably lowered by regulatory authorities barring high-risk drivers and by drivers with advancing diabetic complications who voluntarily stop driving.

Hypoglycaemia

Hypoglycaemia while driving can interfere with driving skills by causing cognitive dysfunction, even during relatively asymptomatic mild hypoglycaemia. Driving performance often becomes impaired at blood glucose concentrations of 3.4–3.8 mmol/L, and deteriorates further at lower levels. Problems included poor road positioning, driving too fast, inappropriate braking and 'crashes' caused by stopping suddenly. In the UK, the Driver and Vehicle Licensing Agency (DVLA) does not distinguish between types of diabetes, and the restrictions are based on the use of insulin as therapy. Judgement and insight can become impaired during hypoglycaemia, and some drivers describe episodes of irrational and compulsive behaviour while hypoglycaemic at the wheel. Hypoglycaemia also causes potentially dangerous mood changes, including irritability and anger. In addition, asymptomatic hypoglycaemia impairs visual information processing and contrast sensitivity, particularly in poor visibility, which may diminish driving performance. Poor perception of hypoglycaemia is also dangerous. Many drivers with diabetes subjectively overestimate their current blood glucose level and feel competent to drive when they are actually hypoglycaemic.

All drivers with insulin-treated diabetes should keep some fast-acting carbohydrate in the vehicle. Each car journey, no matter how short, should be planned in advance to anticipate possible risk of hypoglycaemia, such as traffic delays. It is advisable to check blood glucose levels before and during long journeys, and to take frequent rest and meals. If hypoglycaemia occurs during driving, the car should be stopped in a safe place, and the engine switched off before consuming some glucose. In the UK, the patient should vacate the driver's seat and remove the keys from the ignition, as a charge can be brought for driving while under the influence of a drug (insulin) even if the car is stationary. Because cognitive function is slow to recover after hypoglycaemia, driving should not be resumed for at least 45 minutes after blood glucose has returned to normal. Many features of hypoglycaemia resemble alcohol intoxication, and semi-conscious hypoglycaemic diabetic drivers are sometimes arrested on the assumption that they are drunk. Drivers with insulin-treated diabetes should therefore carry a card or identity bracelet stating the diagnosis. Individuals with newly diagnosed insulin-treated diabetes may have to stop driving temporarily until their glycaemic control is stable. Sulphonylureas are the only group of oral antidiabetic drugs that may cause hypoglycaemia while driving, and people treated with these agents should be informed of this possibility.

Visual impairment

In the UK, monocular vision is accepted for driving, provided that the person meets the minimum legal requirement. The patient must be able to read a number plate with letters 8.9 cm high at a distance of 30 m (corrected if necessary). This corresponds to a distance visual acuity of around 6/10 on the Snellen chart. The number plate test:

- is poorly reproducible under clinical conditions
- does not assess visual fields
- does not assess night vision
- does not assess the ability to see moving objects.

All of these may be severely reduced by retinal ischaemia in preproliferative retinopathy, while visual field loss can be caused by extensive laser photocoagulation for diabetic retinopathy or macular oedema. Cataracts often accentuate glare from headlights, and in such cases driving in the dark should be avoided.

Eye screening is a crucial part of assessing medical fitness to drive. Pupillary dilatation for fundoscopy or retinal photography temporarily reduces visual acuity, particularly if the usual binocular visual acuity is 6/9 or worse. Patients should be told not to drive for at least 2 hours after the use of mydriatics. The driving regulatory authority may request perimetry to assess visual fields.

Most European countries restrict vocational (group 2) driving licences for people with insulin-treated diabetes. These include category C licences for large goods vehicles (LGV; previously called heavy goods vehicles) weighing over 7500 kg, and category D licences for passenger-carrying vehicles (PCV; previously called public service vehicles), or those with more than 17 seats.

Oral antidiabetic medication is not a bar to vocational driving licences in the UK. In practice, however, many public transport companies restrict the employment of drivers with T2DM who take sulphonylureas; metformin or exenatide treatment is not a contraindication, but medical assessment is usually necessary.

Outside Europe, the regulations in different countries range from a complete ban to no restriction other than a medical examination for prospective or current drivers who require insulin. In the USA, the Federal Highways Administration (FHWA) prohibits drivers with insulin-treated diabetes from driving commercial motor vehicles across state borders.

Aircraft pilot licences

The UK Civil Aviation Authority does not allow individuals with diabetes treated with insulin or sulphonylureas to fly commercial aircraft or to work as air traffic controllers. Private pilot licences can be issued to individuals with diabetes taking sulphonylureas (provided they have a safety licence endorsement), but not insulin.

The European Union has discussed introducing common airworthiness regulations for pilots with medical disorders.

PSYCHOLOGICAL IMPACT OF DIABETES

The diagnosis of diabetes carries a major emotional impact for many patients, their immediate family and possible carers. The precise nature of this for an individual will depend on many factors including the patient's age, type of diabetes, treatment, type of self-monitoring required, comorbidities (including complications of diabetes) and employment.

Important psychological factors will have a bearing not only on the initial reaction to the diagnosis but also on the patient's success in managing the disease in the longer term. These will include the patient's personality, temperament, health beliefs, cultural or religious beliefs, psychological state, intelligence, occupation and philosophical attitudes.

Such factors may influence the response to diabetes education, which aims to equip the patient with the knowledge and means to self-manage the disorder wherever possible. However, it can be quite surprising how little some diabetic patients take 'on board' in terms of making changes when they have been diagnosed with a chronic and potentially serious illness. There are clearly barriers to change that we do not fully understand.

Generally offering a sympathetic approach, tailored to the individual as appropriate, is required from the diabetes health-care team. From an anecdotal point of view, the patient who deals with the diagnosis very poorly initially will usually in time come to terms with the diagnosis and its implications. The process, common to the diagnosis of any chronic disease, has been compared with mourning.

INFLUENCE OF PSYCHOSOCIAL FACTORS ON DIABETES CONTROL

Studies investigating the relationships among psychological and social variables and diabetes outcomes are generally cross-sectional in nature, rather than longitudinal, and often fail to report pre-diagnosis baseline data. The patients recruited into trials from diabetes clinics are usually not newly diagnosed. In addition, they often do not have significant comorbid medical problems. Most outcomes are reported over relatively short periods, whereas diabetes is a lifelong condition. Furthermore, conclusions about using interventions in different ethnic groups may be problematic because of their lack of representation in the research.

Psychological and social factors impact on the ability of people with diabetes to manage their condition. Whether the burden of managing diabetes causes psychological and social problems, or vice versa, remains unclear.

The following factors are associated with poorer control in children and young people with type 1 diabetes:

- aspects of family functioning including conflict, lack of cohesiveness and openness
- depression
- anxiety
- maternal distress
- eating disorders
- behavioural problems.

The following factors are associated with poorer control in adults with type 1 diabetes:

- clinical depression and subclinical levels of mood disruption
- anxiety
- eating disorders.

Depression is more common in people with diabetes than in the general population. The presence of cardiovascular complications is often associated with a higher prevalence of depression and lower quality of life. Remission of depression is often associated with an improvement in glycaemic control.

Tip box

Regular assessment of a broad range of psychological and behavioural problems in children and adults with type 1 diabetes is recommended:
- in children this should include eating disorders, behavioural, emotional and family functioning problems
- in adults this should include anxiety, depression and eating disorders.

SCREENING FOR PSYCHOLOGICAL DISTRESS

The majority of patients cope well, some remaining remarkably stoical in the face of considerable problems. However, higher rates of depression have been recorded in adults with diabetes and may occur particularly in those with serious chronic tissue complications, notably sight-threatening retinopathy and cardiovascular disease. Overall, however, the prevalence of depression is similar to that observed in other chronic diseases. Psychosocial pressures are often cited by patients as a reason for their failure (as they may see it) to attain or sustain glycaemic targets. The identification of serious psychiatric disturbance such as depression with suicidal intent demands an expert psychiatric opinion. Self-administered insulin overdose can have catastrophic consequences, either by causing death or by inflicting permanent intellectual or cognitive impairment. Chronic psychoses, habitual drug abuse or alcoholism may place considerable obstacles in the path to successful self-management.

Tip box

Depression is more common in patients with diabetes mellitus.

Health-care professionals who are involved in the treatment of significant psychological problems in children and adults with diabetes should refer to the standard guidelines. Cognitive behavioural therapy (CBT) is a psychological treatment that attempts to find links between the person's feelings and the beliefs that underpin their distress. CBT, psychotherapy programmes and coping skills training are useful in treating depression in patients with diabetes. However, CBT is possibly less effective in patients with complications.

Antidepressant therapy with a selective serotonin reuptake inhibitor (SSRI) is a useful treatment in depressed patients with diabetes and may improve glycaemic control; however, tricyclic antidepressants may adversely affect metabolic control. Continued antidepressant treatment for 1 year after recovery may prevent recurrence of depression.

Healthcare professionals should:

- on those occasions where significant psychosocial problems are identified, try to explain the link between these and poorer diabetes control. If possible, it is good practice also to give written information.
- be mindful of the burden caused by psychosocial problems such as clinical and subclinical levels of depression when setting goals and adjusting complex treatment regimens. Patients are less able to make substantial changes to their lives during difficult times.

People with diabetes (or parents/guardians) should:

- try to speak to their general practitioner or diabetes team if they feel they (or their children) have significant psychosocial issues such as those detailed in this section

- be aware that many psychosocial problems make diabetes self-care more difficult, and also that many difficulties can be successfully treated with the right help.

Depression can be assessed using simple questions regarding mood and enjoyment of day-to-day activities using self-completed measures or via a more intensive clinical interview (normally carried out by psychologists or psychiatrists).

Some symptoms of diabetes overlap with symptoms of common psychological problems. This can make identification of psychological problems more difficult and can lead to false positives when using screening tools designed for the use within the general population.

There is no evidence showing how to assess psychological problems reliably and validly in young people or adults with diabetes. Screening tools that have been validated and are widely used to assess general psychological distress in the general population are widely used in adults or young people with diabetes. The Hospital Anxiety and Depression Scale (HADS) is the most widely used self-report screening tool for adults with medical conditions, including diabetes in the UK. The HADS is short (14 items) and screens for both anxiety and depression.

Some self-report screening tools have also been assessed in people with diabetes. These include the Beck Depression Inventory (BDI), the Centre for Epidemiological Studies Depression Scale (CES-D) and the Patient Health Questionnaire (PHQ-9). These are relatively short (21, 20 and 9 items respectively) and could be completed by most patients in a clinic setting within 10–15 minutes. There are other reliable validated measures of general psychological distress in relation to diabetes, including the PAID (Problem Areas In Diabetes) Scale and the WHO-5 Well-Being Index.

There are no validated tools to screen for eating disorders in people with diabetes.

Tip box

Health-care professionals should be aware of cultural differences in type/presentation of psychological problems in people from different ethnic communities living with diabetes, and facilitate appropriate psychological/emotional support.

Health professionals working in diabetes should have sufficient levels of consulting skills to be able to identify psychological problems and to decide whether or not referral to specialist services is required.

EFFECT OF PSYCHOLOGICAL INTERVENTIONS ON DIABETES OUTCOMES

Children and adolescents with type 1 diabetes

Most interventions, particularly in children and adolescents with diabetes, appear to have only a small effect on glycaemic outcomes but a more substantial effect on psychosocial function. Family interventions in children and adolescents (including educational and psychological components) have a larger improvement in glycaemic control.

Tip box

Health-care professionals working with adults and children with diabetes should refer those with significant psychological problem to services or colleagues with an expertise in this area.

APPENDIX 6.1. PRINCIPLES OF DIETARY PLANNING IN CHILDREN WITH DIABETES

1. Eat a well balanced diet, with daily energy intake distributed as follows:
   - Carbohydrate 50–55% (sucrose intake up to 10% total energy)
   - Fat 30–35% (up to 20% monounsaturated fat; $< 10\%$ polyunsaturated fat; $< 10\%$ saturated fat and trans fatty acids; n-3 fatty acids 0.15 g/day)
   - Protein 10–15%.
2. If possible, eat meals and snacks at the same time each day.
3. Use snacks to prevent and treat hypoglycaemia (avoid overtreatment):
   - Young children often have a mid or late morning snack
   - Most people will have a mid or late afternoon snack
   - Many children require a bedtime snack, particularly if the bedtime blood glucose is below 130 mg/dL (7 mmol/L) or if they have been active during the day.
4. Gauge energy intake to maintain appropriate weight and body mass index:
   - Overinsulinization leads to 'forced' snacking, excess food intake and promotes excessive weight gain
   - Eating disorders are common in teenage girls with diabetes.
5. Recommended fibre intake for children older than 1 year: 2.8–3.4 g/MJ; children older than 2 years should eat = (age in years + 5) g fibre/day.

6. Avoid foods high in sodium that may increase the risk of hypertension; target salt intake – to less than 6 g/day.

7. Avoid excessive protein intake.

8. Children with diabetes have the same vitamin and mineral requirements as other healthy children.

9. There is no evidence of harm from an intake of artificial sweeteners in doses not exceeding acceptable daily intakes.

10. Specially labelled diabetic foods are not recommended because they are expensive, unnecessary, often high in fat and may contain sweeteners with laxative effects. These include the sugar alcohols such as sorbitol.

11. Although alcohol intake is generally prohibited in youth, teenagers continue to experiment with and sometimes abuse alcohol. Alcohol may induce prolonged hypoglycaemia in young people with diabetes (up to 16 hours after drinking). Carbohydrate should be eaten before, during and/or after alcohol intake. It may be also necessary to lower the insulin dose, particularly if exercise is performed during or after drinking (e.g. dancing).

12. Approximately 10% of patients with type 1 diabetes have serological evidence of coeliac disease. Those with positive intestinal biopsy or symptomatic have to be treated with a gluten-free diet (GFD). Products derived from wheat, rye, barley and triticale are eliminated and replaced with potato, rice, soy, tapioca, buckwheat and perhaps oats. Most of the children are asymptomatic but the long-term consequences of untreated coeliac autoimmunity appear to warrant a GFD.

APPENDIX 6.2. CHECKLIST FOR PROVISION OF INFORMATION TO WOMEN WITH GDM

Pre-pregnancy

● Discuss pregnancy planning with women with diabetes of childbearing age at their annual review.

● Advise women with diabetes who are planning pregnancy that they will be referred to a pre-pregnancy multidisciplinary clinic and outline the benefits of multidisciplinary management.

● Provide information on the risks of diabetes to both mother and the fetus.

● Explain why a review of glycaemic control is necessary. Suggest that they should aim for a glycated haemoglobin (HbA1c) level of $<7.0\%$ (53 mmol/mol) for 3 months prior to pregnancy.

● Advise that folic acid 5 mg (available on prescription only) should be taken for 3 months prior to conception and until the end of week 12 of pregnancy.

- Offer lifestyle advice, for example on stopping smoking, alcohol consumption and exercise.
- Explain about the need for a review with the dietitian.
- Explain that a review of all medication will be necessary when planning a pregnancy and offer advice on which medications may need to be stopped, the reasons behind stopping and what the alternatives are.
- Provide contact telephone numbers.

Pregnancy
- Ensure that the principles of the Keeping Childbirth natural and Dynamic (KCND) initiative are maintained where possible.
- Advise women with diabetes who are pregnant that they will be referred to a joint diabetes antenatal clinic (where available) and outline the benefits of multidisciplinary management.
- Explain that a review of all medication will be necessary when pregnant and offer advice on which medications may need to be stopped, the reasons behind stopping and the alternatives available.
- Advise women about the risks of hypoglycaemia, how to recognize the warning signs and symptoms and what treatment they may require. Ensure they have a glucagon kit and know how and when to use it.
- Advise that during pregnancy tight glycaemic control is necessary and they will need to monitor their blood glucose more often. Be clear about the targets that need to be achieved.
- Offer advice about sick day rules and planning for periods of illness (even minor) that may cause hyperglycaemia. These may include:
  - what to do with insulin or tablets
  - appropriate food to maintain blood glucose levels
  - how often to measure blood glucose and when to check for ketones
  - when to contact the diabetes team and contact numbers.
- Explain about the need for a review with the dietitian.
- Offer lifestyle advice, for example on stopping smoking, alcohol consumption and exercise.
- Offer advice on safe driving and ensure that women inform the DVLA and their insurance company if they are starting on insulin.
- Inform women about the risk of retinopathy and advise that they will have retinal screening during each trimester. Explain what screening involves and what treatment to expect if retinopathy is found.
- Provide contact telephone numbers.

REFERENCES, BIBLIOGRAPHY & FURTHER READING

Section 1

Alberti, K.G.M.M., Zimmet, P.Z., for the WHO consultations, 1998. Definition, diagnosis and classification of diabetes mellitus and its complications. Part 1. Diagnosis and classification of diabetes mellitus. Provisional report of a WHO consultation. Diabet. Med. 15, 539–553.

American Diabetes Association, 2011. Diagnosis and classification of diabetes mellitus. Diabetes Care 34 (Suppl. 1), S62–S69.

Buchholz, S., Morrow, A.F., Coleman, P.L., 2008. Atypical antipsychotic induced diabetes mellitus: an update on epidemiology and postulated mechanisms. Intern. Med. J. 38, 602–606.

DECODE Study Group, 2003. Gender difference in all-cause and cardiovascular mortality related to hyperglycaemia and newly-diagnosed diabetes. Diabetologia 46, 608–617.

Expert Committee on the Diagnosis and Classification of Diabetes Mellitus, 1997. Report of the expert committee on the diagnosis and classification of diabetes mellitus. Diabetes Care 20, 1183–1197.

Expert Committee Report on the Diagnosis of Diabetes, 2009. The role of glycated haemoglobin (A1C) assay in the diagnosis of diabetes in non-pregnant persons. Diabetes Care 32, 1327–1334.

Fourlanos, S., Dotta, F., Greenbaum, C.J., et al., 2005. Latent autoimmune diabetes in adults (LADA) should be less latent. Diabetologia 48, 2206–2212.

Franks, S., 2006. Diagnosis of polycystic ovary syndrome: in defence of the Rotterdam criteria. J. Clin. Endocrinol. Metab. 91, 786–789.

International Diabetes Federation (IDF), 2006. The IDF Consensus Worldwide Definition of the Metabolic Syndrome. International Diabetes Federation, Brussels.

International Diabetes Federation, 2009. Diabetes Atlas, fourth ed. International Diabetes Federation.

Kahn, R., Buse, J., Ferrannini, E., et al., American Diabetes Association, European Association for the Study of Diabetes, 2006. The metabolic syndrome: time for a critical appraisal: joint statement from the American Diabetes Association and the European Association for the Study of Diabetes. Diabetes Care 28, 2289–2304.

Kotronen, A., Westerbacka, J., Bergholm, R., et al., 2007. Liver fat in metabolic syndrome. J. Clin. Endocrinol. Metab. 92, 3490–3497.

Kotronen, A., Yki-Jarvinen, H., 2008. Fatty liver: a novel component of the metabolic syndrome. Arterioscler. Thromb. Vasc. Biol. 28, 27–38.

Lammi, N., Blomstedt, P.A., Moltchanova, E., et al., 2008. Marked temporal increase in the incidence of type 1 and type 2 diabetes among young adults in Finland. Diabetologia 51, 897–899.

Lanng, S., Thornsteinsson, B., Nerup, Koch, C., 2001. Diabetes mellitus in cystic fibrosis: effect of insulin therapy on lung function and infections. Acta Paediatr. 90, 515–519.

Li, G., Zhang, P., Wang, J., et al., 2008. The long-term effect of lifestyle interventions to prevent diabetes in the China Da Qing Diabetes Prevention Study: a 20-year follow-up study. Lancet 371, 1783–1789.

Lindström, J., Louheranta, A., Mannelin, M., et al., 2003. The Finnish Diabetes Prevention Study (DPS): lifestyle intervention and 3-year result on diet and physical activity. Diabetes Care 26, 3230–3236.

Littorin, B., Sundkvist, G., Hagopian, W., et al., 1999. Islet cell and glutamic acid decarboxylase antibodies present at diagnosis of diabetes predict the need for insulin treatment: a cohort study in young adults whose disease was initially labelled as type 2 or unclassifiable diabetes. Diabetes Care 22, 409–412.

Moczulski, D.K., Greszczak, W., Gawlik, B., 2001. Role of hemochromatosis C282Y and H63D mutations in *HFE* gene in development of type 2 diabetes and diabetic nephropathy. Diabetes Care 24, 1187–1191.

Mohan, V., Farooq, S., Deepa, M., 2008. Prevalence of fibrocalculous pancreatic diabetes in Chennai in South India. JOP 9, 489–492.

Niederau, C., 1999. Diabetes mellitus in hemochromatosis. Z. Gastroenterol 1 (Suppl.) 22–32.

Pan, X.R., Li, G.W., Hu, Y.H., et al., 1997. Effects of diet and exercise in preventing NIDDM in people with impaired glucose tolerance. The Da Qing IGT and Diabetes Study. Diabetes Care 20, 537–544.

Pang, T.T., Narendran, P., 2008. Addressing insulin resistance in type 1 diabetes. Diabet. Med. 25, 1015–1024.

Patterson, C.C., Dahlquist, G., Gyurus, E., et al., EURODIAB Study Group, 2009. Incidence trends for childhood type 1 diabetes in Europe during 1989–2003 and predicted new cases 2005–20: a multicentre prospective registration study. Lancet 373, 2027–2033.

Reaven, G., 1988. Banting lecture 1988: Role of insulin resistance in human disease. Diabetes 37, 1595–1607.

Rewers, M., Zimmet, P., 2004. The rising tide of childhood type 1 diabetes: what is the elusive environmental trigger? Lancet 364, 1645–1647.

Robert, J.J., Mosnier-Pudar, H., 2000. Diagnosis and treatment of diabetes in adult patients with cystic fibrosis. Rev. Mal. Respir. 17, 798–801.

The Rotterdam ESHRE/ASRM-Sponsored PCOS Consensus Workshop Group, 2004. Revised 2003 consensus on diagnostic criteria and long-term health risks related to polycystic ovary syndrome (PCOS). Hum. Reprod. 19, 41–47.

Tuomilehto, J., Lindström, J., Eriksson, J.G., et al., 2001. Prevention of type 2 diabetes mellitus by changes in lifestyle among subjects with impaired glucose intolerance. N. Engl. J. Med. 344, 1343–1350.

Wild, S., Roglic, G., Green, A., Sicree, R., King, H., 2004. Global prevalence of diabetes: estimates for the year 2000 and projections for 2030. Diabetes Care 27, 1047–1053.

World Health Oranization (WHO) Consultation, 2006. Definition and Diagnosis of Diabetes Mellitus and Intermediate Hyperglycaemia. WHO, Geneva.

Section 2

American Diabetes Association, 2011. Diagnosis and classification of diabetes mellitus. Diabetes Care 34 (Suppl. 1), S62–S69.

Bilous, R., Donnelly, R., 2010. Handbook of Diabetes, fourth ed. Wiley-Blackwell, Chichester.

Brand-Miller, J., Hayne, S., Petocz, P., et al., 2003. Low-glycemic index diets in the management of diabetes: a meta-analysis of randomized controlled trials. Diabetes Care 26, 2261–2267.

Channon, S.J., Huws-Thomas, M.V., Rollnick, S., et al., 2007. A multicenter randomized controlled trial of motivational interviewing in teenagers with diabetes. Diabetes Care 30, 1390–1395.

DAFNE Study Group, 2002. Training in flexible, intensive insulin management to enable dietary freedom in people with type 1 diabetes: dose adjustment for normal eating (DAFNE) randomised controlled trial. BMJ 325, 746.

Deakin, T., McShane, C.E., Cade, J.E., et al., 2005. Group based training for self management strategies in people with type 2 diabetes mellitus. Cochrane Database Syst. Rev. 2, CD003417.

Deakin, T.A., Cade, J.E., Williams, R., et al., 2006. Structured patient education: the diabetes X-PERT Programme makes a difference. Diabet. Med. 23, 944–954.

Diabetes, U.K., What to expect on a regular basis. Online. Available at: http://www.diabetes.org.uk/Guide-to-diabetes/What_care_to_expect/From_your_healthcare_team/What_to_expect_on_a_regular_basis (accessed June 2011).

Duckworth, W., Abraira, C., Moritz, T., et al., 2009. Glucose control and vascular complications in veterans with type 2 diabetes. N. Engl. J. Med. 360, 129–139.

Duke, S.A., Colagiuri, S., Colagiuri, R., 2009. Individual patient education for people with type 2 diabetes mellitus. Cochrane Database Syst. Rev. 1, CD005268.

Fagot-Campagna, A., Narayan, K.M., Imperatore, G., 2001. Type 2 diabetes in children. Br. Med. J. 322, 377–378.

Gaede, P., Lund-Andersen, H., Parving, H.H., et al., 2008. Effect of a multifactorial intervention on mortality in type 2 diabetes. N. Engl. J. Med. 358, 580–591.

George, J.T., Valdovinos, A.P., Russell, I., et al., 2008. Clinical effectiveness of a brief educational intervention in type 1 diabetes: results from the BITES (Brief Intervention in Type 1 diabetes, Education for Self-efficacy) trial. Diabet. Med. 25, 1447–1453.

Gerstein, H.C., Miller, M.E., Byington, R.P., et al., Action to Control Cardiovascular Risk in Diabetes Study Group, 2008. Effects of intensive glucose lowering in type 2 diabetes. N. Engl. J. Med. 358, 2545–2569.

Hill-Briggs, F., Gemmell, L., 2007. Problem solving in diabetes self management and control: a systematic review of the literature. Diabetes Educ. 33, 1032–1050.

Holman, R.R., Paul, S.K., Bethel, M.A., et al., 2008. 10-year follow-up of intensive glucose control in type 2 diabetes. N. Engl. J. Med. 359, 1577–1589.

Hovorka, R., 2005. Continuous glucose monitoring and closed-loop systems. Diabet. Med. 23, 1–12.

Howard, A.A., Arnsten, J.H., Gourevitch, M.N., 2004. Effect of alcohol consumption on diabetes mellitus: a systematic review. Ann. Intern. Med. 140, 211–219.

Jacobs-van der Bruggen, M.A., Van Baal, P.H., Hoogenveen, R.T., et al., 2009. Cost-effectiveness of lifestyle modification in diabetic patients. Diabetes Care 32, 1453–1458.

Juvenile Diabetes Research Foundation Continuous Glucose Monitoring Study Group, 2009. The effect of continuous glucose monitoring in well-controlled type 1 diabetes. Diabetes Care 32, 1378–1383.

Karamanous, B., Thanopoulou, A., Angelico, F., et al., 2002. Nutritional habits in the Mediterranean Basin: the macronutrient composition of diet and its relation with the traditional Mediterranean diet. Multicentre study of the Mediterranean Group for the Study of Diabetes (MGSD). Eur. J. Clin. Nutr. 56, 983–991.

Koppes, L.L., Dekker, J.M., Hendriks, H.F., et al., 2006. Metaanalysis of the relationship between alcohol consumption and coronary heart disease and mortality in type 2 diabetic patients. Diabetologia 49, 648–652.

Manson, J.E., Rimm, E.B., Stampfer, M.J., et al., 1991. Physical activity and incidence of non-insulin dependent diabetes mellitus in women. Lancet 338, 774–778.

Nathan, D.M., Buse, J.B., Davidson, M.B., et al., 2009. Medical management of hyperglycaemia in type 2 diabetes mellitus: a consensus algorithm for the initiation and adjustment therapy. Consensus statement from the American Diabetes Association and the European Association for the Study of Diabetes. Diabetologia 52, 17–30.

National Institute for Clinical Excellence (NICE), 2008. Type 1 Diabetes in Adults: NICE Guidance. NICE, London.

National Institute for Clinical Excellence (NICE), 2008. Diabetes Type 2 (update): NICE Guidance. NICE, London.

Patel, A., MacMahon, S., Chalmers, J., et al., ADVANCE Collaborative Group, 2008. Intensive blood glucose control and vascular outcomes in patients with type 2 diabetes. N. Engl. J. Med. 358, 2560–2572.

Sarol, Jr., J.N., Nicodemus, Jr., N.A., Tan, K.M., et al., 2005. Selfmonitoring of blood glucose as part of a multi-component therapy among non-insulin requiring type 2 diabetes patients: a metaanalysis (1966–2004). Curr. Med. Res. Opin. 21, 173–184.

Schachinger, H., Hegar, K., Hermanns, N., et al., 2005. Randomized controlled clinical trial of Blood Glucose Awareness Training (BGATIII) in Switzerland and Germany. J. Behav. Med. 28, 587–594.

Snoek, F.J., Van Der Ven, N.C.W., Twisk, J.W.R., et al., 2008. Cognitive behavioural therapy (CBT) compared with blood glucose awareness training (BGAT) in poorly controlled type 1 diabetic patients: long-term effects on HbA1c moderated by depression. A randomized controlled trial. Diabet. Med. 25, 1337–1342.

Suarez, L., Barrett-Connor, E., 1984. Interaction between cigarette smoking and diabetes mellitus in the prediction of death attributed to cardiovascular disease. Am. J. Epidemiol. 120, 670–675.

Thomas, D.E., Elliot, E.J., Naughton, G.A., 2006. Exercise for type 2 diabetes mellitus. Cochrane Database Syst. Rev. 3, CD002968.

Turner, R., 1998. Effect of intensive blood-glucose control with sulphonylureas or insulin compared with conventional treatment and risk of complications in patients with type 2 diabetes (UKPDS 33). Lancet 352, 837–853.

Turner, R., 1998. Effect of intensive blood-glucose control with metformin on complications in overweight patients with type 2 diabetes (UKPDS 34). Lancet 352, 854–865.

Winkley, K., Ismail, K., Landau, S., et al., 2006. Psychological interventions to improve glycaemic control in patients with type 1 diabetes: systematic review and meta-analysis of randomised controlled trials. Br. Med. J. 333, 65.

Section 3

Amori, R.E., Lau, J., Pittas, A.G., 2007. Efficacy and safety of incretin therapy in type 2 diabetes: systematic review and meta-analysis. JAMA 298, 194–206.

Barnard, K.D., Lloyd, C.E., Skinner, T.C., 2007. Systematic literature review: quality of life associated with insulin pump use in type 1 diabetes. Diabet. Med. 24, 607–617.

Bartley, P.C., Bogoev, M., Larsen, J., et al., 2008. Long-term efficacy and safety of insulin detemir compared to Neutral Protamine Hagedorn insulin in patients with type 1 diabetes using a treat-to-target basal-bolus regimen with insulin aspart at meals: a 2-year, randomized, controlled trial. Diabet. Med. 25, 442–449.

Belsey, J., Krishnarajah, G., 2008. Glycaemic control and adverse events in patients with type 2 diabetes treated with metformin + sulphonylurea: a meta-analysis. Diabetes Obes. Metab. 1 (Suppl. 1), 1–7.

Bolen, S., Wilson, L., Vassy, J., et al., 2007. Comparative Effectiveness and Safety of Oral Diabetes Medications for Adults With Type 2 Diabetes. Agency for Healthcare Research and Quality, Rockville, MD. Online. Available at: http://effectivehealthcare.ahrq.gov/ehc/products/6/39/ OralFullReport.pdf (accessed 05.01.2010).

Bolen, S., Feldman, L., Vassy, J., et al., 2007. Systematic review: comparative effectiveness and safety of oral medications for type 2 diabetes mellitus. Ann. Intern. Med. 147, 386–399.

Buse, J.B., Rosenstock, J., Sesti, G., et al., 2009. Liraglutide once a day versus exenatide twice a day for type 2 diabetes: a 26-week randomised, parallel-group, multinational, open-label trial (LEAD-6). Lancet 374, 39–47.

Canadian Agency for Drugs and Technologies in Health, 2009. Systematic Review of Use of Blood Glucose Test Strips for the Management of Diabetes Mellitus. Optimal Therapy Report – COMPUS, Ottawa. Online. Available at: http://cadth.ca/media/pdf/BGTS_SR_Report_of_Clinical_ Outcomes.pdf (accessed January 2012).

Davies, M., Dixon, S., Currie, C.J., et al., 2001. Evaluation of a hospital diabetes specialist nursing service: a randomized controlled trial. Diabet. Med. 18, 301–307.

DeFronzo, R.A., Ratner, R.E., Han, J., et al., 2005. Effects of exenatide (exendin-4) on glycemic control and weight over 30 weeks in metformin-treated patients with type 2 diabetes. Diabetes Care 28, 1092–1100.

DeFronzo, R.A., Hissa, M.N., Garber, A.J., et al., 2009. The efficacy and safety of Saxagliptin when added to metformin therapy in patients with inadequately controlled type 2 diabetes with metformin alone. Diabetes Care 32, 1649–1655.

Diabetes Control and Complications Trial Research Group, 1993. The effect of intensive treatment of diabetes on the development and progression of long-term complications in insulin-dependent diabetes mellitus. N. Engl. J. Med. 329, 977–986.

Diabetologia, M.A., Meininger, G., Sheng, D., et al., 2007. Efficacy and safety of the dipeptidyl peptidase-4 inhibitor, sitagliptin, compared with the sulfonylurea, glipizide, in patients with type 2 diabetes inadequately controlled on metformin alone: a randomized, double-blind, non-inferiority trial. Diabetes Obes. Metab. 9, 194–205.

Dormandy, J.A., Charbonnel, B., Eckland, D.J., et al., 2005. Secondary prevention of macrovascular events in patients with type 2 diabetes in the PROactive Study (PROspective pioglitAzone Clinical Trial In macroVascular Events): a randomised controlled trial. Lancet 366, 1279–1289.

Erdmann, E., Dormandy, J.A., Charbonnel, B., et al., 2007. The effect of pioglitazone on recurrent myocardial infarction in 2445 patients with type 2 diabetes and previous myocardial infarction: results from the PROactive (PROactive 05) Study. J. Am. Coll. Cardiol. 49, 1772–1780.

Eurich, D.T., McAlister, F.A., Blackburn, D.F., et al., 2007. Benefits and harms of antidiabetic agents in patients with diabetes and heart failure: systematic review. Br. Med. J. 335, 497–501.

Funnell, M.M., Brown, T.L., Childs, B.P., et al., 2011. National standards for diabetes self-management education. Diabetes Care 34, S89–S96.

Goke, B., Hershon, K., Kerr, D., et al., 2008. Efficacy and safety of vildagliptin monotherapy during 2-year treatment of drug-naive patients with type 2 diabetes: comparison with metformin. Horm. Metab. Res. 40, 892–895.

Goudswaard, A.N., Furlong, N.J., Valk, G.D., et al., 2004. Insulin monotherapy versus combinations of insulin with oral hypoglycaemic agents in patients with type 2 diabetes mellitus. Cochrane Database Syst. Rev. 4, CD003418.

Heine, R.J., Van, G.L.F., Johns, D., et al., 2005. Exenatide versus insulin glargine in patients with suboptimally controlled type 2 diabetes: a randomized trial. Ann. Intern. Med. 143, 559–569.

Hermansen, K., Kipnes, M., Luo, E., et al., 2007. Efficacy and safety of the dipeptidyl peptidase-4 inhibitor, sitagliptin, in patients with type 2 diabetes mellitus inadequately controlled on glimepiride alone or on glimepiride and metformin. Diabetes Obes. Metab. 9, 733–745.

Inzucchi, S.E., 2002. Oral antihyperglycemic therapy for type 2 diabetes: scientific review. JAMA 287, 360–372.

Jeitler, K., Horvath, K., Berghold, A., et al., 2008. Continuous subcutaneous insulin infusion versus multiple daily insulin injections in patients with diabetes mellitus: systematic review and meta-analysis. Diabetologia 51, 941–951.

Lago, R.M., Singh, P.P., Nesto, R.W., 2007. Congestive heart failure and cardiovascular death in patients with prediabetes and type 2 diabetes given thiazolidinediones: a meta-analysis of randomised clinical trials. Lancet 370, 1129–1136.

Loveman, E., Frampton, G.K., Clegg, A.J., 2008. The clinical effectiveness of diabetes education models for type 2 diabetes: a systematic review. Health Technol. Assess 12, 1–116, iii.

Mannucci, E., Monami, M., Lamanna, C., et al., 2008. Pioglitazone and cardiovascular risk. A comprehensive metaanalysis of randomized clinical trials. Diabetes Obes. Metab. 10, 1221–1238.

Meinert, C.L., Knatterud, G.L., Prout, T F., et al., 1970. A study of the effects of hypoglycemic agents on vascular complications in patients with adult-onset diabetes. II. Mortality results. Diabetes 19, (Suppl.), 789–830.

Monami, M., Marchionni, N., Mannucci, E., 2009. Long-acting insulin analogues vs. NPH human insulin in type 1 diabetes. A metaanalysis. Diabetes Obes. Metab. 11, 372–378.

Moretto, T.J., Milton, D.R., Ridge, T.D., et al., 2008. Efficacy and tolerability of exenatide monotherapy over 24 weeks in antidiabetic drug-naive patients with type 2 diabetes: a randomized, double-blind, placebo-controlled, parallel-group study. Clin. Ther. 30, 1448–1460.

National Institute for Health and Clinical Excellence (NICE), Type 2 Diabetes – Newer Agents (partial update of CG66):NICE clinical guideline CG87. Online Available at: http://www.nice.org.uk/CG87 (accessed August 2010)..

Nauck, M., Stöckmann, F., Ebert, R., et al., 1986. Reduced incretin effect in type 2 (non-insulin-dependent) diabetes. Diabetologia 29, 46–52.

Newman, S.P., Cooke, D., Casbard, A., et al., 2009. A randomised controlled trial to compare minimally invasive glucose monitoring device with conventional monitoring in the management of insulin-treated diabetes mellitus (MITRE). Health Technol. Assess 13, iii–iv, ix–xi, 1–194.

O'Kane, M.J., Bunting, B., Copeland, M., et al., 2008. Efficacy of self monitoring of blood glucose in patients with newly diagnosed type 2 diabetes (ESMON study): randomised controlled trial. Br. Med. J. 336, 1174–1177.

Pankowska, E., Blazik, M., Dziechciarz, P., et al., 2009. Continuous subcutaneous insulin infusion vs. multiple daily injections in children with type 1 diabetes: a systematic review and meta-analysis of randomized control trials. Pediatr. Diabetes 10, 52–58.

Pickup, J.C., Sutton, A.J., 2008. Severe hypoglycaemia and glycaemic control in type 1 diabetes: meta-analysis of multiple daily insulin injections compared with continuous subcutaneous insulin infusion. Diabet. Med. 25, 765–774.

Richter, B., Bandeira-Echtler, E., Bergerhoff, K., et al., 2006. Pioglitazone for type 2 diabetes mellitus. Cochrane Database Syst. Rev. 4, CD006060.

Richter, B., Bandeira-Echtler, E., Bergerhoff, K., et al., 2008. Dipeptidyl peptidase-4 (DPP-4) inhibitors for type 2 diabetes mellitus. Cochrane Database Syst. Rev. 2, CD006739.

Rosenstock, J., Aguilar-Salinas, C., Klein, E., et al., 2009. Effect of saxagliptin monotherapy in treatment-naive patients with type 2 diabetes. Curr. Med. Res. Opin. 25, 2401–2411.

Saenz, A., Fernandez-Esteban, I., Mataix, A., et al., 2005. Metformin monotherapy for type 2 diabetes mellitus. Cochrane Database Syst. Rev. 3, CD002966.

Scottish Study Group for the Care of the Young with Diabetes, 2006. A longitudinal observational study of insulin therapy and glycaemic control in Scottish children with type 1 diabetes: DIABAUD 3. Diabet. Med. 23, 1216–1221.

Siebenhofer, A., Plank, J., Berghold, A., et al., 2006. Short acting insulin analogues versus regular human insulin in patients with diabetes mellitus. Cochrane Database Syst. Rev. 2, CD003287.

Singh, S.R., Ahmad, F., Lal, A., et al., 2009. Efficacy and safety of insulin analogues for the management of diabetes mellitus: a meta-analysis. Can. Med. Assoc. J. 180, 385–397.

Tzoulaki, I., Molokhia, M., Curcin, V., et al., 2009. Risk of cardiovascular disease and all cause mortality among patients with type 2 diabetes prescribed oral antidiabetes drugs: retrospective cohort study using UK general practice research database. Br. Med. J. 339, b4731.

Van de Laar, F.A., Lucassen, P.L., Akkermans, R.P., et al., 2005. Alpha-glucosidase inhibitors for type 2 diabetes mellitus. Cochrane Database Syst. Rev. 2, CD003639.

Section 4

Alberti, K.G., 1977. Low-dose insulin in the treatment of diabetic ketoacidosis. Arch. Intern. Med. 137, 1367–1376.

American Diabetes Association Workgroup on Hypoglycemia, 2005. Defining and reporting hypoglycemia in diabetes. Diabetes Care 28, 1245–1249.

Banarer, S., Cryer, P.E., 2003. Sleep-related hypoglycemia-associated autonomic failure in type 1 diabetes: reduced awakening from sleep during hypoglycemia. Diabetes 52, 1195–1203.

Cryer, P.E., 2005. Mechanisms of hypoglycemia-associated autonomic failure and its component syndromes in diabetes. Diabetes 54, 3592–3601.

Cryer, P.E., 2008. The barrier of hypoglycemia in diabetes. Diabetes 57, 3169–3176.

Davis, S., Alonso, M.D., 2004. Hypoglycemia as a barrier to glycemic control. J. Diabetes Complications 18, 60–68.

DeRosa, M.A., Cryer, P.E., 2004. Hypoglycemia and the sympathoadrenal system: neurogenic symptoms are largely the result of sympathetic neural, rather than adrenomedullary, activation. Am. J. Physiol. Endocrinol. Metab. 287, E32–E41.

Diabetes Control and Complications Trial Research Group, 1997. Hypoglycemia in the Diabetes Control and Complications Trial. Diabetes 46, 271–286.

Diabetes Control and Complications Trial/Epidemiology of Diabetes Interventions and Complications Study Research Group, 2007. Long-term effect of diabetes and its treatment on cognitive function. N. Engl. J. Med. 356, 1842–1852.

Donnelly, L.A., Morris, A.D., Frier, B.M., et al., 2005. Frequency and predictors of hypoglycemia in type 1 and insulin-treated type 2 diabetes: a population-based study. Diabet. Med. 22, 749–755.

Eledrisi, M.S., Alshanti, M.S., Shah, M.F., et al., 2006. Overview of the diagnosis and management of diabetic ketoacidosis. Am. J. Med. Sci. 331, 243–251.

English, P., Williams, G., 2004. Hyperglycaemic crises and lactic acidosis in diabetes mellitus. Postgrad. Med. J. 80, 253–261.

Fall, P.J., Szerlip, H.M., 2005. Lactic acidosis: from sour milk to septic shock. J. Intensive Care Med. 20, 255–271.

Fanelli, C.G., Epifano, L., Rambotti, A.M., et al., 1993. Meticulous prevention of hypoglycemia normalizes the glycemic thresholds and magnitude of most of neuroendocrine responses to, symptoms of, and cognitive function during hypoglycemia in intensively treated patients with short-term IDDM. Diabetes 42, 1683–1689.

Fong, Y.M., Marano, M.A., Moldawer, L.L., et al., 1990. The acute splanchnic and peripheral tissue metabolic response to endotoxin in humans. J. Clin. Invest. 85, 1896–1904.

Geddes, J., Schopman, J.E., Zammitt, N.N., et al., 2008. Prevalence of impaired awareness of hypoglycemia in adults with type 1 diabetes. Diabet. Med. 25, 501–504.

Henderson, J.N., Allen, K.V., Deary, I.J., et al., 2003. Hypoglycemia in insulin-treated type 2 diabetes: frequency, symptoms and impaired awareness. Diabet. Med. 20, 1016–1021.

Hermanns, N., Kulzer, B., Kubiak, T., et al., 2007. The effect of an education programme (HyPOS) to treat hypoglycaemia problems in patients with type 1 diabetes. Diabetes Metab. Res. Rev. 23, 528–538.

Holstein, A., Egberts, E.H., 2003. Risk of hypoglycemia with oral antidiabetic agents in patients with type 2 diabetes. Exp. Clin. Endocrinol. Metab. 111, 405–414.

Kitabchi, A.E., Umpierrez, G.E., Murphy, M.B., et al., 2006. Hyperglycemic crises in adult patients with diabetes: a consensus statement from the American Diabetes Association. Diabetes Care 29, 2739–2748.

Kitabchi, A.E., Umpierrez, G.E., Fisher, J.N., et al., 2008. Thirty years of personal experience in hyperglycemic crises: diabetic ketoacidosis and hyperglycemic hyperosmolar state. J. Clin. Endocrinol. Metab. 93, 1541–1552.

Lalau, J.D., 2010. Lactic acidosis induced by metformin: incidence, management and prevention. Drug Saf. 33, 727–740.

Langouche, L., Vander Perre, S., Wouters, P.J., et al., 2007. Effect of intensive insulin therapy on insulin sensitivity in the critically ill. J. Clin. Endocrinol. Metab. 92, 3890–3897.

Leese, G.P., Wang, J., Broomhall, J., et al., DARTS/MEMO Collaboration, 2003. Frequency of severe hypoglycemia requiring emergency treatment in type 1 and type 2 diabetes: a population based study of health service resource use. Diabetes Care 26, 1176–1180.

Mitrakou, A., Ryan, C., Veneman, T., et al., 1991. Hierarchy of glycemic thresholds for counterregulatory hormone secretion, symptoms and cerebral dysfunction. Am. J. Physiol. Endocrinol. Metab. 260, E67–E74.

Moller, N., Foss, A.C., Gravholt, C.H., et al., 2005. Myocardial injury with biomarker elevation in diabetic ketoacidosis. J. Diabetes Complications 19, 361–363.

Moller, N., Jensen, M.D., Rizza, R.A., et al., 2006. Renal amino acid, fat and glucose metabolism in type 1 diabetic and non-diabetic humans: effects of acute insulin withdrawal. Diabetologia 49, 1901–1908.

Rachoin, J.S., Weisberg, L.S., McFadden, C.B., 2010. Treatment of lactic acidosis: appropriate confusion. J. Hosp. Med. 5, E1–E7.

Rossetti, P., Porcellati, F., Bolli, G.B., et al., 2008. Prevention of hypoglycemia while achieving good glycemic control in type 1 diabetes. Diabetes Care 31 (Suppl. 2), S113–S120.

Sandoval, D.A., Aftab Guy, D.L., Richardson, M.A., et al., 2004. Effects of low and moderate antecedent exercise on counterregulatory responses to subsequent hypoglycemia in type 1 diabetes. Diabetes 53, 1798–1806.

Schwartz, N.S., Clutter, W.E., Shah, S.D., et al., 1987. Glycemic thresholds for activation of glucose counterregulatory systems are higher than the threshold for symptoms. J. Clin. Invest. 79, 777–781.

Stentz, F.B., Umpierrez, G.E., Cuervo, R., et al., 2004. Proinflammatory cytokines, markers of cardiovascular risks, oxidative stress, and lipid peroxidation in patients with hyperglycemic crises. Diabetes 53, 2079–2086.

UK Hypoglycemia Study Group, 2007. Risk of hypoglycemia in type 1 and 2 diabetes: effects of treatment modalities and their duration. Diabetologia 50, 1140–1147.

Vernon, C., Letourneau, J.L., 2010. Lactic acidosis: recognition, kinetics, and associated prognosis. Crit. Care Clin. 26, 255–283.

Waller, S.L., Delaney, S., Strachan, M.W.J., 2007. Does an integrated care pathway enhance the management of diabetic ketoacidosis? Diabet. Med. 24, 359–363.

Wolfsdorf, J., Glaser, N., Sperling, M.A., 2006. Diabetic ketoacidosis in infants, children, and adolescents: a consensus statement from the American Diabetes Association. Diabetes Care 29, 1150–1159.

Wright, A.D., Cull, C.A., MacLeod, K.M., et al., UKPDS Group, 2006. Hypoglycemia in type 2 diabetic patients randomized to and maintained on monotherapy with diet, sulfonylurea, metformin or insulin for 6 years from diagnosis: UKPDS 73. J. Diabetes Complications 20, 395–401.

Section 5

Adam, D.J., Beard, J.D., Cleveland, T., et al., 2005. Bypass versus angioplasty in severe ischaemia of the leg (BASIL): multicentre, randomised controlled trial. Lancet 366, 1925–1934.

Adler, A.I., Boyko, E.J., Ahroni, J.H., et al., 1999. Lower-extremity amputation in diabetes. The independent effects of peripheral vascular disease, sensory neuropathy, and foot ulcers. Diabetes Care 22, 1029–1035.

Al-Khoury, S., Afzali, B., Shah, N., et al., 2006. Anaemia in diabetic patients with chronic kidney disease – prevalence and predictors. Diabetologia 49, 1183–1189.

Amato, L., Paolisso, G., Cacciatore, F., et al., 1996. Non-insulin-dependent diabetes mellitus is associated with a greater prevalence of depression in the elderly. The Osservatorio Geriatrico of Campania Region Group. Diabetes Metab. 22, 314–318.

Anon, 1998. Early worsening of diabetic retinopathy in the Diabetes Control and Complications Trial. Arch. Ophthalmol. 116, 874–886.

Backonja, M., Beydoun, A., Edwards, K.R., et al., 1998. Gabapentin for the symptomatic treatment of painful neuropathy in patients with diabetes mellitus: a randomized controlled trial. JAMA 280, 1831–1836.

Beck, R.W., Edwards, A.R., Aiello, L.P., et al., 2009. Diabetic Retinopathy Clinical Research Network. Three-year follow-up of a randomized trial comparing focal/grid photocoagulation and intravitreal triamcinolone for diabetic macular edema. Arch. Ophthalmol. 127, 245–251.

Blume, P.A., Walters, J., Payne, W., et al., 2008. Comparison of negative pressure wound therapy using vacuum-assisted closure with advanced moist wound therapy in the treatment of diabetic foot ulcers: a multicenter randomized controlled trial. Diabetes Care 31, 631–636.

Cannon, C.P., McCabe, C.H., Belder, R., et al., 2002. Design of the Pravastatin or Atorvastatin Evaluation and Infection Therapy (PROVE IT)-TIMI 22 trial. Am. J. Cardiol. 89, 860–861.

Chaturvedi, N., Sjolie, A.K., Stephenson, J.M., et al., 1998. Effect of lisinopril on progression of retinopathy in normotensive people with type 1 diabetes. The EUCLID Study Group. EURODIAB Controlled Trial of Lisinopril in Insulin-Dependent Diabetes Mellitus. Lancet 351, 28–31.

Chaturvedi, N., Porta, M., Klein, R., et al., DIRECT Programme Study Group, 2008. Effect of candesartan on prevention (DIRECT-Prevent 1) and progression (DIRECT-Protect 1) of retinopathy in type 1 diabetes: randomised, placebo-controlled trials. Lancet 372, 1394–1402.

Colhoun, H.M., Betteridge, D.J., Durrington, P.N., et al., 2004. Primary prevention of cardiovascular disease with atorvastatin in type 2 diabetes in the Collaborative Atorvastatin Diabetes Study (CARDS): multicentre randomised placebo-controlled trial. Lancet 364, 685–696.

Collins, R., Armitage, J., Parish, S., et al., Heart Protection Study Collaborative Group, 2003. MRC/BHF Heart Protection Study of cholesterol-lowering with simvastatin in 5963 people with diabetes: a randomised placebo-controlled trial. Lancet 361, 2005–2016.

Crawford, F., Inkster, M., Kleijnen, J., et al., 2007. Predicting foot ulcers in patients with diabetes: a systematic review and meta-analysis. Q. J. Med. 100, 65–86.

Daly, E.J., Trivedi, M.H., Raskin, P., et al., 2007. Screening for depression in a diabetic outpatient population. Int. J. Psychiatry Clin. Prac. 11, 268–272.

Davis, M.D., Fisher, M.R., Gangnon, R.E., et al., 1998. Risk factors for high-risk proliferative diabetic retinopathy and severe visual loss: Early Treatment Diabetic Retinopathy Study Report #18. Invest. Ophthalmol. Vis. Sci. 39, 233–252.

de Galan, B.E., Perkovic, V., Ninomiya, T., et al., 2009. Lowering blood pressure reduces renal events in type 2 diabetes. J. Am. Soc. Nephrol. 20, 883–892.

Eijkelkamp, W.B., Zhang, Z., Remuzzi, G., et al., 2007. Albuminuria is a target for renoprotective therapy independent from blood pressure in patients with type 2 diabetic nephropathy: post hoc analysis from the Reduction of Endpoints in NIDDM with the Angiotensin II Antagonist Losartan (RENAAL) trial. J. Am. Soc. Nephrol. 18, 1540–1546.

Fong, D.S., Strauber, S.F., Aiello, L.P., et al., Writing Committee for the Diabetic Retinopathy Clinical Research Network, 2007. Comparison of the modified Early Treatment Diabetic Retinopathy Study and mild macular grid laser photocoagulation strategies for diabetic macular edema. Arch. Ophthalmol. 125, 469–480.

Gaede, P., Vedel, P., Parving, H.H., et al., 1999. Intensified multifactorial intervention in patients with type 2 diabetes mellitus and microalbuminuria: the Steno type 2 randomised study. Lancet 353, 617–622.

Gregg, J.A., Callaghan, G.M., Hayes, S.C., et al., 2007. Improving diabetes self-management through acceptance, mindfulness, and values: a randomized controlled trial. J. Consult. Clin. Psychol. 75, 336–343.

Gupta, A., Gupta, V., Thapar, S., et al., 2004. Lipid-lowering drug atorvastatin as an adjunct in the management of diabetic macular edema. Am. J. Ophthalmol. 137, 675–682.

Hansen, H.P., Tauber-Lassen, E., Jensen, B.R., et al., 2002. Effect of dietary protein restriction on prognosis in patients with diabetic nephropathy. Kidney Int. 62, 220–228.

Hardy, K.J., Furlong, N.J., Hulme, S.A., et al., 2007. Delivering improved management and outcomes in diabetic kidney disease in routine clinical care. Br. J. Diabetes Vasc. Dis. 7, 172–178.

Holt, R.I.G., Cockram, C.S., Flyvbjerg, A., et al., 2010. Textbook of Diabetes, fourth ed. Wiley-Blackwell, Oxford.

Hurley, R.W., Lesley, M.R., Adams, M.C., et al., 2008. Pregabalin as a treatment for painful diabetic peripheral neuropathy: a meta-analysis. Reg. Anesth. Pain Med. 33, 389–394.

Ismail, K., Winkley, K., Rabe-Hesketh, S., 2004. Systematic review and meta-analysis of randomised controlled trials of psychological interventions to improve glycaemic control in patients with type 2 diabetes. Lancet 363, 1589–1597.

Jeffcoate, W., Lima, J., Nobrega, L., 2000. The Charcot foot. Diabet. Med. 17, 253–258.

Jerums, G., Panagiotopoulos, S., Premaratne, E., et al., 2008. Lowering of proteinuria in response to antihypertensive therapy predicts improved renal function in late but not in early diabetic nephropathy: a pooled analysis. Am. J. Nephrol. 28, 614–627.

Jin, H.M., Pan, Y., 2007. Renoprotection provided by losartan in combination with pioglitazone is superior to renoprotection provided by Losartan alone in patients with type 2 diabetic nephropathy. Kidney Blood Press. Res. 30, 203–211.

Karamanos, B., Porta, M., Songini, M., et al., 2000. Different risk factors of microangiopathy in patiens with type 1 diabetes mellitus of short versus long duration. The EURODIABIDDM Complications Study. Diabetologia 43, 348–355.

Keech, A.C., Mitchell, P., Summanen, P.A., et al., 2007. Effect of fenofibrate on the need for laser treatment for diabetic retinopathy (FIELD study): a randomised controlled trial. Lancet 370, 1687–1697.

Klein, B.E., Moss, S.E., Klein, R., 1990. Effect of pregnancy on progression of diabetic retinopathy. Diabetes Care 13, 34–40.

Kohner, E.M., Aldington, S.J., Stratton, I.M., et al., 1998. United Kingdom Prospective Diabetes Study, 30: diabetic retinopathy at diagnosis of non-insulin-dependent diabetes mellitus and associated risk factors. Arch. Ophthalmol. 116, 297–303.

Krishnan, S., Nash, F., Baker, N., et al., 2008. Reduction in diabetic amputations over 11 years in a defined UK population: benefits of multidisciplinary team work and continuous prospective audit. Diabetes Care 31, 99–101.

Leese, G.P., Reid, F., Green, V., et al., 2006. Stratification of foot ulcer risk in patients with diabetes: a population-based study. Int. J. Clin. Pract. 60, 541–545.

Leese, G.P., Boyle, P., Feng, Z., et al., 2008. Screening uptake in a well-established diabetic retinopathy screening program: the role of geographical access and deprivation. Diabetes Care 31, 2131–2135.

Leese, G.P., Nathwani, D., Young, M.J., et al., 2009. Good practice guidance for the use of antibiotics in patients with diabetic foot ulcers. Diabetic. Foot J. 12, 62–78.

Lipsky, B.A., Baker, P.D., Landon, G.C., et al., 1997. Antibiotic therapy for diabetic foot infections: comparison of two parenteral-to-oral regimens. Clin. Infect. Dis. 24, 643–648.

Lustman, P.J., Clouse, R.E., Nix, B.D., et al., 2006. Sertraline for prevention of depression recurrence in diabetes mellitus: a randomized, double-blind, placebo-controlled trial. Arch. Gen. Psychiatry 63, 521–529.

MacKinnon, M., Shurraw, S., Akbari, A., et al., 2006. Combination therapy with an angiotensin receptor blocker and an ACE inhibitor in proteinuric renal disease: a systematic review of the efficacy and safety data. Am. J. Kidney Dis. 48, 8–20.

Malmberg, K., Norhammar, A., Wedel, H., et al., 1999. Glycometabolic state at admission: important risk marker of mortality in conventionally treated patients with diabetes mellitus and acute myocardial infarction: long-term results from the Diabetes and Insulin-Glucose Infusion in Acute Myocardial Infarction (DIGAMI) study. Circulation 99, 2626–2632.

Malmberg, K., Ryden, L., Wedel, H., et al., 2005. Intense metabolic control by means of insulin in patients with diabetes mellitus and acute myocardial infarction (DIGAMI 2): effects on mortality and morbidity. Eur. Heart J. 26, 650–661.

Mann, J.F., Schmieder, R.E., McQueen, M., et al., 2008. Renal outcomes with telmisartan, ramipril, or both, in people at high vascular risk (the

ONTARGET study): a multicentre, randomised, double-blind, controlled trial. Lancet 372, 547–553.

Mauer, M., Zinman, B., Gardiner, R., et al., 2009. Renal and retinal effects of enalapril and losartan in type 1 diabetes. N. Engl. J. Med. 361, 40–51.

Meloni, C., Morosetti, M., Suraci, C., et al., 2002. Severe dietary protein restriction in overt diabetic nephropathy: benefits or risks? J. Ren. Nutr. 12, 96–101.

Misra, A., Bachmann, M.O., Greenwood, R.H., et al., 2009. Trends in yield and effects of screening intervals during 17 years of a large UK community-based diabetic retinopathy screening programme. Diabet. Med. 26, 1040–1047.

Mulhauser, I., Bender, R., Bolt, U., et al., 1996. Cigarette smoking and progression of retinopathy and neuropathy in type 1 diabetes. Diabet. Med. 13, 536–543.

National Institute for Health and Clinical Excellence (NICE), 2008. Early Identification and Management of Chronic Kidney Disease in Adults in Primary and Secondary Care. NICE Clinical Guideline 73. NICE, London. Online. Available at: http://www.nice.org.uk/nicemedia/live/12069/42117/42117.pdf (accessed January 2011).

National Prescribing Centre (NPC), 2011. NICE updates its guidance on management of hypertension. MeReC Rapid Review. Number 4470, Online. Available at: http://www.npc.nhs.uk/rapidreview/?p4470 (accessed 14.12.2011).

Olson, J.A., Strachan, F.M., Hipwell, J.H., et al., 2003. A comparative evaluation of digital imaging, retinal photography and optometrist examination in screening for diabetic retinopathy. Diabet. Med. 20, 528–534.

Peters, E.J., Lavery, L.A., 2001. Effectiveness of the diabetic foot risk classification system of the International Working Group on the Diabetic Foot. Diabetes Care 24, 1442–1447.

Price, C.P., Newall, R.G., Boyd, J.C., 2005. Use of protein : creatinine ratio measurements on random urine samples for prediction of significant proteinuria: a systematic review. Clin. Chem. 51, 1577–1586.

Robins, S.J., Collins, D., McNamara, J.R., et al., 2008. Body weight, plasma insulin, and coronary events with gemfibrozil in the Veterans Affairs High-Density Lipoprotein Intervention Trial (VAHIT). Atherosclerosis 196, 849–855.

Rowe, N.G., Mitchell, P.G., Cumming, R.G., et al., 2000. Diabetes, fasting blood glucose and age-related cataract: the Blue Mountains Eye Study. Ophthalmic Epidemiol. 7, 103–114.

Royal College of Ophthalmologists, 1998. The Provision of Low Vision Care. The Royal College of Ophthalmologists, London.

Sarnak, M.J., Levey, A.S., Schoolwerth, A.C., et al., 2003. Kidney disease as a risk factor for development of cardiovascular disease: a statement from the American Heart Association Councils on Kidney in Cardiovascular Disease, High Blood Pressure Research, Clinical Cardiology, and Epidemiology and Prevention. Hypertension 4, 1050–1065.

Scottish Intercollegiate Guidelines Network (SIGN), 2006. Diagnosis and Management of Peripheral Arterial Disease. SIGN Publication No. 89.

SIGN, Edinburgh. Online. Available at: http://www.sign.ac.uk/guidelines/
fulltext/89/index.html (accessed January 2011).

Scottish Intercollegiate Guidelines Network (SIGN), 2007. Management of
Stable Angina. SIGN Publication No. 96. SIGN, Edinburgh. Online.
Available at: http://www.sign.ac.uk/ guidelines/fulltext/96/index.html
(accessed 06.01.2010).

Scottish Intercollegiate Guidelines Network (SIGN), 2007. Risk Estimation
and the Prevention of Cardiovascular Disease. SIGN Publication No. 97.
SIGN, Edinburgh. Online. Available at: http://www.sign.ac.uk/guidelines/
fulltext/97/index.html (accessed May 2011).

Scottish Intercollegiate Guidelines Network (SIGN), 2008. Management of
Patients with Stroke or TIA: Assessment, Investigation, Immediate
Management and Secondary Prevention. SIGN Publication No. 108.
SIGN, Edinburgh. Online. Available at: http://www.sign.ac.uk/guidelines/
fulltext/108/index.html (accessed January 2011).

Selby, P.L., Young, M.J., Boulton, A.J., 1994. Bisphosphonates: a new
treatment for diabetic Charcot neuroarthropathy? Diabet. Med. 11, 28–31.

Sen, K., Misra, A., Kumar, A., et al., 2002. Simvastatin retards progression of
retinopathy in diabetic patients with hypercholesterolemia. Diabetes Res.
Clin. Pract. 56, 1–11.

Sever, P.S., Poulter, N.R., Dahlof, B., et al., 2005. Reduction in
cardiovascular events with atorvastatin in 2532 patients with type 2
diabetes: Anglo-Scandinavian Cardiac Outcomes Trial–lipid-lowering
arm (ASCOT-LLA). Diabetes Care 28, 1151–1157.

Shepherd, J., Barter, P., Carmena, R., et al., 2006. Effect of lowering LDL
cholesterol substantially below currently recommended levels in patients
with coronary heart disease and diabetes: the Treating to New Targets
(TNT) study. Diabetes Care 29, 1220–1226.

Singh, N., Armstrong, D.G., Lipsky, B.A., 2005. Preventing foot ulcers in
patients with diabetes. JAMA 293, 217–228.

So, W.Y., Kong, A.P., Ma, R.C., et al., 2006. Glomerular filtration rate,
cardiorenal end points, and all-cause mortality in type 2 diabetic patients.
Diabetes Care 29, 2046–2052.

Solberg, Y., Rosner, M., Belkin, M., 1998. The association between cigarette
smoking and ocular diseases. Surv. Ophthalmol. 42, 535–547.

Sukhija, R., Bursac, Z., Kakar, P., et al., 2008. Effect of statins on the
development of renal dysfunction. Am. J. Cardiol. 101, 975–979.

Sultan, A., Gaskell, H., Derry, S., et al., 2008. Duloxetine for painful diabetic
neuropathy and fibromyalgia pain: systematic review of randomized trials.
BMC Neurol. 8, 29.

Talbot, F., Nouwen, A., 2000. A review of the relationship between depression
and diabetes in adults: is there a link? Diabetes Care 23, 1556–1562.

Turner, R.C., Millns, H., Neil, H.A., et al., 1998. Risk factors for coronary
artery disease in non-insulin dependent diabetes mellitus. United Kingdom
Prospective Diabetes Study (UKPDS:23). Br. Med. J. 316, 823–828.

UK Prospective Diabetes Study Group, 1998. Tight blood pressure control and
risk of macrovascular and microvascular complications in type 2 diabetes:
UKPDS 38. Br. Med. J. 317, 703–713.

Valk, G.D., Kriegsman, D.M., Assendelft, W.J., 2001. Patient education for preventing diabetic foot ulceration. Cochrane Database Syst. Rev. 4, CD001488.

West, D.S., DiLillo, V., Bursac, Z., et al., 2007. Motivational interviewing improves weight loss in women with type 2 diabetes. Diabetes Care 30, 1081–1087.

Wong, M., Chung, J.W.Y., Wong, T.K., 2007. Effects of treatments for symptoms of painful diabetic neuropathy: systematic review. BMJ 335, 87.

Younis, N., Broadbent, D.M., Harding, S.P., et al., 2003. Incidence of sight-threatening retinopathy in type 1 diabetes in a systematic screening programme. Diabet. Med. 20, 758–765.

Younis, N., Broadbent, D.M., Vora, J.P., et al., 2003. Incidence of sight-threatening retinopathy in patients with type 2 diabetes in the Liverpool Diabetic Eye Study: a cohort study. Lancet 361, 195–200.

Young, M.J., McCardle, J.E., Randall, L.E., et al., 2008. Improved survival of diabetic foot ulcer patients 1995–2008: possible impact of aggressive cardiovascular risk management. Diabetes Care 31, 2143–2147.

Section 6

ACE/ADA Task Force on Inpatient Diabetes, 2006. American College of Endocrinology and American Diabetes Association consensus statement on inpatient diabetes and glycemic control: a call to action. Diabetes Care 29, 1955–1962.

American Diabetes Association, 2009. Standards of medical care in diabetes. Diabetes Care 32 (Suppl. 1), S13–S61.

Australasian Paediatric Endocrine Group for the Department of Health and Ageing, 2005. Clinical Practice Guidelines: Type 1 Diabetes in Children and Adolescents. Australian Government and National Health and Medical Research Council.

Bantle, J.P., Wylie-Rosett, J., Albright, A.L., et al., 2008. Nutrition recommendations and interventions for diabetes: a position statement of the American Diabetes Association. Diabetes Care 31 (Suppl. 1), S61–S78.

Bartsocas, C., 2007. From adolescence to adulthood: the transition from child to adult care. Diabetes Voice 52, 15–17.

Buchwald, H., Estok, R., Fahrbach, K., et al., 2009. Weight and type 2 diabetes after bariatric surgery: systematic review and meta-analysis. Am. J. Med. 122, 248–256.

Clarke, W., Jones, T., Rewers, A., et al., 2008. Assessment and management of hypoglycemia in children and adolescents with diabetes. Pediatr. Diabetes 9, 165–174.

Clinical Resource Efficiency Support Team (CREST), 2006. Safe and Effective Use of Insulin in Secondary Care: Recommendations for Treating Hyperglycaemia in Adults. Online. Available at: http://www.gain-ni.org/library/guidelines/insulin.pdf (accessed January 2012).

Cox, D.J., Gonder-Frederick, L.A., Kovatchev, B., et al., 2000. Progressive hypoglycemia's impact on driving simulation performance. Diabetes Care 23, 163–170.

Crowther, C.A., Hiller, J.E., Moss, J.R., et al., 2005. Effect of treatment of gestational diabetes mellitus on pregnancy outcomes. N. Engl. J. Med. 352, 2477–2486.

Diabetes, U.K., Collation of Inpatient Experiences 2007. Online. Available at: http://www.diabetes.org.uk/Professionals/Publications-reports-and-resources/Reports-statistics-and-case-studies/Reports/Collation-of-inpatient-Experiences-2007/ (accessed January 2012)..

Donaghue, K.C., Chiarelli, F., Trotta, D., et al., 2007. ISPAD clinical practice consensus guidelines 2006–2007: Microvascular and macrovascular complications. Pediatr. Diabetes 8, 163–170.

Dunger, D.B., Sperling, M.A., Acerini, C.L., et al., 2004. European Society for Paediatric Endocrinology/Lawson Wilkins Pediatric Endocrine Society consensus statement on diabetic ketoacidosis in children and adolescents. Pediatrics 113, e133–e140.

Eaton, W.W., Armenian, H., Gallo, J., et al., 1996. Depression and risk for onset of type II diabetes. A prospective populatiaon-based study. Diabetes Care 19, 1097–1102.

Edge, J.A., Jakes, R.W., Roy, Y., et al., 2006. The UK case–control study of cerebral oedema complicating diabetic ketoacidosis in children. Diabetologia 49, 2002–2009.

Ellenberg, M., 1984. Diabetes and female sexuality. Women Health 9, 75–79.

Enzlin, P., Mathieu, C., Van Den, B.A., et al., 2002. Sexual dysfunction in women with type 1 diabetes: a controlled study. Diabetes Care 25, 672–677.

European Diabetes Working Party for Older People (EDWPOP), 2004. Clinical Guidelines for Type 2 Diabetes Mellitus. Online Available at: http://instituteofdiabetes.org/wp-content/themes/IDOP/other/diabetes_guidelines_for_older_people.pdf (accessed January 2012).

Fonseca, V., Seftel, A., Denne, J., et al., 2004. Impact of diabetes mellitus on the severity of erectile dysfunction and response to treatment: analysis of data from tadalafil clinical trials. Diabetologia 47, 1914–1923.

Frier, B.M., 2007. Living with hypoglycaemia. In: Frier, B.M., Fisher, M. (Eds.), Hypoglycaemia in Clinical Diabetes. second ed. John Wiley, Chichester, pp. 309–332.

Gazzaruso, C., Solerte, S.B., Pujia, A., et al., 2008. Erectile dysfunction as a predictor of cardiovascular events and death in diabetic patients with angiographically proven asymptomatic coronary artery disease: a potential protective role for statins and 5-phosphodiesterase inhibitors. J. Am. Coll. Cardiol. 51, 2040–2044.

Govier, F., Potempa, A.J., Kaufman, J., et al., 2003. A multicenter, randomized, double-blind, crossover study of patient preference for tadalafil 20 mg or sildenafil citrate 50 mg during initiation of treatment for erectile dysfunction. Clin. Ther. 25, 2709–2723.

Guerin, A., Nisenbaum, R., Ray, J.G., 2007. Use of maternal GHb concentration to estimate the risk of congenital anomalies in the offspring of women with prepregnancy diabetes. Diabetes Care 30, 1920–1925.

Guideline Development Group, 2008. Management of diabetes from preconception to the postnatal period: summary of NICE guidance. Br. Med. J. 336, 714–717.

Holt, R.I.G., 2008. Antipsychotics, metabolic side effects and the elderly. Geriatr. Med. 38, 399–402.

Holt, R.I.G., Cockram, C.S., Flyvbjerg, A., et al., 2010. Textbook of Diabetes, fourth ed. Wiley- Blackwell, Oxford.

International Association of Diabetes and Pregnancy Study Groups Consensus Panel, 2010. International Association of Diabetes and Pregnancy Study Groups recommendations on the diagnosis and classification of hyperglycemia in pregnancy. Diabetes Care 33, 676–682.

Kamel, H.K., Morley, J.E., 2001. Metabolic risk factors and their treatment. In: Sinclair, A.J., Finucane, P. (Eds.), Diabetes in Old Age. Wiley, Chichester, pp. 187–198.

Korenman, S.G., Viosca, S.P., 1992. Use of a vacuum tumescence device in the management of impotence in men with a history of penile implant or severe pelvic disease. J. Am. Geriatr. Soc. 40, 61–64.

Latif, K.A., Freire, A.X., Kitabchi, A.E., et al., 2002. The use of alkali therapy in severe diabetic ketoacidosis. Diabetes Care 25, 2113–2114.

Lonnen, K.F., Powell, R.J., Taylor, D., et al., 2008. Road traffic accidents and diabetes: insulin use does not determine risk. Diabet. Med. 25, 578–584.

Lundin, C., Danielson, E., Ohrn, I., 2007. Handling the transition of adolescents with diabetes: participant observations and interviews with care providers in pediatric and adult diabetes outpatient clinics. Int. J. Integr. Care 7, 1–10.

Ma, R.C., So, W.Y., Yang, X., et al., 2008. Erectile dysfunction predicts coronary heart disease in type 2 diabetes. J. Am. Coll. Cardiol. 51, 2045–2050.

McAlister, F.A., Majumdar, S.R., Blitz, S., et al., 2005. The relation between hyperglycemia and outcomes in 2,471 patients admitted to the hospital with community-acquired pneumonia. Diabetes Care 28, 810–815.

McCrindle, B.W., Urbina, E.M., Dennison, B.A., et al., 2007. Drug therapy of high-risk lipid abnormalities in children and adolescents: a scientific statement from the American Heart Association Atherosclerosis, Hypertension, and Obesity in Youth Committee, Council of Cardiovascular Disease in the Young, with the Council on Cardiovascular Nursing. Circulation 115, 1948–1967.

McDonagh, J., Viner, R., 2006. Lost in transition? Between paediatric and adult services. Br. Med. J. 332, 435–436.

McGill, M., 2002. How do we organize smooth, effective transfer from paediatric to adult diabetes care? Horm. Res. 57 (Suppl. 1), 66–68.

Metzger, B.E., Lowe, L.P., Dyer, A.R., et al., 2008. Hyperglycemia and adverse pregnancy outcomes. N. Engl. J. Med. 358, 1991–2002.

Moghissi, E.S., Korytkowski, M.T., DiNardo, M., et al., American Association of Clinical Endocrinologists, American Diabetes Association, 2009. American Association of Clinical Endocrinologists and American Diabetes Association consensus statement on inpatient glycemic control. Diabetes Care 32, 1119–1131.

National Diabetes Support Team, Improving Emergency and Inpatient Care for People with Diabetes 2008. Online. Available at: http://www.diabetes. nhs.uk/document.php?o=219 (accessed 18.01.2010)..

National Institute for Health and Clinical Excellence (NICE), 2008. Diabetes in Pregnancy: Management of Diabetes and its Complications from Pre-conception to the Postnatal Period. NICE Clinical Guideline 63. Developed by the National Collaborating Centre for Women's and children's Health. NICE, London. Online. Available at: http://www.nice.org.uk/nicemedia/pdf/CG63NICEGuideline.pdf (accessed January 2012).

Newman, H.F., Northup, J.D., 1981. Mechanism of human penile erection: an overview. Urology 17, 399–408.

Ng, Y.C., Jacobs, P., Johnson, J.A., 2001. Productivity losses associated with diabetes in the US. Diabetes Care 24, 257–261.

Nicolosi, A., Glasser, D.B., Moreira, E.D., et al., 2003. Prevalence of erectile dysfunction and associated factors among men without concomitant diseases: a population study. Int. J. Impot. Res. 15, 253–257.

O'Neill, S., Gill, G.V., 2000. Variation in licensing authority standards for diabetic taxi drivers in the United Kingdom. Driving and Employment Working Party of the British Diabetic Association. Occup. Med. 50, 19–21.

Peele, P.B., Lave, J.R., Songer, T.J., 2002. Diabetes in employer-sponsored health insurance. Diabetes Care 25, 1964–1968.

Pegge, N.C., Twomey, A.M., Vaughton, K., et al., 2006. The role of endothelial dysfunction in the pathophysiology of erectile dysfunction in diabetes and in determining response to treatment. Diabet. Med. 23, 873–878.

Rajfer, J., Aronson, W.J., Bush, P.A., et al., 1992. Nitric oxide as a mediator of relaxation of the corpus cavernosum in response to nonadrenergic, noncholinergic neurotransmission. N. Engl. J. Med. 326, 90–94.

Rowan, J.A., Hague, W.M., Gao, W., et al., 2008. Metformin versus insulin for the treatment of gestational diabetes. N. Engl. J. Med. 358, 2003–2015.

Scottish Intercollegiate Guidelines Network (SIGN), 2010. Management of Diabetes: A National Clinical Guideline. SIGN Publication No. 116. SIGN, Edinburgh. Online. Available at:http://www.sign.ac.uk/pdf/sign116.pdf (accessed January 2012).

Shamloul, R., Ghanem, H., Fahmy, I., et al., 2005. Testosterone therapy can enhance erectile function response to sildenafil in patients with PADAM: a pilot study. J. Sex. Med. 2, 559–564.

Sinclair, A.J., 2001. Issues in the initial management of type 2 diabetes. In: Sinclair, A.J., Finucane, P. (Eds.), Diabetes in Old Age. second ed. Wiley, Chichester, pp. 155–164.

Singh, R., Press, M., 2007. Employment in working age men with diabetes mellitus. Pract. Diab. Int. 24, 75–77.

Sjöström, L., Narbro, K., Sjöström, C.D., et al., 2007. Effects of bariatric surgery on mortality in Swedish obese subjects. N. Engl. J. Med. 357, 741–752.

Stene, L.C., Barriga, K., Hoffman, M., et al., 2006. Normal but increasing hemoglobin A1c levels predict progression from islet autoimmunity to overt type 1 diabetes: Diabetes Autoimmunity Study in the Young (DAISY). Pediatr. Diabetes 7, 247–253.

Stork, A.D.M., Van Haeften, T.W., Veneman, T.F., 2006. Diabetes and driving: desired data, research methods and their pitfalls, current knowledge, and future research. Diabetes Care 29, 1942–1949.

Strachan, M.W.J., Deary, I.J., Ewing, F.M.E., et al., 1997. Is type 2 (non-insulin-dependent) diabetes mellitus associated with an increased risk of cognitive dysfunction? Diabetes Care 20, 438–445.

Umpierrez, G.E., Isaacs, S.D., Bazargan, N., et al., 2002. Hyperglycemia: an independent marker of in-hospital mortality in patients with undiagnosed diabetes. J. Clin. Endocrinol. Metab. 87, 978–982.

Urbach, S., LaFranchi, S., Lambert, L., et al., 2005. Predictors of glucose control in children and adolescents with type 1 diabetes mellitus. Pediatr. Diabetes 6, 69–74.

Von Korff, M., Katon, W., Lin, E.H.B., et al., 2005. Work disability among individuals with diabetes. Diabetes Care 28, 1326–1332.

Waclawski, E.R., 1989. Employment and diabetes: a survey of the prevalence of diabetic workers known by occupation physicians, and the restrictions placed on diabetic workers in employment. Diabet. Med. 6, 16–19.

Wagner, G., Montorsi, F., Auerbach, S., et al., 2001. Sildenafil citrate (Viagra) improves erectile function in elderly patients with erectile dysfunction: a subgroup analysis. J. Gerontol. A. Biol. Sci. Med. Sci. 56, M113–M119.

Wolfsdorf, J., Glaser, N., Sperling, M.A., 2006. Diabetic ketoacidosis in infants, children, and adolescents: a consensus statement from the American Diabetes Association. Diabetes Care 29, 1150–1159.

INDEX

Note: Page numbers followed by *f* indicate figures and *t* indicate tables.